Clinical Simulation *for* Health Care Professionals

Clinical Simulation *for* Health Care Professionals

Audrey L. Zapletal, OTD, OTR/L, CLA
Thomas Jefferson University, East Falls Campus, Philadelphia, Pennsylvania

Joanne M. Baird, PhD, OTR/L, CHSE, FAOTA
University of Pittsburgh, Pittsburgh, Pennsylvania

Tracy Van Oss, DHSc, MPH, OTR/L, FAOTA, CHSE
Quinnipiac University, Hamden, Connecticut

Maureen M. Hoppe, EdD, MA, OTR/L, CPAM, CHSE
College of Saint Mary, Omaha, Nebraska

Jean E. Prast, OTD, MSOT, OTRL, CHSE
Saginaw Valley State University, University Center, Michigan

E. Adel Herge, OTD, OTR/L, FAOTA
Thomas Jefferson University, Philadelphia, Pennsylvania

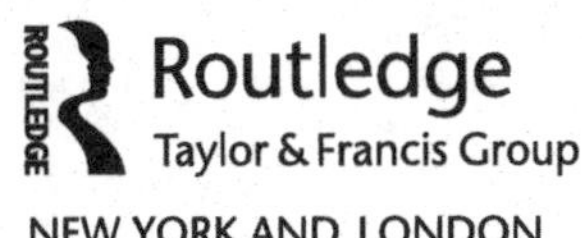

NEW YORK AND LONDON

Instructors: *Clinical Simulation for Health Care Professionals* includes ancillary materials specifically available for faculty use. Please visit http://www.routledge.com/9781630917357 to obtain access.

First published in 2022 by SLACK Incorporated

Published 2024 by Routledge
605 Third Avenue, New York, NY 10058

and by Routledge
4 Park Square, Milton Park, Abingdon, Oxon OX14 4RN

Routledge is an imprint of the Taylor & Francis Group, an informa business

Library of Congress Control Number: 2022934086

Cover Artist: Lori Shields

ISBN: 9781630917357 (pbk)
ISBN: 9781003523161 (ebk)

DOI: 10.4324/9781003523161

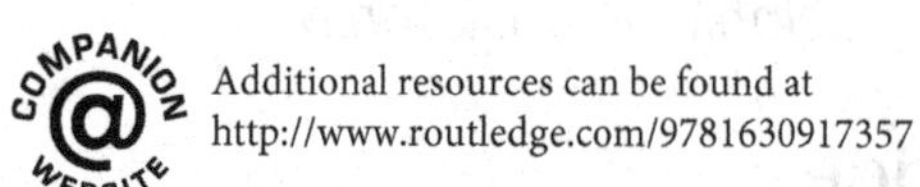

Dedication

We would like to dedicate this book to those who mentored each of us in the world of simulation. A special thank you goes to Janice P. Burke, PhD, OTR/L, FAOTA for planting seeds, nurturing growth, and inspiring innovations that set the motions to bring this dedicated team of simulation educators together.

We would also like to thank our families for supporting us as we took on this exciting adventure, our colleagues for asking questions and taking on new endeavors, our academic leaders for their ongoing encouragement, and (most importantly) to our students for trusting us with their preparation to become future occupational therapists and health professionals.

We are grateful for the support of SLACK Incorporated, specifically Brien Cummings, for his support, positivity, leadership, and helping us move this vision into fruition. We started pre-pandemic, and his continued support and involvement was critical. We believe this is one of the first manuals outside of nursing and medicine to address best practices for using simulation in health professional education and training.

Note About the Book

The book is divided into 35 sections—including the Table of Contents, Foreword, Introduction, the chapters, appendices, and special sections identified as Kern's Steps. The Kern's Model for Curriculum Development is used as the foundation for implementing simulation into a curriculum/course. For those unfamiliar with this process, the "steps" are explained as the process of creating a simulation unfolds. (Kern's Model is reproduced with permission from Thomas, P. A., Kern, D. E., Hughes, M. T., & Chen, B. Y. [Eds.]. *Curriculum development for medical education: A six-step approach* [3rd ed., p. 7]. Johns Hopkins University Press; 2015.)

Contents

Instructors: *Clinical Simulation for Health Care Professionals* includes ancillary materials specifically available for faculty use. Please visit http://www.routledge.com/9781630917357 to obtain access.

About the Authors

Audrey L. Zapletal, OTD, OTR/L, CLA is an Assistant Professor in the Department of Occupational Therapy in the College of Rehabilitation Sciences at Thomas Jefferson University. She serves as the Director for the Master of Science in Occupational Therapy Program at the East Falls campus. She received her bachelor's degree in Occupational Therapy from Boston University's Sargent College, her master's degree from Thomas Jefferson University, and her occupational therapy doctorate from the University of Southern California's Chan Division of Occupational Science and Occupational Therapy. Her clinical experiences vary from pediatric private practice, early intervention, and intensive care nurseries/homes to adult-based medical settings. Her teaching experiences include foundational course work such as neuroanatomy to pediatric and adult interventions courses, program development, and leadership. She received the Fred and Sadye Abrams Award for Excellence in Laboratory Teaching from Thomas Jefferson University. Her current research interests include the use of simulation in health professional education, interprofessional education, and cultural compatibility professional development training for faculty, staff, administrators, and students. She has written publications and presentations focused on best practice in andragogy, including instructional design, and on the use of simulation in occupational therapy education at national and international venues.

Joanne M. Baird, PhD, OTR/L, CHSE, FAOTA is an Associate Professor in the Department of Occupational Therapy at the University of Pittsburgh. She received her bachelor's degree in Occupational Therapy from the University of Pittsburgh, her master's degree in Occupational Therapy from the University of Southern California, and returned to the University of Pittsburgh to receive her doctorate in Rehabilitation Science. Her clinical background includes extensive experience with the mental health and pediatric and geriatric populations across the health care continuum in a variety of national and regional sites. Dr. Baird is a Fellow with the American Occupational Therapy Association (AOTA) and has received numerous teaching awards. She is a certified health care simulation educator, and her research interests include experiential learning and the use of simulation to promote clinical reasoning in graduate education. She developed the simulation curricula for entry-level and post-professional clinical education in occupational therapy at the University of Pittsburgh, serves as a simulation consultant for prelicensure rehabilitation programs, and is a nationally invited speaker for simulation education and development. She has examined the use of near-peer facilitation in occupational therapy graduate programs.

Tracy Van Oss, DHSc, MPH, OTR/L, FAOTA, CHSE is a Clinical Professor in the Occupational Therapy Department at Quinnipiac University. Dr. Van Oss received a Doctor of Health Science degree from Nova Southeastern University, a master's degree in Public Health and a Bachelor of Science degree in Corporate Communication from Southern Connecticut State University, and has a degree in Occupational Therapy from Quinnipiac University. Her credentials also include being a Community Health Education Specialist (CHES), and she has earned the AOTA Specialty Certification in Environmental Modification (SCEM). She received the AOTA International Service Award in 2020. She is a Certified Healthcare Simulation Educator (CHSE) and incorporates simulation and other experiential experiences into the occupational therapy curriculum. Dr. Van Oss is a Fellow with AOTA and has numerous publications and presentations.

Maureen M. Hoppe, EdD, MA, OTR/L, CPAM, CHSE is an Associate Professor in the Occupational Therapy Department at the College of Saint Mary. She received her Bachelor of Science in Occupational Therapy at Creighton University, her master's degree in Health Education from the University of Nebraska in Omaha, as well as her doctorate in Education with a focus in health professions at the College of Saint Mary. Dr. Hoppe also obtained a graduate certificate of specialization in gerontology from University of Nebraska Omaha. She has clinical experience in a variety of practice settings, including inpatient rehabilitation, outpatient, and skilled nursing facilities. Dr. Hoppe is a certified health care simulation educator with research interests in interprofessional education, clinical simulation, and experiential learning to enhance student learning and preparation for transition to practice. She has published and presented nationally and internationally on clinical simulation in health profession education and fieldwork preparation.

Jean E. Prast, OTD, MSOT, OTRL, CHSE is an Associate Professor in the Occupational Therapy Program at Saginaw Valley State University. She received her bachelor's and master's degrees in Occupational Therapy from Saginaw Valley State University, and her doctorate in Occupational Therapy from Rocky Mountain University of Health Professions. She has clinical experience in a variety of settings, including inpatient acute care, outpatient, primary care, and community-based practice. Her specialty areas include neurology, program development, fieldwork education, simulation, and interprofessional education and practice. She is a certified health care simulation educator and currently serves as the Interprofessional Education Coordinator for the College of Health and Human Services. She is actively involved in the development and implementation of simulations and interprofessional education in the college, occupational therapy curriculum, and community. Her research interests include interprofessional education, simulation, and transformative learning to facilitate professional growth in preparation for practice. She has published and presented on the topic of interprofessional education and simulation at national and international levels.

E. Adel Herge, OTD, OTR/L, FAOTA is Professor in the Department of Occupational Therapy at Thomas Jefferson University. She is Director of the BSMS Occupational Therapy Program on the Center City campus and Program Coordinator for the BS-OTD Program on the East Falls campus. Dr. Herge received her bachelor's in Special Education/Elementary Education from Cabrini College, her certificate in Occupational Therapy and Master of Science in Occupational Therapy from Thomas Jefferson University, and her doctorate in Occupational Therapy from Chatham University. When the University Simulation Program was expanded to include health professions students, Dr. Herge served as Director of Health Professions Simulation and supported faculty as they developed, implemented, and evaluated simulation in graduate programs in occupational therapy, physical therapy, and radiological sciences for couples and families. She continues to integrate simulation in her course work with undergraduate and graduate students and serves as lead faculty for an interprofessional simulation program. Dr. Herge is a Fellow with AOTA.

Contributing Authors

Chalia Bellis, MS, OTR/L
(Chapter 14 and Appendix I)

Dennis Brown, DrPH, MPH, PA-C
(Appendices C and D)
Program Director and
Associate Clinical Professor
Physician Assistant Program
University of New England
Portland, Maine

Madeleine Clements, MS, OTR/L
(Chapter 14 and Appendix I)
Thomas Jefferson University
Philadelphia, Pennsylvania

Leslie Cody, MS, OTR/L
(Chapter 2)
Binghamton, New York

Victoria L. B. Grieve, PharmD
(Chapter 10 and Appendices E and F)
Assistant Professor
School of Pharmacy
University of Pittsburgh
Pittsburgh, Pennsylvania

Andrea L. Hergenroeder, PhD, PT
(Appendix G)
Department of Physical Therapy
University of Pittsburgh
Pittsburgh, Pennsylvania

Victoria Hornyak, PT, DPT
(Appendix G)
Department of Physical Therapy
University of Pittsburgh
Pittsburgh, Pennsylvania

Carole Ivey, PhD, OTR/L, FAOTA
(Appendix H)
Virginia Commonwealth University
Richmond, Virginia

Pari Kumar, OTD, OTR/L
(Chapter 11 and Appendix I)
Cadia Healthcare Silverside
Wilmington, Delaware

Jennifer A. Merz, OTD, OTR/L
(Chapter 11 and Appendix I)
Thomas Jefferson University
Philadelphia, Pennsylvania

Susan Norkus, PhD, ATC
(Appendix A)
Department of Rehabilitation, Health and Wellness
Quinnipiac University
Hamden, Connecticut

John M. O'Donnell, DrPH, MSN, RN, CRNA, CHSE, FSSH, FAANA (Foreword)
Professor and Chair
Department of Nurse Anesthesia
Director, Nurse Anesthesia Program
University of Pittsburgh
Pittsburgh, Pennsylvania
Senior Associate Director, WISER
Treasurer, Society for Simulation in Healthcare

Jaime Smiley, MS, OTR/L
(Appendix H)
Vice President of Therapy and Fitness
Retirement Unlimited Inc.
Roanoke, Virginia
Adjunct Professor
Department of Occupational Therapy
Virginia Commonwealth University
Richmond, Virginia

Foreword

Simulation as an educational method in health care has exploded over the past 2 decades with more than 15,000 papers in print and penetration into every health care educational domain. As I look back on my health care career, which began in nursing in 1983 when I took a position as a surgical oncology nurse to my current role as a Department Chair and Director of a Nurse Anesthesia Program, I am struck by the paradigm shift in our collective approach to the preparation of the next generation of health care providers. My bachelor's program prepared me with an excellent knowledge base, but very little hands-on or immersive educational experiences. My experience in my master's program in anesthesia had a little more hands-on training, but was still primarily focused on the apprenticeship model of "see-one, do-one." My doctoral program in epidemiology had a number of screen-based and table-top simulations, but again many of these were abstract or conceptual in nature and not designed for immediate application. In hindsight, there were good reasons for the lack of robust, practical simulations in these educational programs—my teachers simply did not have the tools or techniques at the time to engage in what we now appreciate are best practices in simulation teaching and learning. These include prebriefing, debriefing, deliberate practice, curriculum integration, and meaningful feedback to name a few. In fact, in 1994, when I began working in simulation education at the University of Pittsburgh with Dr. John Schaefer (the founding Director of the Winter Institute for Simulation Education and Research, or WISER), there was really only one textbook (Gaba et al., 1994) that provided us with meaningful guidance on how to design, implement, and evaluate simulation educational activities for anesthesia providers. Many of us who were early adopters of simulation as an educational method were essentially "inventing" the new field of health care simulation … which has now grown exponentially over the past 26 years to the point where the term "simulationist" is now a legitimate descriptor of the role of dedicated health care educators across the world. Quoting my friend Amitai Ziv, MD (2003), the founder of the Israeli National Simulation Center (MSR), health care simulation is not just an important component of our work, it is an "ethical imperative."

I am especially excited with this new textbook, *Clinical Simulation for Health Care Professionals*. First, I am impressed that the text shares my philosophy that our efforts as educators should be guided by educational best practices that embrace this basic premise within a sound educational and theoretical construct, such as the Kern's Model for Curriculum Development. Through my faculty development efforts locally, nationally, and internationally, I have come to understand that one of the great needs in the health care simulation community is accessible resources for new as well as experienced educators that allow them to use their precious time most efficiently. This text has been designed to serve as a practical guide with real examples of simulation designs and approaches across multiple educational domains. Finally, and perhaps most importantly, this text has an underlying theme that the most important outcome of our simulation work is not just in the improvement of our course participants but in their ability to translate these skills downstream into improvements in the quality and safety of delivered care—a truly patient-centric focus.

—John M. O'Donnell, DrPH, MSN, RN, CRNA, CHSE, FSSH, FAANA

Reference

Gaba, D., Fish, K., & Howard, S. (1994). *Crisis management in anesthesiology.* Churchill Livingstone.

FOREWORD

Introduction

This book is the result of a "blind date" arranged by Audrey, who recognized that we all shared a passion for simulation and were working independently to develop rigorous programs. That blind-date led to a good, old-fashioned conference call (no video back then!), which resulted in multiple collaborations on presentations, publications, and research...and ultimately amazing friendships and this book. We believe, and research supports, that well-designed simulation used to complement the education of a health professional has a positive impact on performance in the clinical setting. Therefore, using simulation effectively and safely in your educational setting is critical to a learner's development. We also know that, perhaps outside of nursing and medicine, simulation is under-utilized in prelicensure health care education. Likely because simulation in the health professions (professionals working in health care outside of nursing and medicine) does not have the strong history and background that it does in medicine, and thus many are unsure how to begin. This book is meant to change that.

If you are new to simulation education or have not had formal simulation education training—many have not—there are multiple factors to consider when creating and implementing simulation experiences. This workbook was written to meet the need for educators to become familiar with these factors and develop the skills required to create dynamic learning environments that mimic clinical practice in a safe manner. This book answers questions about the "when, where, why, what, and how" of simulation use. It opens with evidence supporting the use of simulation in a health professional curriculum followed by step-by-step (chapter-by-chapter) "recipes" to create robust simulation experiences within your curriculum or at your facility.

Just as with any endeavor, there is a pathway for success. Successful simulations start with best practices. This book is based on best practices for simulation education, based on evidence and designed to ensure positive outcomes. These include methods to create, design, and implement simulation. For example, because creating a simulation program is a process, Kern's Model for Curriculum Development was specifically chosen as a framework for simulation implementation (Khamis et al., 2016). The International Association for Medical Education's Best Evidence in Medical Education (Issenberg et al., 2005, Motola et al., 2013) and the International Nursing Association in Clinical Simulation and Learning (2021) are used as guidelines for simulation creation and design.

Remember that while great things can be accomplished with simulation education, it does come with the potential for harm. When designing your simulation experiences, it is imperative that these best practice guidelines are kept at the forefront of your planning and implementation because the safety of everyone involved is imperative. Everyone involved in the simulation (learners, facilitators, faculty, standardized patients, others) immerses themselves into this fabricated-yet-realistic world. Physical and psychological states are tested and—within the educational setting—we (i.e., faculty) are responsible. You will learn methods to ensure that your simulations are rigorously developed and contain components designed to ensure the psychological safety of those involved.

Also keep in mind that simulation is an investment. Just as with most investments, there is a cost and a potential for a return on your investment. Cost does not necessarily refer to direct costs/finances: the cost of your time is valuable, too. Planning a simulation takes time, effort, and skill. We have included information about simulation on a shoestring budget and ways to ensure the longevity of your simulation program by assessing outcomes. This investment can have a huge pay-off: it is critical for the learner's success in the simulation ... and in clinical practice.

Book Notes

All authors have extensive expertise in simulation use, and each were independently trained and have experience within their own institution and practices. This diversity has been leveraged to provide rigor with chapters written by the individuals who have the most expertise in the content discussed.

This volume was written as a workbook. Thus, you will note a repetition of key concepts to validate your understanding throughout. There are also sidebars with guiding/application questions within many chapters and worksheets at the end of many chapters. These are meant to assist you with your design, creation, development, implementation, and assessment plans.

A word about … words. This workbook was written to introduce readers to the educational modality of simulation with the goal of rigorous implementation, thus, we often refer to the terms, "simulation", "simulation education," and "simulation experience" interchangeably, although they are defined in the book and these terms have specific definitions within the world of simulation (Lioce et al., 2020). We also refer to "students" and "learners" interchangeably.

Simulation education has experienced a great deal of attention as technology and remote/distance education have grown exponentially recently. This has resulted in an explosion of new research and data. We have updated best practice standards where appropriate and have remained true to rigor by citing proven and reproducible research. We encourage you to explore emerging data to determine what is effective and feasible. We are learning more everyday about how newer models of education and technology can complement each other.

We are excited to share our love for simulation with you. Simulation is an art and science, integrating the worlds of education, your health profession, and the performing arts into one single experience. To play a role in the simulation requires the learner to arrive trained and prepared. As the faculty member your role is the director, planning from the beginning for the learners' journey in your curriculum to the training activities needed for their clinical performance (and beyond!). Feedback and debriefing (the most important simulation elements) are completed after the performance to further enhance your learner's knowledge, skill, and professional development. Enjoy how your production unfolds, and your learners will thank you for this experience.

As they say in the theater, break a leg!

References

INACSL Standards Committee. (2021). Healthcare Simulation Standards of Best Practice. *Clinical Simulation in Nursing, 58,* 66. https://doi.org/10.1016/j.ecns.2021.08.018

Issenberg, S. B., McGaghie, W. C., Petrusa, E. R., Gordon, D. L., & Scalese, R. J. (2005). Features and uses of high-fidelity medical simulations that lead to effective learning: A BEME systematic review. *Medical Teacher, 27*(1), 10–28. https://doi.org/10.1080/01421590500046924

Khamis, N. N., Satava, R. M., Alnassar, S. A., & Kern, D. E. (2016). A stepwise model for simulation-based curriculum development for clinical skills, a modification of the six-step approach. *Surgical Endoscopy,* 279-287. https://doi.org/10.1007/s00464-015-4206x

Lioce, L. (Ed.), Lopreiato, J. (Founding Ed.), Downing, D., Chang, T. P., Robertson, J. M., Anderson, M., Diaz, D. A., Spain, A. E. (Assoc. Eds.), & the Terminology and Concepts Working Group. (2020). Healthcare simulation dictionary (2nd ed.). *Agency for Healthcare Research and Quality,* Publication No. 20-0019. https://doi.org/10.23970/simulationv2

Motola, I., Devine, L. A., Chung, H. S., Sullivan, J. E., & Issenberg, S. B. (2013). Simulation in healthcare education: A best evidence practical guide. AMEE Guide No. 82. *Medical Teacher, 35*(10), e1511-30. https://doi.org/10.3109/0142159X.2013.818632

1

Introduction to Simulation
Evidence

Joanne M. Baird, PhD, OTR/L, CHSE, FAOTA
E. Adel Herge, OTD, OTR/L, FAOTA

Learning Objectives

1. Describe simulation education and its use in health care education.
2. Describe current trends in rehabilitation simulation education.
3. Apply Miller's pyramid to simulation in rehabilitation education.

What Is Simulation?

Simulation refers to set of conditions that includes a person and/or devices that attempts to present evaluation problems realistically. The participant is expected to respond to the situation as they would under natural circumstances (McGaghie, 1999). In a clinical simulation, health care professional learners practice skills in a safe environment without posing risk to real patients (Herge et al., 2013). The simulation environment is learner-centered, not patient-centered, allowing learners to practice skills, receive feedback, and even "do over" in a safe and guided environment (McDougall, 2015). In a simulation, educators can create specific scenarios that may or may not be possible in a clinical setting (Issenberg et al., 1999).

Interest in and use of clinical simulation has increased in health profession education in the past decade. A number of important factors that drive education may be contributing to this new interest. These include:

- *Current Clinical Practice:* Changes in the health care delivery system require entry level practitioners to be prepared for the challenges of current practice, including caring for medically complex patients (Coker-Bolt, 2010; Vogel et al., 2009) and working in interprofessional teams (Bright et al., 2017). Simulation provides learners the opportunity to practice skills in safe,

Zapletal, A. L., Baird, J. M., Van Oss, T., Hoppe, M. M., Prast, J. E., & Herge, E. A. *Clinical Simulation for Health Care Professionals* (pp. 1-6).

realistic settings prior to caring for real patients. Interprofessional simulation has also been used to help develop learner skills in communication and collaboration in preparation for team-based care (King et al., 2014; Kraft et al., 2013; Shoemaker et al., 2011).

- *Active Learning:* Active learning strategies help learners break the "illusion of understanding" (Svinicki & McKeachie, 2011, p. 190). When learners are required to apply concepts that they learned in a classroom setting, they have a better understanding of what they truly know and what they need to practice. This simple realization increases learner motivation to become involved in their own learning process (Svinicki & McKeachie, 2011). Participating in a carefully constructed simulation experience provides learners with opportunities to practice skills such as critical thinking (Vyas et al., 2011), decision making (Guhde, 2010), and therapeutic communication (Velde et al., 2009).
- *Advances in Technology:* Technological advances have contributed to the development of lifelike equipment, such as human patient simulators, that contribute to a sense of realism in the simulation when combined with a carefully constructed scenario (Hwang & Bencken, 2008). Use of simulation technology has the potential to improve a learner's technical skills, which can lead to enhanced patient care (Ghobrial et al., 2015).
- *Effective Assessment:* Carefully constructed simulation scenarios can be used to effectively assess a learner's ability to perform specific skills (Pugh, 2008). As health professions consider a competency-based system of educating the next generation, simulation could be useful to objectively measure the learner's abilities (Boulet & Durning, 2018).
- *Proven Method:* Evidence clearly demonstrates that simulation is an effective teaching/learning method. Simulation training has led to improvements in the learner's knowledge and performance of technical skills for safe, effective patient care (Bethea et al., 2014; Herge et al., 2013; Wu & Shea, 2009); increased student comfort and confidence in completing procedures (Dearmon et al., 2013; Ohtake et al., 2013; Silberman et al., 2013; Thomas & Mackey, 2012); and enhanced development of cultural competence and humility (Rutledge et al., 2008).

Simulation in Contemporary Health Care Education

The United States Medical Licensing Examination (USMLE) includes simulated patient encounters to assess the clinical skills of medical students (Pugh, 2008). The Accreditation Council for Graduate Medical Education identifies six domains of clinical competence, and simulations are used to assess knowledge, skills, and attitudes in these domains (Scalese et al., 2008). Some professions recognize the value of simulation as part of continuing education. For example, the American Board of Anesthesiology formally includes simulation as a weighted category to maintain board certification (Rothkrug & Mahboobi, 2020).

Health professions have also integrated simulation into their curricula. Physical therapy education utilizes simulation with standardized patients (SPs) to instruct students in specific technical skills (Black & Marcoux, 2002; Smith et al., 2012), facilitate development of clinical reasoning (Shoemaker et al., 2009; Shoemaker et al., 2011), and enhance interpersonal skills (Lewis et al., 2008). Program simulators are used to teach students manual therapy mobilization (Chang et al., 2007; Van Zoest et al., 2007). Simulation is also used to prepare students for practice in high stakes in environments such as acute care (Silberman et al., 2013), and to increase students' confidence before transitioning from the academic setting to clinical practice (Wright et al., 2018).

Physical therapy has studied the use of simulated learning environments compared to traditional clinical education (Blackstock et al., 2013; Mori et al., 2015; Watson et al., 2012). Both studies were multisite, randomized controlled trials with large sample sizes. Both studies found no difference in student outcomes between simulated learning environments and typical clinical education (Mori et al., 2015). Use of simulated learning environments can be resource intensive and long-term data about translation to practice is not currently available. Additional investigation is needed to determine the feasibility of using simulation to replace clinical education however this is an idea worth considering (Mori et al., 2015; Pritchard et al., 2016).

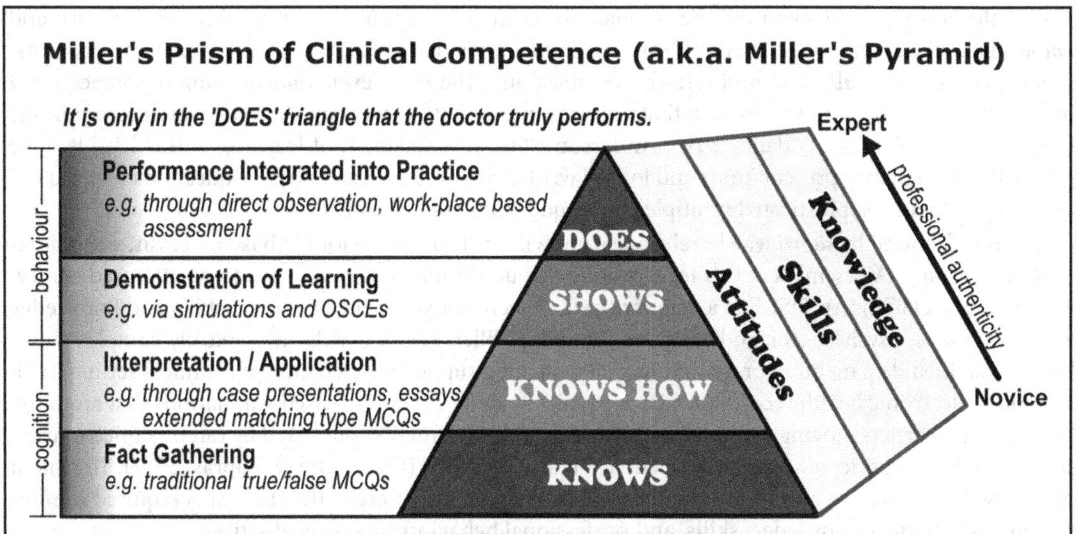

Figure 1-1. Miller's prism of clinical competence (a.k.a. Miller's pyramid). (Adapted by R. Mehay and R. Burns, 2009. In R. Mehay [Ed.], *The Essential Handbook for GP Training and Education* [Chapter 29, p. 414]. Reproduced with permission.)

Various forms of simulation including task trainers, human patient simulators and SPs have been used to instruct students in speech and language pathology in technical and nontechnical skills related to pediatric and adult disorders (MacBean et al., 2013). Baylor et al. (2017) demonstrated that SPs can accurately portray adult voice disorders. Human patient simulators were used to teach and assess specific manual skills, such as tracheostomy management to practicing clinicians (Baker et al., 2008).

Occupational therapy uses simulation to enhance a learner's skills in clinical reasoning, data gathering, and goal setting (Gibbs et al., 2017; Velde et al., 2009); professional communication (Vegni et al., 2010; Velde et al., 2009); understanding of mental illness (Merryman, 2010; Ozelie & Panfil, 2018); and performance of technical skills as part of evaluation (Herge et al., 2013) and intervention (Baird et al., 2015; Castillo, 2011; Van Oss et al., 2013). Simulation is also used to prepare students for clinical practice (Ozelie & Both, 2016; Shoemaker et al., 2011; Wu & Shea, 2009).

Occupational therapy education has begun exploring the use of simulation as a replacement for traditional clinical education. Imms et al. (2018) conducted a multisite, randomized controlled trial and compared student outcomes between students who spent 40 hours in a simulated clinical placement vs. those who spent 40 hours in a traditional clinical placement. The researchers discovered no significant differences between the two student groups. These findings suggest that carefully designed simulation may be a substitute for traditional clinical education (Imms et al., 2018). Again, this may be an idea worth investigating.

Miller's Prism of Clinical Competence

Simulation has been associated with many educational theories (see Chapter 5). One educational model especially well-suited to simulation in rehabilitation is Miller's Prism of Clinical Competence, also referred to as Miller's Pyramid (Figure 1-1).

This model links simulation education to rehabilitation education very well as it seamlessly fits into existing professional models of classroom education, followed by mentored and supervised clinical practice, and then ongoing professional development. Miller's Prism is comprised of four learning levels organized from novice to expert. In each of these levels the learner's competency is considered for three domains: knowledge, skills, and attitudes.

At the bottom of the pyramid, the emphasis is on the novice learner who gathers facts to learn and ***know,*** much like traditional classroom learning and lectures that are assessed with pencil and paper assessments, e.g., true/false and multiple choice questions. The next level, ***knowing how,*** is characterized by a higher level of cognitive learning that requires interpretation and application—words recognizable from Bloom's Taxonomy (Adams, 2015; Anderson, 2001)). Assessment of learning at this level is done primarily through case presentations and longer written answers such as essays or questions that require matching, although sophisticated multiple choice questions may also be used.

This is followed by ***showing,*** whereby a learner will shift to a behaviorally based assessment to demonstrate learning. Assessment at this level is done through simulation or an objective structured clinical examination (OSCE). An OSCE is a standardized, objective assessment of clinical skills and knowledge across cognitive, psychomotor, and affective domains (Miller, 1990). OSCEs are typically complex simulations that include a manikin or SP and may also include supportive elements of a clinical setting, such as a mock electronic health record. OSCEs are typically done as station-based simulations that are time-limited, with learners moving from station to station and assessments completed by raters trained to use a standard scoring rubric; peer-reviewed feedback is also provided (Ogunyemi & Dupras, 2017). The intent of an OSCE is to present a situation similar to the clinic setting, whereby the student is required to *show* or demonstrate their knowledge, skills, and professional behaviors in a clinical setting.

The top level in this model is performance or ***does.*** At this level the learner has integrated their skills into practice patterns and is able to function independently (Miller, 1990). The highest point of the pyramid or prism reflects the practitioner who has achieved a level of expertise.

The model acknowledges several things, including that multiple assessment measures are necessary to ascertain a learner's mastery of the profession as knowledge itself is not sufficient for clinical competence (Miller, 1990). The model also acknowledges the rigor of objective paper-and-pencil methods to assess knowledge and the reality that this type of assessment is far removed from a successful client interaction. Answering a question or writing about a manual skill does not reflect conquering that skill or possessing that ability (Scalese et al., 2008).

At the other end of the assessment spectrum, supervised clinical practice also has disadvantages, including potentially jeopardizing client safety and an inability to assure the consistent and reproducible situations needed to repeatedly practice a skill to a level of competency (Miller, 1990; Scalese et al., 2008).

Simulation offers a solution to these limitations. Simulation has the advantages of marrying client safety, standardization, and reproducibility with the opportunity for manual practice in a realistic environment. Simulations used to demonstrate learning, such as the OSCEs, have been used in formative and summative manners and have been adopted for medical training to assess a wide variety of learning outcomes (Patrício et al., 2013).

References

Adams, N. (2015). Bloom's taxonomy of cognitive learning objectives. *Journal of the Medical Library Association, 103*(3), 152-153. Retrieved from https://www.ncbi.nlm.nih.gov/pmc/articles/PMC4511057/

Anderson, L. W., & Krathwohl, D. R., (Eds.). (2001). *A taxonomy for learning, teaching, and assessing: A revision of Bloom's taxonomy of educational objectives.* Allyn & Bacon.

Baird, J. M., Raina, K. D., Rogers, J. C., O'Donnell, J., Terhorst, L., & Holm, M. B. (2015). Simulation strategies to teach patient transfers: Self efficacy by strategy. *American Journal of Occupational Therapy, 69*(S2). https://doi.org/10.5014/ajot.2015.018705

Baker, C., Pulling, C., McGraw, R., Dagnone, J. D., Hopkins-Rosseel, D., & Medves, J. (2008). Simulation in interprofessional education for patient-centered collaborative care. *Journal of Advanced Nursing, 64*(4). https://doi.org/10.1111/j.1365-2648.2008.04798.x

Baylor, C., Burns, M. I., Struijk, J., Herron, L., Mach, H., & Yorkston, K. (2017). Assessing the believability of standardized patients trained to portray communication disorders. *American Journal of Speech-Language Pathology, 26*(3), 791-805. https://doi.org/1044/2017_AJSLP-16-0068

Bethea, D. P., Castillo, D. C., & Harvison, N. (2014). Use of simulation in occupational therapy education: Way of the future? *American Journal of Occupational Therapy, 68,* S32-S39. https://doi.org/10.5014/ajot.2014.012716

Black, B. & Marcoux, B. C. (2002). Feasibility of using standardized patients in a physical therapy education program: A pilot study. *Journal of Physical Therapy Education, 16*(2), 49-56. https://doi.org/10.1097/00001416-200207000-00008

Blackstock, F. C., Watson, K. M., Morris, N. R., Jones, A., Wright, A., McMeeken, J. M., Rivett, D. A., O'Connor, V., Peterson, R. F., Haines, T., Watson, G., & Jull, G. A. (2013). Simulation can contribute a part of cardiorespiratory physiotherapy clinical education: Two randomized trials. *Simulation in Healthcare, 8*(1), 32-42. https://doi.org/10.1097/SIH.0b013e318273101a

Boulet, J. R. & Durning, S. J. (2018). What we measure ... and what we should measure in medical education. *Medical Education, 53*(1), 86-94. https://doi.org/10.1111/medu.13652

Bright, B., Austin, B., Garn, C., Glass, J., & Sample, S. (2017). Identification of interprofessional practice and application to achieve patient outcomes of health care providers in the acute care setting. *Journal of Interprofessional Education & Practice, 9*, 108-114. https://doi.org/10.1016/j.xjep.2017.09.003

Castillo, D. C. (2011). Experiences in a simulated hospital: Virtual training in occupational therapy. *OT Practice, 16*(22), 21-24. Retrieved from https://www.researchgate.net/publication/289628458_Experiences_in_a_simulated_hospital_Virtual_training_in_occupational_therapy

Chang, J. Y., Chang, G. L., Chien, C. J. Chung, K. C., & Hsu, A. T. (2007). Effectiveness of two forms of feedback on training of a joint mobilization skill by using a joint t*ranslation simulator. Physical Therapy, 87*(4), 418-430. https://doi.org/10.2522/ptj.20060154

Coker-Bolt, P. (2010). Effects of an experiential learning program on the clinical reasoning and critical thinking skills of occupational therapy students. *Journal of Allied Health, 39*(4). Retrieved from https://www.ncbi.nlm.nih.gov/pubmed/21184024

Dearmon, V., Graves, R. J., Hayden, S., Mulekar, M. S., Lawrence, S. M., Jones, L., Smith, K. K., & Farmer, J. E. (2013). Effectiveness of simulation-based orientation of baccalaureate nursing students preparing for their first clinical experience. *Journal of Nursing Education, 51*(2). https://doi.org/10.3928/01484834-20121212-02

Ghobrial, G. M., Hamade, Y. J., Bendok, B. R., & Harrop, J. S. (2015). Technology and simulation to improve patient safety. *Neurosurgery Clinics of North America, 26*(2), 239-243. https://doi.org/10.1016/j.nec.2014.11.002

Gibbs, D. M., Dietrich, M., & Dagnan, E. (2017). Using high fidelity simulation to impact occupational therapy student knowledge, comfort, and confidence in acute care. *The Open Journal of Occupational Therapy, 5*(1). https://doi.org/10.15453/2168-6408.1225

Guhde, J. (2010). Using online exercises and patient simulation to improve students' clinical decision-making. *Nursing Education Perspectives, 31*(6). https://www.ncbi.nlm.nih.gov/pubmed/21280447

Herge, E. A., Lorch, A., DeAngelis, T., Vause-Earland, T., Mollo, K. & Zapletal, A. (2013). The standardized patient encounter: A dynamic approach to prepare professional healthcare students for the workplace. *Journal of Allied Health, 42*(4), 229-235. Retrieved from https://www.ncbi.nlm.nih.gov/pubmed/24326920

Hwang, J. C. F., & Bencken, B. (2008). Integrating simulation with existing clinical educational programs. In R. R. Kyle & W. B. Murray (Eds.), *Clinical simulation: Operations, engineering, and management* (pp. 85-87). Academic Press.

Imms, C., Froude, E., Mang Ye Chu, E., Sheppard, L., Darzins, S., Guinea, S., Gospodarevskaya, E., Carter, R., Symmons, M. A., Penman, M., Nicola-Richmond, K., Hunt, S. G., Gribble, N., Ashby, S., & Mathieu, E. (2018). Simulated versus traditional occupational therapy placements: A randomised controlled trial. *Australian Occupational Therapy Journal, 65*(6), 556-564. https://doi.org/10.1111/1440-1630.12513

Issenberg, S. B., McGaghie, W. C., Hart, I. R., Mayer, J. W., Felner, J. M., Petrusa, E. R., Waugh, R. A., Brown, D. D., Safford, R. R., Gessner, I. H., Gordon, D. L., & Ewy, G.A. (1999). Simulation technology for health care professional skills training and assessment. *Journal of the American Medical Association, 282*(9), 861-866. https://doi.org/10.1001/jama.282.9.861

King, S., Carbonaro, M., Greidanus, E., Ansell, D., Foisy-Doll, C., & Magus, S. (2014). Dynamic and routine interprofessional simulations: Expanding the use of simulation to enhance interprofessional competencies. *Journal of Allied Health, 43*(3), 169-175. Retrieved from https://www.ncbi.nlm.nih.gov/pubmed/25194064

Kraft, S., Wise, H. H., Jacques, P. F., & Burik, J. K. (2013). Discharge planning simulation: Training the interprofessional team for the future workplace. *Journal of Allied Health, 43*(3). Retrieved from https://www.ncbi.nlm.nih.gov/pubmed/24013249

Lewis, M., Bell, J., & Asghar, A. (2008). Use of simulated patients in development of physiotherapy students' interpersonal skills. *International Journal of Therapy and Rehabilitation, 15*(5), 221-227. https://doi.org/10.12968/ijtr.2008.15.5.29234

MacBean, N., Theodoros, D., Davidson, B., & Hill, A. E. (2013). Simulated learning environments in speech-language pathology: An Australian response. *International Journal of Speech-Language Pathology, 15*(3), 345-357. https://doi.org/10.3109/17549507.2013.779024

McDougall, E. M. (2015). Simulation in education for health care professionals. *British Columbia Medical Journal, 57*(1), 444-448. Retrieved from https://www.bcmj.org/articles/simulation-education-health-care-professionals

McGaghie, W. C. (1999) Simulation in health professional competence assessment: Basic considerations. In A. Tekian, C. H. McGuire, & W. C. McGaghie (Eds), *Innovative simulations for assessing professional competence* (pp. 7-22). Department of Medical Education, University of Illinois Chicago.

Merryman, M. B. (2010). Effects of simulated learning and facilitated debriefing on student understanding of mental illness. *Occupational Therapy in Mental Health, 26*(1), 18-31. https://doi.org/10.1080/01642120903513933

Miller, G. (1990). The assessment of clinical skills/competence/performance. *Journal of the Association of American Medical Colleges, 65*(9), 63–67. https://doi.org/10.1097/00001888-199009000-00045

Mori, B., Carnahan, H., & Herold, J. (2015). Use of simulation learning experiences in physical therapy entry-to-practice curricula: A systematic review. *Physiotherapy Canada, 67*(2), 194-202. https://doi.org/10.3138/ptc.2014-40E

Ogunyemi, D., & Dupras, D. (2017). Does an objective structured clinical examination fit your assessment toolbox? *Journal of Graduate Medical Education, 9,* 771-772. https://doi.org/10.4300/JGME-D-17-00655.1

Ohtake, P. J., Lazarus, M., Schillo, R., & Rosen, M. (2013). Simulation experience enhances physical therapist student confidence in managing a patient in critical care environment. *Physical Therapy, 93*(2). https://doi.org/10.2522/ptj.20110463

Ozelie, R., & Both, C. (2016). High-fidelity simulation in occupational therapy curriculum: Impact on level II fieldwork performance. *The Open Journal of Occupational Therapy, 4*(4). https://doi.org/10.15453/2168-6408.1242

Ozelie, R., & Panfil, P. (2018). Hearing voices simulation: Impact on occupational therapy students. *The Open Journal of Occupational Therapy, 6*(4). https://doi.org/10.15453/2168-6408.1452

Patrício, M. F., Julião, M., Fareleira, F., & Carneiro, A. V. (2013). Is the OSCE a feasible tool to assess competencies in undergraduate medical education? *Medical Teacher, 35,* 503-514. https://doi.org/10.3109/0142159X.2013.774330

Pritchard, S. A., Blackstock, F. C., Nestel, D., & Keating, J. L. (2016). Simulated patients in physical therapy education: Systematic review and meta-analysis. *Physical Therapy, 96*(9), 1342-1353. https://doi.org/10.2522/ptj.20150500

Pugh, C. M. (2008). Simulation and high-stakes testing. In R. R. Kyle. & W. B. Murray (Eds.), *Clinical simulation: Operations, engineering, and management* (pp. 655-666). Academic Press.

Rothkrug, A., & Mahboobi, S. (2020). *Simulation training and skill assessment in anesthesiology.* StatPearls Publishing. Retrieved August 9, 2020, from https://www.ncbi.nlm.nih.gov/books/NBK557711/

Rutledge, C. M., Barham, P., Wiles, L., Benjamin, R. S., Eaton, P., & Palmer, K. (2008). Integrative simulation: A novel approach to educating culturally competent nurses. *Contemporary Nurse, 28*(1-2), 119-128. https://doi.org/10.5172/conu.673.28.1-2.119

Scalese, R. J., Obeso, V. T., & Issenberg, S. B (2008). Simulation technology for skills training and competency assessment in medical education. *Journal of General Internal Medicine, 23*(1), 46-49. https://doi.org/10.1007/s11606-007-0283-4

Shoemaker, M. J., Beasley, J., Cooper, M., Perkins, R., Smith, J., & Swank, C. (2011). A method for providing high-volume interprofessional simulation encounters in physical and occupational therapy education programs. *Journal of Allied Health, 40*(1), 15-21. Retrieved from https://www.ncbi.nlm.nih.gov/pubmed/21399842

Shoemaker, M. J., Riemersma, I., Perkins, R. (2009). Use of high fidelity human simulation to teach physical therapist decision-making skills for the intensive care setting. *Cardiopulmonary Physical Therapy Journal, 20*(1), 13-18. https://doi.org/10.1097/01823246-200920010-00003

Silberman, N. J., Panzarella, K. J., & Melzer, B. A. (2013). Using human simulation to prepare physical therapy students for acute care clinical practice. *Journal of Allied Health, 41*(1), 25-32. Retrieved from https://www.ncbi.nlm.nih.gov/pubmed/23471282

Smith, N., Prybylo, S., & Conner-Kerr, T. (2012). Using simulation and patient role play to teach electrocardiographic rhythms to physical therapy students. *Cardiopulmonary Physical Therapy Journal, 23*(1). https://doi.org/10.1097/01823246-201223010-00007

Svinicki, M., & McKeachie, W. J. (2011). *McKeachie's teaching tips.* (pp. 190). Cengage Learning.

Thomas, C., & Mackey, E. (2012). Influence of a clinical simulation elective on baccalaureate nursing student clinical confidence. *Journal of Nursing Education, 51*(4). https://doi.org/10.3928/01484834-20120224-03.

Van Oss, T., Perez, J., & Hartmann, K. (2013). Making mistakes virtually: Simulation helps students practice occupational therapy. OT Practice, 15-17.

Van Zoest, G. G., Staes, F. F., & Stappaerts, K. H. (2007). Three-dimensional manual contact force evaluation of graded perpendicular push force delivery by second-year physiotherapy students during simple feedback training. *Journal of Manipulative and Physiological Therapeutics, 30*(6), 438-439. https://doi.org/10.1016/j.jmpt.2007.06.001

Velde, B. P., Lane, H., & Clay, M. (2009). Hands on learning: The use of simulated clients in intervention cases. *Journal of Allied Health, 38*(1), 17-21. Retrieved from https://www.ncbi.nlm.nih.gov/pubmed/19753408

Vegni, E., Mauri, E., D'Apice, M., & Moja, E. A. (2010). A quantitative approach to measure occupational therapist-client interactions: A pilot study. *Scandinavian Journal of Occupational Therapy, 17*(3), 217-224. https://doi.org/10.3109/11038120903147956

Vogel, K. A., Geelhoed, M., Grice, K. O., & Murphy D. (2009). Do occupational therapy and physical therapy curricula teach critical thinking skills? *Journal of Allied Health, 38*(3), 152-7. Retrieved from https://www.ncbi.nlm.nih.gov/pubmed/19753426

Vyas, D., Ottis, E. J., & Caligiuri, F. J. (2011). Teaching clinical reasoning and problem-solving skills using human patient simulation. *American Journal of Pharmaceutical Education, 75*(9), 189. https://doi.org/10.5688/ajpe759189

Watson, K., Wright, A., Morris, N., McKeeken, J., Rivett, D., Blackstock, F., Jones, A., Haines, T., O'Connor, V., Watson, G., Peterson, R., & Jull, G. (2012). Can simulation replace part of clinical time? Two parallel randomised controlled trials. *Medical Education, 46*(7), 657-667. https://doi.org/10.1111/j.1365-2923.2012.04295.x

Wright, A., Moss, P., Dennis, D. M., Harrold, M., Levy, S., Furness, A. L., & Reubenson, A. (2018). The influence of a full-time, immersive simulation-based clinical placement on physiotherapy student confidence during the transition to clinical practice. *Advances in Simulation, 3*(3). https://doi.org/10.1186/s41077-018-0062-9

Wu, R., & Shea, C. (2009). Using simulations to prepare OT students for ICU practice. *American Occupational Therapy Association, Inc., Education Special Interest Section Quarterly, 19*(4), 1-4.

Section I

Introduction to Kern's Model

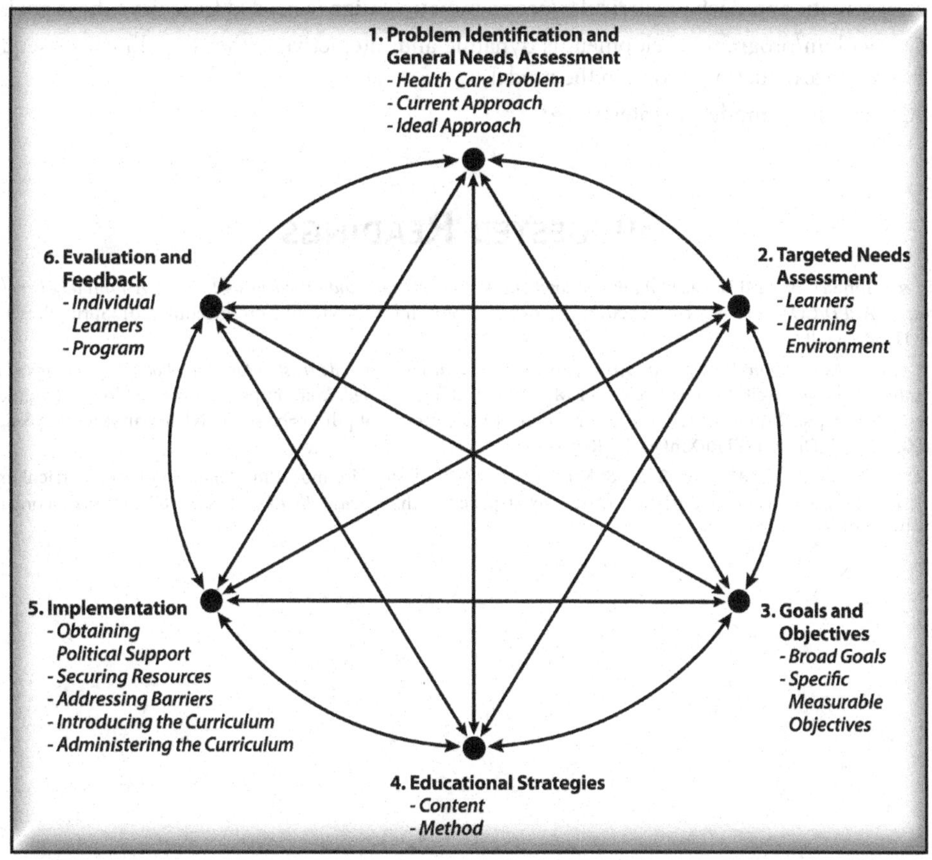

- Kern's six-step model is designed to integrate simulation into a curriculum/program using simulation design that is applicable across disciplines.
- Simulation is an educational methodology and not a specified curriculum or program. Like any educational tool, it must be used effectively.
- To be effective, simulation must be "built in" rather than "bolted on" to a program, course, and/or curriculum.
- Simulation should be integrated and conform to academic, clinical, and/or accreditation requirements.
- Simulation should reflect discipline specific knowledge, skills, and abilities of learners.
- Simulation experiences should be created using best practice guidelines.

- This workbook is organized into sections that correspond with each of these six steps to provide a guide for curricular/programmatic simulation integration.
- Each section begins with an overview of the next step for curricular/programmatic integration to ensure that simulation is used to the best advantage.
- This model views curriculum/program development as a type of scholarly activity and a method for change at the level of the institution/organization.
- A curriculum/program should be planned but never static and always reflective of a discipline's best practice.
- The Kern's Model is based on several underlying assumptions:
  - Educational programs have goals, although not all may be explicitly stated.
  - Health care educators are obligated to meet the needs of learners, clients, and society.
  - Health care educators should be held accountable for the outcomes of their learning interventions.
  - A systematic approach to curricular/programmatic design is needed to achieve these goals.
  - Curriculum/program development is dynamic and interactive, rather than linear or sequential, hence the articulating arrows in the model.
  - All steps in the model are interrelated.

Suggested Readings

Farnan, J., & Schindler, N. (2013). *Curriculum development and evaluation guide resident as teacher: A mutually beneficial arrangement APPD/COMSEP pre course 2013.* Retrieved from: https://www.appd.org/meetings/2013SpringPresentations/PCWS1Handout.pdf

Kern, D. E. (2014). *Curriculum development: An essential educational skill, a public trust, a form of scholarship, an opportunity for organizational change.* Weill Cornell College of Medicine, Qatar. Retrieved from: https://dnnyqetna.blob.core.windows.net/portals/15/Six-Step%20Approach%20to%20Curriculum%20Development.pdf?sr=b&si=DNNFileManagerPolicy&sig=9sAOUX/lzfZQsN6QKLOpWJ46YLRuXmQwOghR7ptxnFw=

Khamis, N. N., Satava, R. M., Alnassar, S. A., & Kern, D. E. (2016). A stepwise model for simulation-based curriculum development for clinical skills, a modification of the six-step approach. *Surgical Endoscopy,* 279-287. https://doi.org/10.1007/s00464-015-4206x

KERN'S MODEL STEP 1
PROBLEM IDENTIFICATION AND GENERAL NEEDS ASSESSMENT

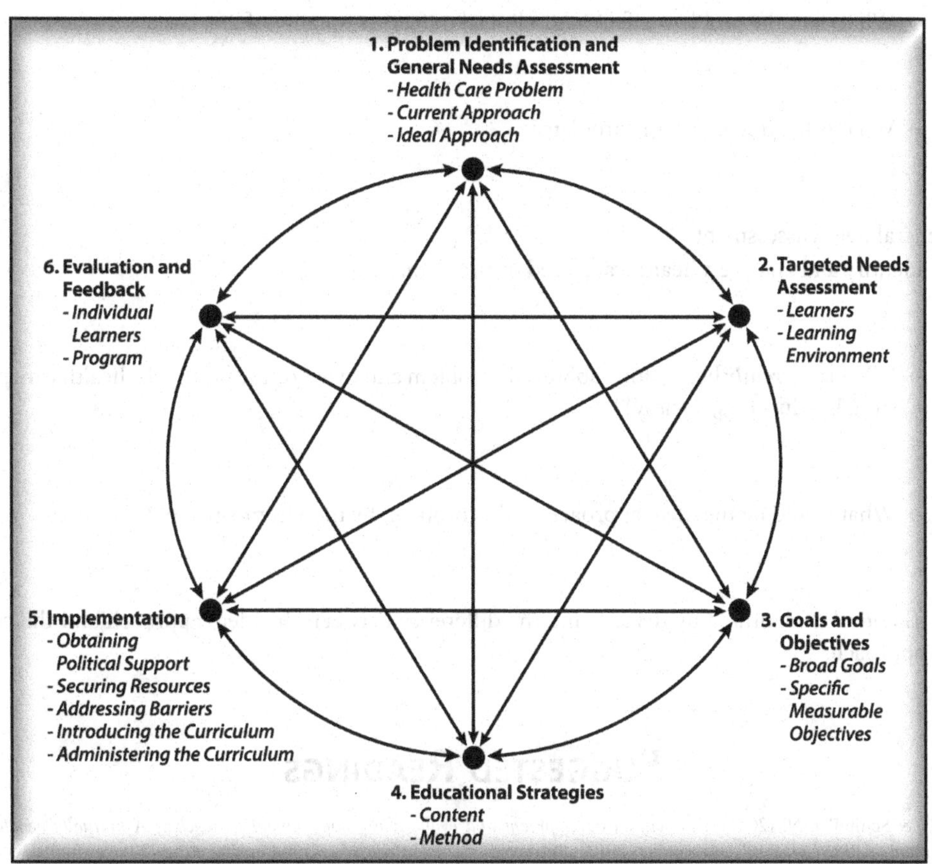

- The first step in Kern's Model is designed to build a rationale for the curriculum/program.
- Problem identification and general needs assessment refers to a larger scale review, done at the international, national, or regional level.
- This might include a literature review, consultations with experts, or reviews of other resources, such as health statistics, accreditation information, professional organization documents.
- The purpose of this step is to ground simulation within the curriculum/program and ensure that it generalizes into the needs of the clients or populations served, which in turn will focus educational and evaluation strategies and approaches.

- Another purpose is to ensure that curriculum/program developers build upon what already exists, so duplication of effort is eliminated. "Work smarter not harder."
- This step will provide a foundation to establish meaningful objectives for the simulations.

- Problem identification:
  - Identify an area of the curriculum/program to develop or refine.

    → Whom does the problem affect (e.g., clients, society, health care professionals, learners)?

    → What does the problem affect (e.g., clinical outcomes, quality of life, costs, satisfaction, work)?

    → What is the impact of this problem?

- General needs assessment:
  - Identify and analyze a health care need or problem.

    → What is ***currently*** being done about this problem and by whom (e.g., clients, health care professionals, educators, society)?

    → What would be the ***ideal*** approach to this problem by these same groups?

  - The ***need*** is identified by discovering the difference between the ideal approach and the current approach.

Suggested Readings

Farnan, J., & Schindler, N. (2013). *Curriculum development and evaluation guide resident as teacher: A mutually beneficial arrangement APPD/COMSEP pre course 2013.* Retrieved from: https://www.appd.org/meetings/2013SpringPresentations/PCWS1Handout.pdf

Kern, D. E. (2014). *Curriculum development: An essential educational skill, a public trust, a form of scholarship, an opportunity for organizational change.* Weill Cornell College of Medicine, Qatar. Retrieved from: https://dnnyqetna.blob.core.windows.net/portals/15/Six-Step%20Approach%20to%20Curriculum%20Development.pdf?sr=b&si=DNNFileManagerPolicy&sig=9sAOUX/lzfZQsN6QKLOpWJ46YLRuXmQwOghR7ptxnFw=

Khamis, N. N., Satava, R. M., Alnassar, S. A., & Kern, D. E. (2016). A stepwise model for simulation-based curriculum development for clinical skills, a modification of the six-step approach. *Surgical Endoscopy,* 279-287. https://doi.org/10.1007/s00464-015-4206x

2

Evidence for Linking Simulation Instructional Methods With Clinical Experiences

E. Adel Herge, OTD, OTR/L, FAOTA
Leslie Cody, MS, OTR/L
Audrey L. Zapletal, OTD, OTR/L, CLA

Learning Objectives

1. Demonstrate how simulation modalities can be used to enhance clinical and professional skills in the workplace.
2. Showcase evidence that supports the use of simulation modalities for particular skill sets.

Kern's Model of Program Development

The content in this chapter articulates Step 1 of Kern's Model: Problem Identification and General Needs Assessment. Information in this chapter contributes to the development of simulation in a curriculum or program that serves the needs of clients or populations based on input from external resources and/or community partners. This is the basis for the rationale for the program, which should include a review of evidence.

Zapletal, A. L., Baird, J. M., Van Oss, T., Hoppe, M. M., Prast, J. E., & Herge, E. A. *Clinical Simulation for Health Care Professionals* (pp. 11-25).

Introduction

Simulation encounters create opportunities for learners to practice and/or enhance skills in a supportive environment that imitates clinical practice without compromising patient safety (Braude et al., 2015; Maran & Glavin, 2003). Simulation has proven to be effective in building learners' technical and nontechnical skills (Braude et al., 2015; Riem et al., 2012). Simulation training complements other educational methods, such as didactic presentations (Bould & Naik, 2009). The skills practiced in simulation encounters have been shown to transfer to the clinical practice setting (Wayne et al., 2008).

Simulation is a valuable educational methodology in professional education and continuing professional education (Sachdeva, 2016). While a full review of the literature supporting the use of simulation in varied educational settings is beyond the scope of this chapter, the authors will present succinct summaries of selected current evidence supporting the use of simulation in the teaching or expansion of technical and nontechnical skills.

Simulation

Simulation and Educational Curriculums

Simulation has been used in medical, nursing, and health professional education to instruct learners in the technical skills related to their scope of practice. Simulation is integral to medical and nursing education (Bradley, 2006; Hayden et al., 2014; INACSL, 2021; NCSBN, 2020). Occupational therapy education uses simulation to enhance a student's skills in clinical reasoning (Gibbs & Dietrich, 2017; Velde et al., 2009), professional communication (Velde et al., 2009), and technical skills (Van Oss et al., 2013) and to prepare students for clinical practice with underserved populations (Haracz et al., 2015). Physical therapy education has incorporated simulation into educational curriculums to improve the student's communication skills (Riopel et al., 2018), clinical decision making (Johnston, 2018), and comfort and confidence when working in specialized areas such as acute care (Ohtake et al., 2013). Accreditation standards in pharmacy professions include simulation (ACPE, 2016, 2020), and well-designed simulation activities may replace a certain percentage of clinical hours in nursing, physical therapy, and occupational therapy educational programs (ACOTE, 2018; Imms et al., 2017; Larue et al., 2015; Rutherford-Hemming et al., 2016; Watson et al., 2012)

Simulation and Interprofessional Education

Guiding the implementation of interprofessional education (IPE) are four core competencies (Interprofessional Education Collaborative, 2016). These include respecting the value and ethics of all professions, understanding roles and responsibilities of team members, building teams and teamwork skills, and enhancing interprofessional communication. Interprofessional simulation activities have been effective in building teamwork skills (Gardner & Ahmed, 2014; Joyal et al., 2015; Marken et al., 2010).

Simulation and Remediation

In some professional programs, students must complete and sufficiently pass clinical competencies. Students who fail to meet minimal clinical competencies may benefit from a comprehensive approach to remediation. Student failure may occur in either in academic or professional areas (Liu et al., 2016). Academic underachievement may result from a lack of effort on the part of the student, external stressors such as caregiving responsibilities and financial, learning differences, or difficulties with spatial perceptual tasks. Students may lack confidence in their ability to perform non-technical skills expected in the clinical setting (Liu et al., 2016). Students may fail to demonstrate responsible professional behavior, including use of appropriate communication with supervisors, team members, and/or patients/clients.

Nursing education has effectively used simulation in the remediation of students failing to meet clinical competencies (Alinier et al., 2006; Evans & Harder, 2013; Haskvitz & Koop, 2004; Lynn & Twigg, 2011). Video analysis of self-performance is an effective means to self-improvement. Giles and colleagues (2014) demonstrate effective use of simulation with standardized patients and video analysis to help prepare occupational therapy students for their full-time clinical fieldwork. Students completed a simulation encounter that was video recorded, and afterwards, students reviewed the video and analyzed their performance to determine areas of strength and areas in need of improvement.

Simulation and Cultural Awareness and Humility

Cultural awareness, humility and competence are required today's practice. Cultural competemility, the intentional integration of these terms, is a life-long learning endeavour to understand the intersectionality of our consumers in order to meet their unique needs (Campinha-Bacote, 2018). Exposure to populations and communities that differ from the learner is one method to bring attention to how important health professionals must be aware of their own biases in order to deliver client-centered care. Simulation has been effective to bring light to some populations that are impacted by health disparities. Evidence has shown that high-fidelity simulation has been useful in helping students develop an awareness and cultural sensitivity to many populations (Foronda et al., 2018; Greene et al., 2017; Lau et al., 2016; Rutledge et al., 2008; Sales et al., 2013; Sequeira et al., 2012). Table 2-1 provides literature supporting the use of simulation to address cultural competemility.

In Situ Simulation

Simulation has been shown to be effective when used in situ, that is within the natural setting with equipment that is frequently used (Lopreiato et al., 2016; Ostergaard et al., 2011). Simulation encounters in situ often occur during the typical workday with learners who are on duty (Kalaniti, 2014). The learning that occurs in a simulation in an authentic environment is highly relevant and may be stored and retrieved more efficiently (Fialkow et al., 2014; Schmidt & Boshuizen, 1993, as cited in Kalaniti, 2014). Simulations in situ also may reveal systems issues that can be adjusted to allow for more effective team response

Table 2-2 provides additional evidence of how simulation can be used to enhance a variety of skills.

Table 2-3 is an example of clinical experiences. These activities can be incorporated into high-fidelity simulations.

Table 2-1. Example Simulations Addressing Cultural Humility

Reference	Country of Origin	Objective	Focus Population	Type of Simulation Modality (Paper Case, Task Trainer, Manikin, SP)	Other
Bobianski et al., 2016	United States	"The simulation of end-of-life care in a Chinese-American home was scripted with student actors to familiarize students with the concepts of death and dying, as well as integrating cultural considerations in providing such care."	Chinese American individuals	Role play	Nursing students
Leake et al., 2010	United States	"The purpose of the project was to grapple with the challenge of increasing culturally responsive practice in a context of safety and permanency that is defined by American political and cultural values. The learning of cultural competence in the context of a Latino population was evaluated."	Latino individuals	Complex multicharacter role play	Child welfare professionals
Mager & Grossman, 2013	United States	"To increase cultural awareness in nursing students caring for diverse older adults in home care."	Patients with diverse health history, age, culture, religion, dietary preferences, marital status, family involvement, and socio-economic status	Case studies and high-fidelity simulators	Nursing students
Maguire et al., 2017	United States	"To create an experiential educational activity that would both set the tone for, and have a lasting impact on, residents."	Low-income and low-resource clients	Multicharacter role play	Medical interns

(continued)

Table 2-1 (continued). Example Simulations Addressing Cultural Humility

Reference	Country of Origin	Objective	Focus Population	Type of Simulation Modality (Paper Case, Task Trainer, Manikin, SP)	Other
Ndiwane et al., 2017	United States	"To introduce an OSCE with culturally diverse standardized patients to graduate nursing students."	Ethnically diverse	Standardized patients	Nursing students
Paroz et al., 2016	Switzerland	"Testing the feasibility of using simulated patients as a method to improve cultural sensitivity."	Case #1: Sexual orientation, country of origin, religion, and social status Case #2: Country of origin, gender and family dynamics, social inclusion, and lifestyle and nutrition	Simulated patient	Resident doctors
Sales et al., 2013	United States	"To compare three educational interventions (a cultural competence lecture, two written case scenarios, and a simulated patient exercise) to determine the extent to which each intervention enhanced cultural competency."	Racial diversity	Case studies and role play	Pharmacy students
Simones et al., 2010	United States	"To develop a five-bed simulation project to enable nursing students to practice and apply principles related to delegation, supervision, scope of practice, and culturally competent care to enhance students' cultural awareness and sensitivity in the clinical setting."	Diverse racial and ethnic groups	Case scenarios via online learning modules	Nursing students

(continued)

Table 2-1 (continued). Example Simulations Addressing Cultural Humility

Reference	Country of Origin	Objective	Focus Population	Type of Simulation Modality (Paper Case, Task Trainer, Manikin, SP)	Other
Smith & Silk et al., 2011	United States	"To investigate the impact of simulation involving an Arab American Muslim patient on medical students' knowledge, skills, and attitudes regarding culturally competent health care to Arab-American Muslim patients."	Arab American Muslims	Online 30- to 60-minute interactive patient simulation	Osteopathic medicine students Being bilingual was the strongest predictor of success, bilingual students scored higher on all measures than English-only speaking students
Yang et al., 2014	United States	"Evaluated the effectiveness of a poverty simulation in increasing understanding of and attitudes toward poverty and resulting in changes in clinical practice among nursing seniors."	Low-income clients	Role play	Senior community health nursing students Authors recommend doing a poverty simulation earlier in the curriculum

Adapted from Foronda et al., 2018.

Table 2-2. Evidence of Skills Enhanced Through Simulation

	Task Trainer	Human Patient Simulators	Standardized Patient	Hybrid
Teamwork		Gardner & Ahmed, 2014; Marken et al., 2010; Titzer et al., 2012	Joyal et al., 2015; Marken et al., 2010;	Rosen et al., 2008
Communication		Bambini et al., 2009	Borghi et al., 2016; Rickles et al., 2009; Wear & Varley, 2008	Bowyer et al., 2010
Decision Making		Gibbs & Dietrich, 2017; Baird et al., 2015	Haracz et al., 2015; Johnston, 2018; Velde et al., 2009	
Situational Awareness			Giles et al., 2014	
Safe Practice	Barsuk et al., 2009	Ford et al., 2010; Wolf & Gantt, 2008		
Remediation		Haskvitz & Koop, 2004; Lynn & Twigg, 2011	Giles et al., 2014	
Technical Skills	McGaghie et al., 2011	Baird et al., 2015; Ohtake et al., 2013; Van Oss et al., 2013; Wayne et al., 2008		

Table 2-3. Clinical Activities That Can Be Incorporated Into Simulation Encounters

Thomas Jefferson University
Jefferson College of Rehabilitation Sciences
Department of Occupational Therapy
OT 340—Domains of Occupational Therapy Practice

Student Name: ____________________ Due: Upload image to BBL by due date
Site: ______________________________ Date: _______________ Grade: ___/5

Level I Fieldwork Active Learning and Engagement Tool

This tool is designed to be utilized by the fieldwork educator (FWEd) to communicate expectations for active engagement and assist students with developing clinical skills through active learning activities during Level I fieldwork. A collaborative process should be used between the FWEd and the student when identifying which activities should be targeted. It is recommended that additional activities be added to this tool to better meet the needs of each student and fieldwork site. It is important for the FWEd to be aware of where the student is at in the progression of their academic program. It is meant for this tool to be utilized as a tracking form for the student's active participation and completion of assignments while at Level I fieldwork.

(continued)

Table 2-3 (continued). Clinical Activities That Can Be Incorporated Into Simulation Encounters

Occupational Therapy Process Skills	Student Activities (Minimum of 5; 2 points)	Date Initiated and FWEd Initials (1.5 points)	Date Final Review and FWEd Initials (1.5 points)
Evaluation: Developing an Occupational Profile	• Review client chart and provide pertinent details to the FWEd prior to the FWEd starting the evaluation • Complete an interview to obtain the occupational profile • Develop an interview template with questions pertinent to the setting • Articulate the distinct value of occupational therapy to a client and/or family Additional Activities:		
Evaluation: Analyzing Occupational Performance	• Take vital signs • Screen for ROM/MMT • Review a completed evaluation report and identify any additional assessments that could have been utilized • Observe client performance during an evaluation and identify the client's limiting and supporting factors • Administer parts of an assessment tool, score and write up the results Additional Activities:		
Intervention: Developing an Intervention Plan	• Identify and write two goals for a client • Utilizing the professional language from the OTPF-4, identify the main approach and at least two types of occupational therapy interventions with examples to be incorporated into the intervention plan • Bring in a summary of one to two current articles to expand the current types of intervention utilized at the site on a topic suggested by the FWEd Additional Activities:		

(continued)

Table 2-3 (continued). Clinical Activities That Can Be Incorporated Into Simulation Encounters

Occupational Therapy Process Skills	Student Activities (Minimum of 5; 2 points)	Date Initiated and FWEd Initials (1.5 points)	Date Final Review and FWEd Initials (1.5 points)
Intervention: Implementing Interventions	• Review client chart, discuss any pertinent medical status changes with the interprofessional team, and notify the FWEd of any updates prior to starting the session • Assist with putting together written materials for client education • Retrieve all supplies for an intervention session, set up and clean up the room • Explain the intervention plan (developed by the FWEd) for a client in preparation for their session • Observe an intervention session and document on the site-specific documentation system and/or write a SOAP note • Complete an intervention plan and implement it as part of an intervention session under the supervision of the FWEd • Set up, scan the environment, and identify safety concerns for the client prior to transitioning to a new activity • Complete or instruct the FWEd on the steps of a functional transfer Additional Activities:		
Intervention: Reviewing Interventions	• Reflect on an intervention session and identify if the interventions met the client's goals or if they need to be modified and how • Observe an intervention session, review the plan, and update goals based on the client's performance Additional Activities:		
Targeting of Outcomes	• Identify outcome measures utilized by the site Additional Activities:		

(continued)

Table 2-3 (continued). Clinical Activities That Can Be Incorporated Into Simulation Encounters

Occupational Therapy Process Skills	Student Activities (Minimum of 5; 2 points)	Date Initiated and FWEd Initials (1.5 points)	Date Final Review and FWEd Initials (1.5 points)
Clinical Reasoning	• Reflect on a day's events and identify any changes to make for the next visit • Observe a session and identify reasons why the FWEd may have chosen a particular intervention for a client and compare your thoughts with the FWEd Additional Activities:		
Therapeutic Use of Self	• Reflect on your experiences with people who were difficult to communicate with and identify three strategies for communicating with challenging clients • Identify three to four interventions to address one of a client's goals, then collaborate with the client to give choices • Articulate the distinct value of occupational therapy to a client and/or family Additional Activities:		
Activity Analysis	• Choose a piece of equipment or an activity and identify how it could be utilized in at least three different ways to accomplish varying goals • Complete an occupation-based activity analysis through determining occupational demands of an activity that is challenging for a client and utilize this when developing the intervention plan Additional Activities:		

 Occupational Therapy Process Skills obtained from *Occupational Therapy Practice Framework: Domain and Process* (4th ed., AOTA, 2020).

References

Accreditation Council for Occupational Therapy Education. (2018). Accreditation Council for Occupational Therapy Education (ACOTE) Standards and Interpretive Guide. *American Occupational Therapy Association, 72*(Supplement_2), 7212410005p1–7212410005p83. https://doi.org/10.5014/ajot.2018.72S217

Accreditation Council for Pharmacy Education. (2011). *Accreditation standards and guidelines for the professional program in pharmacy leading to the doctor of pharmacy degree.* S2007, Guidelines 2.0, Preamble Addendum, Appendix D. Retrieved from http://www.acpe-accredit.org/pdf/FinalS2007Guidelines2.0.pdf.

Alinier, G., Hunt, B., Gordon, R., & Harwood, C. (2006). Effectiveness of intermediate-fidelity simulation training technology in undergraduate nursing education. *Journal of Advanced Nursing, 54*(3), 359-369. https://doi.org/10.1111/j.1365-2648.2006.03810.x

American Occupational Therapy Association. (2020). Occupational therapy practice framework: Domain and process—fourth edition. *American Journal of Occupational Therapy, 74*(Supplement_2), 7412410010p1–7412410010p87. https://doi.org/10.5014/ajot.2020.74S2001

Baird, J. M., Raina, K. D., Rogers, J. C., O'Donnell, J., & Holm, M. B. (2015). Wheelchair transfer simulations to enhance procedural skills and clinical reasoning. *American Journal of Occupational Therapy, 69*(2), 1-8. https://doi.org/10.5014/ajot.2015.018697

Bambini, D., Washburn, J., & Perkins, R. (2009). Outcomes of clinical simulation for novice nursing students: Communication, confidence, clinical judgment. *Nursing Education Perspectives, 30*(2), 79-82. Retrieved from https://www.ncbi.nlm.nih.gov/pubmed/19476069

Barsuk, J. H., McGaghie, W. C., Cohen, E. R., O'Leary, K. J., & Wayne, D. B. (2009). Simulation-based mastery learning reduces complications during central venous catheter insertion in a medical intensive care unit. *Critical Care Medicine, 37*(10), 2697-2701. https://doi.org/10.1097/00003246-200910000-00003

Bobianski, K., Aselton, P., & Cho, K. S. (2016). Home care simulation to teach culturally based competencies in end-of-life care. *Journal of Nursing Education, 55*(1), 49-52. https://doi.org/10.3928/01484834-20151214-12

Borghi, L., Johnson, I., Barlascini, L., Moja, E. A., & Vegni, E. (2016). Do occupational therapists' communication behaviours change with experience? *Scandinavian Journal of Occupational Therapy, 23*(1), 50-56. https://doi.org/10.3109/11038128.2015.1058856

Bould, M. D., & Naik, V. N. (2009). Teaching how to expect the unexpected: Improving the retention of knowledge for rare clinical events. *Canadian Journal of Anesthesiology, 56*(1), 14-18. https://doi.org/10.1007/s12630-008-9005-6

Bowyer, M. W., Hanson, J. L., Pimentel, E. A., Flanagan, A. K., Rawn, L. M., Rizzo, A. G., Ritter, E., & Lopreiato, J. O. (2010). Teaching breaking bad news using mixed reality simulation. *Journal of Surgical Research, 159*(1), 462-467. https://doi.org/10.1016/j.jss.2008.11.041

Bradley, P. (2006). The history of simulation in medical education and possible future directions. *Medical Education, 40,* 254-262. https://doi.org/10.1111/j1365-2929.2006.02394.x

Braude, P., Reedy, G., Dasgupta, D., Dimmock, V., Jaye, P., & Birns, J. (2015). Evaluation of a simulation training programme for geriatric medicine. *Age and Aging, 44*(4), 677-682. https://doi.org/10.1093/ageing/afv049

Campinha-Bacote, J., (2018). Cultural competemility: A paradigm shift in the cultural competence versus cultural humility debate—Part I. *The Online Journal of Issues in Nursing, 24,*1. https://doi.org/10.3912/OJIN.Vol24No01PPT20

Evans, C. J. & Harder, N. (2013). A formative approach to student remediation. *Nurse Educator, 38*(4), 147-151. https://doi.org/10.1097/NNE.0b013e318296dd0f

Fialkow, M. F., Adams, C. R., Carranza, L., Golden, S. J., Benedetti, T. J., & Fernandez, R. (2014). An in situ standardized patient-based simulation to train postpartum hemorrhage and team skills on a labor and delivery unit. *Simulation in Healthcare, 9*(1), 65-71. https://doi.org/10.1097/SIH.0000000000000007

Ford, D. G., Seybert, A. L., Smithburger, P. L., Kobulinsky, L. R., Samosky, J. T., & Kane-Gill S. L. (2010). Impact of simulation-based learning on medication error rates in critically ill patients. *Intensive Care Medicine, 36*(9), 1526-1531. https://doi.org/10.1007/s00134-010-1860-2

Foronda, C. L., Baptiste, D. L., Pfaff, T., Velez, R., Reinholdt, M., Sanchez, M., & Hudson, K. W. (2018). Cultural competency and cultural humility in simulation-based education: An integrative review. *Clinical Simulation in Nursing, 15,* 42-60. https://doi.org/10.1016/j.ecns.2017.09.006.

Gardner, A. K. & Ahmed, R. A. (2014). Transforming trauma teams through transactive memory: Can simulation enhance performance? *Simulation and Gaming, 45*(3), 356-370. https://doi.org/10.1177%2F1046878114547836

Gibbs, D. M., & Dietrich, M. (2017). Using high fidelity simulation to impact occupational therapy student knowledge, comfort, and confidence in acute care. *The Open Journal of Occupational Therapy, 5*(1), 10. https://doi.org/10.15453/2168-6408.1225

Giles, A. K., Carson, N. E., Breland, H. L., Coker-Bolt, P., & Bowman, P. (2014). Use of simulated patients and reflective video analysis to assess occupational therapy students' preparedness for fieldwork. *American Journal of Occupational Therapy, 68,* 57-66. https://doi.org/10.5014/ajot.2014.685S03

Greene, R. E., Hanley, K., Cook, T. E., Gillespie, C., & Zabar, S. (2017). Meeting the primary care needs of transgender patients through simulation. *Journal of Graduate Medical Education, 9*(3), 380-381.

Haracz, K., Arrighi, G., & Joyce, B. (2015). Simulated patients in a mental health occupational therapy course: A pilot study. *British Journal of Occupational Therapy, 78*(12), 757-766. https://doi.org/10.1177%2F0308022614562792

Haskvitz, L. M., & Koop, E. C. (2004). Students struggling in clinical? A new role for the patient simulator. *Journal of Nursing Education, 43*(4), 181-184. Retrieved from https://www.ncbi.nlm.nih.gov/pubmed/15098913

Hayden, J. K., Smiley, R. A., & Gross, L. (2014). Simulation in nursing education: Current regulations and practices. *Journal of Nursing Regulation, 5*(2), 25-30. https://doi.org/10.1016/s2155-8256(15)30084-3

Imms, C., Chu, E. M. Y., Guinea, S., Sheppard, L., Froude, E., Carter, R., Darzins, S., Ashby, S. Gilbert-Hunt, S., Gribble, N., Nicola-Richmond, K., Penman, M., Gospodarevskaya, E., Mathieu, E., & Symmons, M. (2017). Effectiveness and cost-effectiveness of embedded simulation in occupational therapy clinical practice education: Study protocol for a randomized controlled trial. *Trials, 18*(1), 345. https://doi.org/10.1186/s13063-017-2087-0

Interprofessional Education Collaborative. (2016). *Core competencies for interprofessional collaborative practice: 2016 update.* Interprofessional Education Collaborative.

Johnston, T. E. (2018). Assessment of medical screening and clinical reasoning skills by physical therapy students in a simulated patient encounter. *Internet Journal of Allied Health Sciences and Practice, 16*(2), 10. Retrieved from https://nsuworks.nova.edu/cgi/viewcontent.cgi?article=1735&context=ijahsp

Joyal, K. M., Katz, C., Harder, N., & Dean, H. (2015). Interprofessional education using simulation of an overnight inpatient ward shift. *Journal of Interprofessional Care, 29*(3), 268-270. https://doi.org/10.3109/13561820.2014.944259

Kalaniti, K. (2014). In situ simulation: Let's work, practice, and learn together. *Acta Paediatrica, 103*(12), 1219-1220. https://doi.org/10.1111/apa.12802

Kane-Gill, S. L., & Smithburger, P. L. (2011). Transitioning knowledge gained from simulation to pharmacy practice. *American Journal of Pharmaceutical Education, 75*(10), 210. https://doi.org/10.5688/ajpe7510210

Larue, C., Pepin, J., & Allard, E. (2015). Simulation in preparation or substitution for clinical placement: A systematic review of the literature. *Journal of Nursing Education and Practice, 5*(9), 132-140. https://doi.org/10.5430/jnep.v5n9p132

Lau, P. M. Y., Woodward-Kron, R., Livesay, K., Elliott, K., & Nicholson, P. (2016). Cultural respect encompassing simulation training: Being heard about health through broadband. *Journal of Public Health Research, 5*(1), 657. https://doi.org/10.4081/jphr.2016.657

Leake, R., Holt, K., Potter, C., & Ortega, D. M. (2010). Using simulation training to improve culturally responsive child welfare practice. *Journal of Public Child Welfare, 4*(3), 325-346. https://doi.org/10.1080/15548732.2010.496080

Liu, J., Yucel, K., & Bedi, H. S. (2016). Radiology resident remediation: Five important questions to ask. *American Journal of Roentgenology, 206*(5), 1045-1048. https://doi.org/10.2214/ajr.15.15551

Lopreiato, J. O. (Ed.), Downing, D., Gammon, W., Lioce, L., Sittner, B., Slot, V., Spain, A. E. (Associate Eds.), and the Terminology & Concepts Working Group. (2016). *Healthcare simulation dictionary.* Retrieved from http://www.ssih.org/dictionary

Lynn, M. C., & Twigg, R. D. (2011). A new approach to clinical remediation. *Journal of Nursing Education, 50*(3), 172-175. https://doi.org/10.3928/01484834-20101230-12

Mager, D. R., & Grossman, S. (2013). Promoting nursing students' understanding and reflection on cultural awareness with older adults in home care. *Home Healthcare Now, 31*(10), 582-588. https://doi.org/10.1097/01.nhh.0000436218.64596.b4

Maguire, M. S., Kottenhaun, R., Consiglio-Ward, L., Smalls, A., & Dressler, R. (2017). Using a poverty simulation in graduate medical education as a mechanism to introduce social determinants of health and cultural competency. *Journal of Graduate Medical Education, 9*(3), 386-387. https://doi.org/10.4300/JGME-D-16-00776.1

Maran, N. J., & Glavin, R. J. (2003). Low-to high-fidelity simulation—A continuum of medical education? *Medical Education, 37,* 22-28. https://doi.org/10.1046/j.1365-2923.37.s1.9.x

Marken, P. A., Zimmerman, C., Kennedy, C., Schremmer, R., & Smith, K. (2010). Human simulators and standardized patients to teach difficult conversations to interprofessional health care teams. *American Journal of Pharmaceutical Education, 74*(7), 120. https://doi.org/10.5688/aj7407120

McGaghie, W. C., Issenberg, S. B., Cohen, E. R., Barsuk, J. H., & Wayne, D. B. (2011). Does simulation-based medical education with deliberate practice yield better results than traditional clinical education? A meta-analytic comparative review of the evidence. *Academic Medicine, 86*(6), 706-711. https://doi.org/10.1097/ACM.0b013e318217e119

Ndiwane, A., Koul, O., & Theroux, R. (2014). Implementing standardized patients to teach cultural competency to graduate nursing students. *Clinical Simulation in Nursing, 10*(2). https://doi.org/10.1016/j.ecns.2013.07.002

Ohtake, P. J., Lazarus, M., Schillo, R., & Rosen, M. (2013). Simulation experience enhances physical therapist student confidence in managing a patient in the critical care environment. *Critical Illness Special Series, 93*(2), 216-228. https://doi.org/10.2522/ptj.20110463

Ostergaard, D., Dieckmann, P., & Lippert, A. (2011). Simulation and CRM. *Best Practice and Research Clinical Anaesthesiology, 25*(2), 239-249. https://doi.org/10.1016/j.bpa.2011.02.003

Paroz, S., Daele, A., Viret, F., Vadot, S., Bonvin, R., & Bodenmann, P. (2016). Cultural competence and simulated patients. *The Clinical Teacher, 13*(5), 369-373. https://doi.org/10.1111/tct.12466

Rickles, N. M., Tieu, P., Myers, L., Galal, S., & Chung, V. (2009). The impact of a standardized patient program on student learning of communication skills. *American Journal of Pharmaceutical Education, 73*(1), 4. https://doi.org/10.5688/aj730104

Riem, N., Boet, S., Bould, M. D., Tavares, W., & Naik, V. N. (2012). Do technical skills correlate with non-technical skills in crisis resource management: A simulation study. *British Journal of Anaesthesia, 109*(5), 723-728. https://doi.org/10.1093%2Fbja%2Faes256

Riopel, M. A., Litwin, B., Silberman, N., & Fernandez-Fernandez, A. (2018). Utilizing standardized patient feedback to facilitate professional behavior in physical therapy students: A pilot study. *Internet Journal of Allied Health Sciences and Practice, 16*(3), 4. https://doi.org/10.3138/ptc.2018-04.e

Rosen, M. A., Salas, E., Wilson, K. A., King, H. B., Salisbury, M., Augenstein, J. S., Robinson, D. W., & Birnbach, D. J. (2008). Measuring team performance in simulation-based training: Adopting best practices for healthcare. *Simulation in Healthcare, 3*(1), 33-41. https://doi.org/10.1097/SIH.0b013e3181626276

Rutherford-Hemming, T., Nye, C., & Coram, C. (2016). Using simulation for clinical practice in nurse practitioner education in the United States: A systematic review. *Nurse Education Today, 37*, 128-135. https://doi.org/10.1016/j.nedt.2015.11.006

Rutledge, C. M., Barham, P., Wiles, L., Benjamin, R. S., Eaton, P., & Palmer, K. (2008). Integrative simulation: A novel approach to educating culturally competent nurses. *Contemporary Nurse, 28*(1-2), 119-128. https://doi.org/10.5172/conu.673.28.1-2.119

Sachdeva, A. K. (2016). Continuing professional development in the twenty-first century. *Journal of Continuing Education in the Health Professions, 36*(1), 8-13. https://doi.org/10.1097/CEH.0000000000000107

Sales, I., Jonkman, L., Connor, S., & Hall, D. (2013). A comparison of educational interventions to enhance cultural competency in pharmacy students. *American Journal of Pharmaceutical Education, 77*(4), 76. https://doi.org/10.5688/ajpe77476

Schmidt, H. G., & Boshuizen, H. P. A. (1993). On acquiring expertise in medicine. *Educational Psychology Review, 5*(3), 205-221. https://doi.org/10.1007/BF01323044

Sequeira, G. M., Chakraborti, C., & Panunti, B. A. (2012). Integrating lesbian, gay, bisexual, and transgender (LGBT) content into undergraduate medical school curricula: A qualitative study. *The Ochsner Journal, 12*(4), 379-382.

Simones, J., Wilcox, J., Scott, K., Goeden, D., Copley, D., Doetkott, R., & Kippley, M. (2010). Collaborative simulation project to teach scope of practice. *Journal of Nursing Education, 49*(4), 190-197. https://doi.org/10.3928/01484834-20091217-01

Smith, D. B., & Silk, K. (2011). Cultural competence clinic: An online, interactive, simulation for working effectively with Arab American Muslim patients. *Academic Psychiatry, 35*(5), 312-316. https://doi.org/10.1176/appi.ap.35.5.312

Titzer, J. L., Swenty, C. F., & Hoehn, W. G. (2012). An interprofessional simulation promoting collaboration and problem solving among nursing and allied health professional students. *Clinical Simulation in Nursing, 8*(8), 325-333. https://doi.org/10.1016/j.ecns.2011.01.001

Van Oss, T., Perez, J., & Hartmann, K. (2013). Making mistakes virtually: Simulation helps students practice occupational therapy. *OT Practice*, 15-17.

Velde, B. P., Lane, H., & Clay, M. (2009). Hands on learning: The use of simulated clients in intervention cases. *Journal of Allied Health, 38*(1), 17-21. Retrieved from https://www.ncbi.nlm.nih.gov/pubmed/19753408

Watson, K., Wright, A., Morris, N., McKeeken, J., Rivett, D., Blackstock, F., Jones, A., Haines, T., O'Connor, V., Watson, G., Peterson, R., & Jull, G. (2012). Can simulation replace part of clinical time? Two parallel randomised controlled trials. *Medical Education, 46*(7), 657-667. https://doi.org/10.1111/j.1365-2923.2012.04295.x

Wayne, D. B., Didwania, A., Feinglass, J., Fudala, M. J., Barsuk, J. H., & McGaghie, W. C. (2008). Simulation-based education improves quality of care during cardiac arrest team responses at an academic teaching hospital. *CHEST, 133*(1), 56-61. https://doi.org/10.1378/chest.07-0131

Wear, D., & Varley, J. D. (2008). Rituals of verification: The role of simulation in developing and evaluating empathic communication. *Patient Education and Counseling, 71*(2), 153-156. https://doi.org/10.1016/j.pec.2008.01.005

Wolf, L., & Gantt, L. T. (2008). The use of human patient simulation in ED triage training can improve nursing confidence and patient outcomes. *Journal of Emergency Nursing, 34*(2), 169-171. https://doi.org/10.1016/j.jen.2007.11.005

Yang, K., Woomer, G. R., Agbemenu, K., & Williams, L. (2014). Relate better and judge less: Poverty simulation promoting culturally competent care in community health nursing. *Nurse Education in Practice, 14*(6), 680-685. https://doi.org/10.1016/j.nepr.2014.09.001

Suggested Readings

Ali, J., Adam, R., Sammy, I., Ali, E., & Williams, J. I. (2007). The simulated trauma patient teaching module—Does it improve student performance? *The Journal of Trauma and Acute Care Surgery, 62*(6), 1416-1420. https://doi.org/10.1097/TA.0b013e3180479813

Arif, S., Cryder, B., Mazan, J., Quinones-Boex, A., & Cyganska, A. (2017). Using patient case video vignettes to improve students' understanding of cross-cultural communication. *American Journal of Pharmaceutical Education, 81*(3), 56. https://doi.org/10.5688/ajpe81356

Barrows, H. S. (1968). Simulated patients in medical teaching. *Canadian Medical Association Journal, 98*(14), 674-676. Retrieved from https://www.ncbi.nlm.nih.gov/pubmed/5646104

Barrows, H. S. (1993). An overview of the uses of standardized patients for teaching and evaluating clinical skills. *Academic Medicine, 68*(6), 443-453. https://doi.org/10.1097/00001888-199306000-00002

Bensfield, L. A., Olech, M. J., & Horsley, T. L. (2012). Simulation for high-stakes evaluation in nursing. *Nurse Educator, 37*(2), 71-74. https://doi.org/10.1097/NNE.0b013e3182461b8c

Beyea, S. C., & Kobokovich, L. J. (2004). Human patient simulation: A teaching strategy. *Association of Perioperative Registered Nurses Journal, 80*(4), 738, 741-742. https://doi.org/10.1016/s0001-2092(06)61329-x

Bosek, M. S., Li, S., & Hicks, F. D. (2007). Working with standardized patients: A primer. *International Journal of Nursing Education Scholarship, 4*(1), 16. https://doi.org/10.2202/1548-923X.1437

Bradley, G., Whittington, S., & Mottram, P. (2013). Enhancing occupational therapy education through simulation. *British Journal of Occupational Therapy, 76*(1), 43-46. https://doi.org/10.4276%2F030802213X13576469254775

Butler, K. W., & Veltre, D. E. (2009). Implementation of active learning pedagogy comparing low-fidelity simulation versus high-fidelity simulation in pediatric nursing education. *Clinical Simulation in Nursing, 5*(4), 129-136. https://doi.org/10.1016/j.ecns.2009.03.118

Cannon-Diehl, M. R. (2009). Simulation in healthcare and nursing: State of the science. *Critical Care Nurse, 32*(2), 128-136. https://doi.org/10.1097/CNQ.0b013e3181a27e0f

Cumin, D., Merry, A. F., & Weller, J. M. (2008). Editorial: Standards for simulation. *Journal of the Association of Anaesthetists of Great Britain and Ireland, 63*, 1281-1287. https://doi.org/10.1111/j.1365-2044.2008.05787.x

Dawson, S. (2006). Procedural simulation: A primer. *Journal of Vascular and Interventional Radiology, 17*(2), 205-213. https://doi.org/10.1148/radiol.2411062581

Day, J. A. (1985). Beyond lecture and laboratory in the physical therapy classroom. *Physical Therapy, 65*(8), 1214-1216. https://doi.org/10.1093/ptj/65.8.1214

Doll, J., Packard, K., Furze, J., Huggett, K., Jensen, G., Jorgensen, D., Wilken, M., Chelel, H., & Maio, A. (2013). Reflections from an interprofessional education experience: Evidence for the core competencies for interprofessional collaborative practice. *Journal of Interprofessional Care, 27*(2), 194-196. https://doi.org/10.3109/13561820.2012.729106

Ebbert, D. W., & Connors, H. (2004). Standardized patient experiences: Evaluation of clinical performance and nurse practitioner student satisfaction. *Nursing Education Perspectives, 25*(1), 12-15. Retrieved from https://www.ncbi.nlm.nih.gov/pubmed/15017794

Elman, D., Hooks, R., Tabak, D., Regehr, G., & Freeman, R. (2004). The effectiveness of unannounced standardized patients in the clinical setting as a teaching intervention. *Medical Education, 38*(9), 969-973. https://doi.org/10.1111/j.1365-2929.2004.01919.x

Ericsson, K. A. (2004). Deliberate practice and the acquisition and maintenance of expert performance in medicine and related domains. *Academic Medicine, 79*(10), 70-81. https://doi.org/10.1097/00001888-200410001-00022

Flanagan, B., Nestel, D., & Joseph, M. (2004). Making patient safety the focus: Crisis resource management in the undergraduate curriculum. *Medical Education, 38*(1), 56-66. https://doi.org/10.1111/j.1365-2923.2004.01701.x

Hale, L. S., Lewis, D. K., Eckert, R. M., Wilson, C. M., & Smith, B. S. (2006). Standardized patients and multidisciplinary classroom instruction for physical therapist students to improve interviewing skills and attitudes about diabetes. *Journal of Physical Therapy Education, 20*(1), 22-27. https://doi.org/10.1097/00001416-200601000-00003

Hawkins, K., Todd, M., & Manz, J. (2008). A unique simulation teaching method. *Journal of Nursing Education, 47*(11), 524-527. https://doi.org/10.3928/01484834-20081101-04

Hayward, L. M., Blackmer, B., & Markowski, A. (2006). Standardized patients and communities of practice: A realistic strategy for integrating the core values in a physical therapist education program. *Journal of Physical Therapy Education, 20*(2), 29-37. https://doi.org/10.1097/00001416-200607000-00005

Karkowsky, C. E., & Chazotte, C. (2013). Simulation: Improving communication with patients. *Seminars in Perinatology, 37*(3), 157-160. https://doi.org/10.1053/j.semperi.2013.02.006

Khan, Z., & Kapralos, B. (2017). A low-fidelity serious game for medical-based cultural competence education. *Health Informatics Journal, 25*(3), 1-17. https://doi.org/10.1177/1460458217719562

Maguire, M. S. (2017). Using a poverty simulation in graduate medical education as a mechanism to introduce social determinants of health and cultural competency. *Journal of Graduate Medical Education, 9*(3), 386-387. https://doi.org/10.4300%2FJGME-D-16-00776.1

Makoul, G. (2006). Communication skills: How simulation training supplements experiential and humanist learning. *Academic Medicine, 81*(3), 271-274. https://doi.org/10.1097/00001888-200603000-00018

Mathew, L., Brewer, B., Crist, J. D., & Poedel, R. J. (2017). Designing a virtual simulation case for cultural competence using a community-based participatory research approach. *Nurse Educator, 42*(4), 191-194. https://doi.org/10.1097/NNE.0000000000000338

McGraw, R. C., & O'Connor, H. M. (1999). Standardized patients in the early acquisition of clinical skills. *Medical Education, 33*(8), 572-578. https://doi.org/10.1046/j.1365-2923.1999.00381.x

Ndiwane, A. N., Baker, N., Makosky, A., Reidy, P., & Guarino, A. J. (2017). Use of simulation to integrate cultural humility into advanced health assessment for nurse practitioner students. *Educational Innovations, 56*(9), 567-571. https://doi.org/10.3928/01484834-20170817-11

Overstreet, M. (2008). The use of simulation technology in the education of nursing students. *Nursing Clinics of North America, 43*(4), 593-603. https://doi.org/10.1016/j.cnur.2008.06.009

Parker, B., & Myrick, F. (2010). Transformative learning as a context for human patient simulation. *Journal of Nursing Education, 49*(6), 326-332. https://doi.org/10.3928/01484834-20100224-02

Rash, E. M. (2008). Simulating health promotion in an online environment. *Journal of Nursing Education, 47*(11), 515-517. https://doi.org/10.3928/01484834-20081101-05

Rubin, N. J., & Philp, E. B. (1998). Health care perceptions of the standardized patient. *Medical Education, 32*(5), 538-542. https://doi.org/10.1046/j.1365-2923.1998.00259.x

Rull, G., Rosher, R. B., McCann-Stone, N., & Robinson, S. B. (2006). A simulated couple aging across the four years of medical school. *Teaching and Learning in Medicine, 18*(3), 261-266. https://doi.org/10.1207/s15328015tlm1803_12

Sachdeva, A. K., Wolfson, P. J., Blair, P. G., Gillum, D. R., Gracely, E. J., & Friedman, M. (1997). Impact of a standardized patient intervention to teach breast and abdominal examination skills to third-year medical students at two institutions. *American Journal of Surgery, 173*(4), 320-325. https://doi.org/10.1016/S0002-9610(96)00391-1

Salas, E., Wilson, K., Burke, C. S., & Priest, H. (2005). Using simulation-based training to improve patient safety: What does it take? *Journal on Quality and Patient Safety, 31*(7), 363-371. https://doi.org/10.1016/S1553-7250(05)31049-X

Schwartz, L. R., Fernandez, R., Kouyoumjian, S. R., Jones, K. A., & Compton, S. (2007). A randomized comparison trial of case-based learning versus human patient simulation in medical student education. *Academic Emergency Medicine, 14*(2), 130-137. https://doi.org/10.1197/j.aem.2006.09.052

Seibert, D. C., Guthrie, J. T., & Adamo, G. (2004). Improving learning outcomes: Integration of standardized patients & telemedicine technology. *Nursing Education Perspectives, 25*(5), 232-237. Retrieved from https://www.ncbi.nlm.nih.gov/pubmed/15508562

Sportsman, S., Bolton, C., Bradshaw, P., Close, D., Lee, M., Townley, N., & Watson, M. N. (2009). A regional simulation center partnership: Collaboration to improve staff and students competency. *The Journal of Continuing Education in Nursing, 40*(2), 67-73. https://doi.org/10.3928/00220124-20090201-09

Stimmel, B., Cohen, D., Fallar, R., & Smith, L. (2006). The use of standardized patients to assess clinical competence: Does practice make perfect? *Medical Education, 40*(5), 444-449. https://doi.org/10.1111/j.1365-2929.2006.02446.x

Stillman, P. L., Regan, M. B., Philbin, M., & Haley, H. L. (1990). Results of a survey on the use of standardized patients to teach and evaluate clinical skills. *Academic Medicine, 65*(5), 288-292. https://doi.org/10.1097/00001888-199005000-00002

Triola, M., Feldman, H., Kalet, A. L., Zabar, S., Kachur, E. K., Gillespie, C., Anderson, M., Griesser, C., & Lipkin, M. (2006). A randomized trial of teaching clinical skills using virtual and live standardized patients. *Journal of General Internal Medicine, 21(5), 424-429. https://doi.*org/10.1111/j.1525-1497.2006.00421.x

Ziv, A., Wolpe, P. R., Small, S. D., & Glick, S. (2003). Simulation-based medical education: An ethical imperative. *Academic Medicine, 78*(8), 783-788. https://doi.org/10.1097/00001888-200308000-00006

Zraick, R. I. (2004). Playacting with a purpose: Using standardized patients to assess clinical skills. *The ASHA Leader, 9*(22), 22. https://doi.org/10.1044/leader.FTR5.09102004.22

Kern's Model Step 2
Targeted Needs Assessment

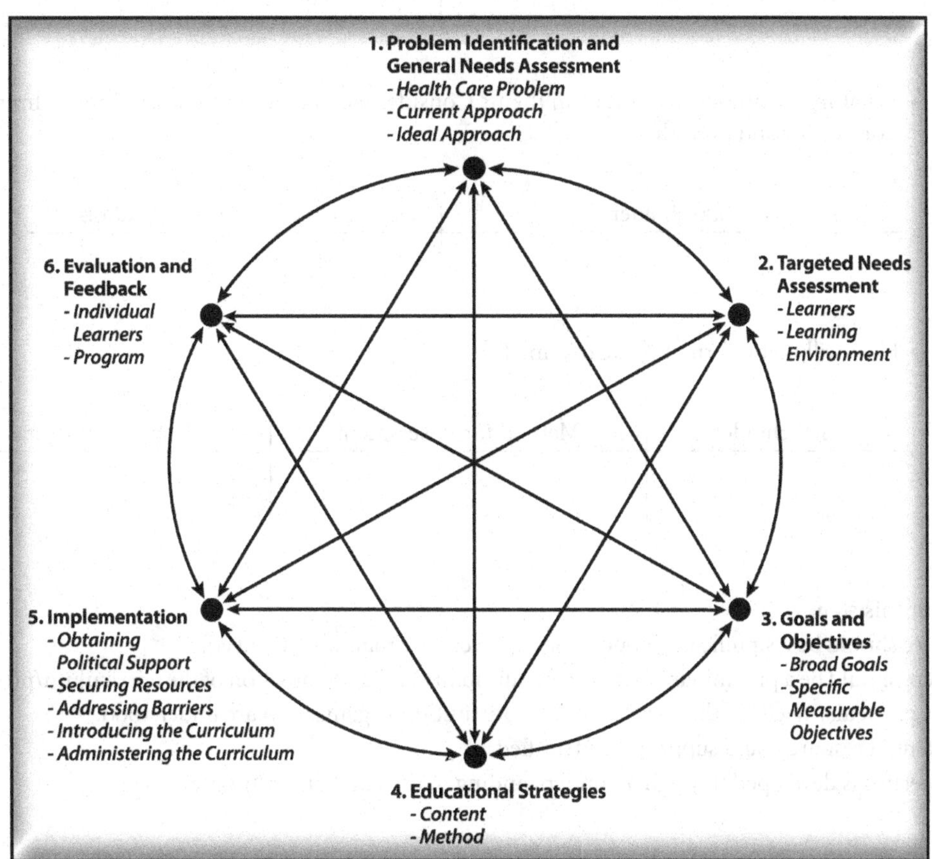

- The purpose of this step is to refine the foundation and ground the curriculum/program in the specific needs of the learners at this institution/organization, which might be different than the needs of learners in general.
- The needs assessment is done at the institutional/organizational level and requires collection of data about the learners and learning environment.
- Data received from the needs assessment will help discover the hidden or informal curriculum/program that is likely influencing behavioral and performance outcomes.
- This step will help integrate simulation activities effectively with the institution's/organization's overall curriculum/program.

- It also identifies stakeholders and involves them in the curriculum/program design process.
- The targeted assessment allows educational strategies to be tailored for specific needs while aligning strategies with resources.

- Identify target audience:
  - Conduct a needs assessment on the learner and learning environment.
  - Consider the methods used and questions to be asked.
    → Who are the learners/stakeholders? Consider previous training and experience.

Learners/Stakeholders	How Are They Impacted by the Problem?

→ What information is needed from them? Consider factors related to institutional administration, policy and procedures.

Stakeholder	Relevant Information

→ How will that information be obtained?

Stakeholder	Method for Assessment	Resources Needed

After this step:

- There should be a significant support for a curricular/programmatic need.
- There should be a preliminary idea of generalizability and dissemination of the curriculum/program.
- The particular needs of the learners and the institution/organization are understood.
- Potential resources and support are identified.
- Expertise is developed through an understanding of the curriculum/program.

Suggested Readings

Farnan, J., & Schindler, N. (2013). *Curriculum development and evaluation guide resident as teacher: A mutually beneficial arrangement APPD/COMSEP pre course 2013.* Retrieved from: https://www.appd.org/meetings/2013SpringPresentations/PCWS1Handout.pdf

Kern, D. E. (2014). *Curriculum development: An essential educational skill, a public trust, a form of scholarship, an opportunity for organizational change.* Weill Cornell College of Medicine, Qatar. Retrieved from: https://dnnyqetna.blob.core.windows.net/portals/15/Six-Step%20Approach%20to%20Curriculum%20Development.pdf?sr=b&si=DNNFileManagerPolicy&sig=9sAOUX/lzfZQsN6QKLOpWJ46YLRuXmQwOghR7ptxnFw=

Khamis, N. N., Satava, R. M., Alnassar, S. A., & Kern, D. E. (2016). A stepwise model for simulation-based curriculum development for clinical skills, a modification of the six-step approach. *Surgical Endoscopy,* 279-287. https://doi.org/10.1007/s00464-015-4206x

3

Clinicians and Educators
A Partnership in Simulation

Jean E. Prast, OTD, MSOT, OTRL, CHSE
Joanne M. Baird, PhD, OTR/L, CHSE, FAOTA

Learning Objectives

1. Define the advantages of simulation as a learning opportunity to best prepare students for clinical practice.
2. Describe how clinical practitioners can contribute to the design and implementation of a simulation experience.

Kern's Model of Program Development

The content in this chapter articulates Step 2 of Kern's Model: Targeted Needs Assessment. Information in this chapter contributes to the creation or modification of a curriculum that prepares students for contemporary clinical practice based upon input from practitioners with expertise in the field. This step identifies stakeholders and involves them in curriculum and course design.

Zapletal, A. L., Baird, J. M., Van Oss, T., Hoppe, M. M., Prast, J. E., & Herge, E. A. *Clinical Simulation for Health Care Professionals* (pp. 29-35).

For health care educators, identifying effective methods for health care training and preparation of students is paramount. Current challenges related to differences and inconsistencies in learning experiences; competition for limited clinical sites; educator and faculty shortages; and the increasing expectations for fast-paced, high-level skills and knowledge of novice clinicians have resulted in an examination of how students are progressed to entry-level professional practice. These discussions have included simulation as an instructional method to meet clinical requirements, with simulation as part of academic training to teach technical and professional skills necessary for practice (Gaba, 2004; Lamb & Harvison, 2017; National Council of State Boards of Nursing, 2014). Simulation has been adopted as a teaching method by multiple health care professions because it does not put patients at harm, is preferred by students, and effectively improves performance in practice areas such as communication, hands-on clinical skills, and patient safety (Bethea et al., 2014; Herge et al., 2013; Lowry, 2016). Research indicates that simulation is most effective when it is realistic and meets the learner's educational needs; thus, there is a need for health care professionals and academic programs to work together to create simulations to prepare students for clinical practice (Lewis et al., 2012; Salas et al., 2005). In this chapter, we will discuss how the skills of clinical educators and health care professionals are ideal for involvement in simulation.

Simulation Partnerships: Academic and Clinical

Although simulations take different forms, the best simulations are created with input from health care professionals, who are subject matter experts, and faculty, who are teaching experts (Salas et al., 2005). Health care professionals are especially well suited to assist with simulation because it requires many of the same skills used in clinical practice. They also have an understanding of the current skills and knowledge needed in clinical health care settings and can create clear, simple tasks that reflect these combinations. The following are examples of how health care professionals can partner with faculty to develop authentic simulations.

Simulation Creation

Creating a simulation involves ensuring its relevance to clinical practice and linking this relevance to what students are expected to learn. This linkage forms an important part of curricular design. Simulation design should be in sync with curricular design, as both are focused on the learning needs of the students. Once these desired outcomes are determined, learning objectives (goals) can be developed to measure performance (Munshi et al., 2015). These objectives should be observable, measurable, and have a range of complexity. Health care professionals have distinct skills that support the development of learning objectives, including goal writing. The goal writing experience of health care professionals can assist faculty to develop learning objectives that optimize simulation outcomes.

Collaboration between health care professionals and faculty, each with different perspectives, ensures that all learning objectives are addressed and takes the realities of clinical practice and recommended educational approaches into consideration (Flood & Robinia, 2014). Health care professionals promote authenticity by ensuring that the simulation replicates events that commonly occur in clinical health care practice. These might include explaining the profession and communicating goals and discharge recommendations to others, encouraging client participation, adjusting the environment for safety, or preparing the environment for intervention.

An example of collaboration would be a simulation to address client assessment. Assessing performance is common in daily practice. Health care professionals are familiar with assessment tools and are able to apply their experience to simulation. In collaboration with faculty, health care professionals can review assessment tools (i.e., standardized or nonstandardized, questionnaire, checklist) to determine what may work best to measure student performance. Health care professionals can evaluate students and take notes to use as teaching points. For example, an observation checklist can be used to track expected interventions, skills, and responses to the simulation. Data from this tool can be used to support students through the clinical reasoning process.

An important component of any learning activity is outcome measurement. Whether in an academic or clinical setting, gathering this information is imperative for growth and change (Scherer et al., 2016). Health care professionals can assist academic programs to develop tools (e.g., surveys, questionnaires, checklists, rubrics, feedback forms) to measure outcomes, rate student performance, or assess specific behaviors and skills. Information from these tools can help with student learning, program development, simulation revisions, and collaboration of involved parties.

Simulation Preparation

Simulation requires careful and thoughtful planning, including when (e.g., class or clinic time) and where (e.g., location, space) it will take place and what resources (e.g., equipment, personnel) are needed. For all simulations, a common theme is the concept of fidelity, which is explored further in Chapter 8. A high level of fidelity means that the simulation has a high level of realism, whereas low-fidelity simulation has a low level of realism. For example, if a simulation to teach a student how to complete an acute care evaluation is done in a classroom setting at a desk and chair, it would be a low-fidelity simulation. That same acute care simulation done in a setting that mimics a hospital room and uses a hospital bed would be high fidelity. High-fidelity simulations are typically more effective instructional methods (Lewis et al., 2012).

Health care professionals can assist the academic program to set up the classroom laboratory environment so that it mimics the clinical practice setting, as well as collect the necessary equipment or tools needed to carry out the simulation. This includes configuring a mock acute care room with a hospital bed, bedside commode, bedside chair, overbed table, telephone, bedside dresser, call light, and associated medical equipment. They can also assist with collecting resources needed to carry out the simulation, which might include borrowing clinic equipment or sharing client education resources.

As education of clients, caregivers, and professionals occurs constantly in clinical practice, health care professionals are well prepared to assist with training standardized patients (SPs) or those fulfilling the patient role. Simulations should be based on realistic clients with varying conditions and life circumstances. Some clinical conditions may be protocol based, while others are more complex. In addition to the clinical conditions of simulation, a client's behavioral responses can vary considerably. Health care professionals can bring their knowledge of these conditions (e.g., signs, symptoms, impairments) and behaviors (e.g., attitudes, adherence, responses) to train SPs for maximum authenticity without sacrificing consistency (Salas et al., 2005).

Simulation Participation

Health care professionals have exclusive perspectives that add value to the didactic education of a student while learning in a safe, controlled environment. SPs need to display realistic behaviors, adequate responses, and movements to depict specific conditions and to interact with the student in a dynamic manner. Health care professionals work with clients daily; therefore, fulfilling the role of an SP by displaying behaviors and simulating signs and symptoms of the condition can offer a sense of realism to the learning experience. While partaking in this role, they can help guide the learning process and provide verbal and written feedback.

Although simulations for an entry-level professional program are often established within an academic setting, there are many opportunities to expand the use of simulation to the clinical setting. Depending on the community and established academic and health care partnerships, simulations can also occur in the health care environment to allow use of onsite resources. This type of simulation is called *in situ* simulation (Lopreiato et al., 2016). Examples include simulations done in an outpatient clinic (including a treatment table, assessment tools, modalities, electronic medical records) or in a hospital setting (i.e., in a designated patient room or unit, using approved medical equipment, incorporating other professionals). Academic programs, health care professionals, and community partners can work together to use resources without affecting client care.

While establishing a high-fidelity simulation is beneficial to student learning, other task-specific simulation activities can be created to prepare students for practice. Health care professionals can support the academic program by training students to use medical equipment commonly seen in specific practice settings (e.g., IV pump, catheter, monitors, drains, ventilators) based on their area of practice and expertise. After familiarity, additional components can be added to create a sense of realism and application to daily practice. For example, a simulation using a standardized client or a role play to identify the proper way to manage the equipment while keeping a client safe.

Health care professionals, especially those with experience as clinical student educators, can assist with the reflective component of simulation, as they often ask students reflective questions before, during, and/or after a client encounter. Once trained in debriefing methods, clinicians can actively engage the student in reflection about specific events and actions to lead a student to identify areas in need of reinforcement and correct areas in need of improvement (Zigmont et al., 2011). Faculty and health care professionals can work together to select the preferred format (e.g., discussion, survey, video) and develop questions to best support student learning during or after a simulation. Using this skill can help to elicit clinical reasoning and critical thinking skills to better prepare students for practice.

Conclusion

Creating a simulation in a safe, controlled, and supportive learning environment can positively affect learning and better prepare students for health care practice (Lewis et al., 2012). Working together, academic programs and health care professionals can better support students in the mastery of clinical skills while learning from their mistakes without causing any harm or risk to an actual client.

Using simulation to promote application of clinical reasoning and analytical skills as part of clinical experiences may help students be better prepared to engage in clinical practice. This may create more effective and efficient health care professionals, thus decreasing the burden placed on clinical educators and clinical sites. Information about using high-fidelity simulation as a teaching method is supported in literature and continues to emerge in various health care professions. One specific example is in the field of occupational therapy, where the use of simulation as part of clinical fieldwork is emerging with benefits to a combination of simulation and clinical fieldwork (Reed, 2016).

Worksheet 3-1
Considerations for Collaboration

Planning the Simulation	*Response*	*Challenges/Barriers*
Who are your current clinical/academic partners? • Identify current community/academic relationships or affiliations		
Who are some potential clinical/academic partners? • Identify health care/educational programs in your area for possible collaboration		
What areas in the learning process do you feel simulation can better support? • Consider student, client, community needs (e.g., interviewing, assessment, interprofessional practice, discharge planning, communication)		
What are the learning needs? • Consider the knowledge and required skills needed for the student • Identify simple tasks that reflect these components		
What is the relevance to education/clinical practice? • Consider realism in preparation for practice • Identify ways to replicate the actual environment and scenario		
What are the learning objectives? • Identify what students are expected to learn • Consider the setting and where the student is in the process (e.g., basic or advanced technical skill development, initial or end phase of service provision)		

(continued)

Worksheet 3-1 (continued)

Considerations for Collaboration

Planning the Simulation	*Response*	*Challenges/Barriers*
What tools are needed to carry out the simulation? • Consider tools to measure outcomes (standardized assessments, observation checklist, surveys, questionnaires, rubrics, feedback forms)		
What resources will you need to plan and carry out the simulation? • Consider when it will happen and where it will take place (e.g., realism) • Identify the tools/resources needed, as well as who has them (e.g., equipment, personnel) • Identify any training needs (e.g., debriefing, verbal/written feedback, SPs, clinical conditions, and behavioral responses)		
What are some additional needs and/or concerns that you have moving forward? • Consider ways to address any needs/concerns identified		

References

Bethea, D. P., Castillo, D. C., & Harvison, N. (2014). Use of simulation in occupational therapy education: Way of the future? *American Journal of Occupational Therapy, 68,* S32-S39. https://doi.org/10.5014/ajot.2014.012716

Flood, L. S., & Robinia, K. (2014). Bridging the gap: Strategies to integrate classroom and clinical learning. *Nurse Education in Practice, 14,* 329-332. https://doi.org/10.1016/j.nepr.2014.02.002

Gaba, D. M. (2004). The future vision of simulation in health care. *Quality & Safety in Health Care, 13,* i2-i10. https://doi.org/10.1136/qshc.2004.009878

Herge, E. A., Lorch, A., DeAngelis, T., Vause-Earland, T., Mollo, K., & Zapletal, A. (2013). The standardized patient encounter: A dynamic educational approach to enhance students' clinical healthcare skills. *Journal of Allied Health, 42*(4), 229-235. Retrieved from https://www.ncbi.nlm.nih.gov/pubmed/24326920

Lamb, A., & Harvison, N. (2017). *2017 Fieldwork (Experiential Learning) Ad Hoc Committee report and recommendations.* Retrieved from https://www.aota.org/~/media/Corporate/Files/EducationCareers/Educators/Fieldwork/AOTA-Fieldwork/residency-for-OTs-considered-by-AOTA-ad-hoc-committee-presentation.pdf

Lewis, R., Strachan, A., & Smith, M. M. (2012). Is high fidelity simulation the most effective method for the development of non-technical skills in nursing? A review of the current evidence. *Open Nursing Journal, 6,* 82-89. https://doi.org/10.2174/1874434601206010082

Lopreiato, J. O. (Ed.), Downing, D., Gammon, W., Lioce, L., Sittner, B., Slot, V., Spain, A. E. (Associate Eds.), and the Terminology & Concepts Working Group. (2016). *Healthcare simulation dictionary.* Retrieved from http://www.ssih.org/dictionary.

Lowry, M. (2016). Improving student nurse skills with simulation. *Nursing Times, 13,* 4-6. Retrieved from https://www.nursingtimes.net/roles/nurse-educators/improving-student-nurse-skills-with-simulation-31-10-2016/

Munshi, F., Lababidi, H., & Alyousef, S. (2015). Low- versus high-fidelity simulations in teaching and assessing clinical skills. *Journal of Taibah University Medical Sciences, 10,* 12-15. https://doi.org/oi: 10.1016/j.jtumed.2015.01.008

National Council of State Boards of Nursing (2014). The NCSBN national simulation study: A longitudinal, randomized, controlled study replacing clinical hours with simulation in prelicensure nursing education. *Journal of Nursing Regulation 5*(2), S3-S50. Retrieved from: https://www.ncsbn.org/JNR_Simulation_Supplement.pdf

Reed, H. (2016). Student responses to the use of simulation in combination with traditional level I fieldwork. *American Journal of Occupational Therapy, 70,* 7011505105p1. https://doi.org/10.5014/ajot.2016.70S1-PO1075

Salas, E., Wilson, K., Burke, C. S., & Priest, H. (2005). Using simulation-based training to improve patient safety: What does it take? *Journal on Quality and Patient Safety, 31*(7), 363-371. https://doi.org/10.1016/S1553-7250(05)31049-X

Scherer, Y., Foltz-Ramos, K., Fabry, D., & Chao, Y.-Y. (2016). Evaluating simulation methodologies to determine best strategies to maximize student learning. *Journal of Professional Nursing, 32,* 349-357. https://doi.org/10.1016/j.profnurs.2016.01.003

Zigmont, J., Kappus, L., & Sudikoff, S. (2011). The 3D model of debriefing: Defusing, discovering, and deepening. *Seminars in Perinatology, 35,* 52-58. https://doi.org/10.1053/j.semperi.2011.01.003

4

Creating Your Simulation

Where Do You Begin? Appreciative Inquiry Approach

E. Adel Herge, OTD, OTR/L, FAOTA

Learning Objectives

1. Establish a vision for integrating clinical simulation into your courses and/or curriculum using an appreciative inquiry approach.
2. Reflect on existing strengths and supports that can facilitate successful implementation of simulation in your course/curriculum.
3. Formulate creative strategies to address identified challenges with implementing clinical simulation in your course/curriculum.

Kern's Model of Program Development

The content in this chapter articulates Step 2 of Kern's Model: Targeted Needs Assessment. Information in this chapter provides a framework for identifying strategies to create a simulation program by leveraging resources. Appreciative inquiry is one method that can be used to align resources with needs.

Zapletal, A. L., Baird, J. M., Van Oss, T., Hoppe, M. M., Prast, J. E., & Herge, E. A. *Clinical Simulation for Health Care Professionals* (pp. 37-43).

Content

Creating a new simulation program or revising an existing simulation can feel like an overwhelming task. Typically, when we approach a challenge such as this, we focus on finding a realistic solution that is feasible given our current situation. While this method is often successful, it can also lead us to focus on barriers we feel powerless to change (e.g., limited budgets, lack of time, scarce resources). This can change our perspective from one of optimistic desire *"I would love to add simulation into my course,"* to abject negativity or hopelessness *"I have no budget for SPs* (standardized patients) *so I will never be able to add simulation into my course."* This can cause us to either abandon the idea altogether or move forward toward the goal with less excitement—cautiously looking for when the next barrier will present itself.

A different way to approach challenges and seek change is using appreciative inquiry (AI). Developed by Cooperrider and Srivastva (1987), AI is a framework for initiating or managing change that focuses on the positive attributes that may fuel change (Dematteo & Reeves, 2011, p. 203). AI has been used in business (Bushe, 1998), health care (Carter et al., 2007; Lind & Smith, 2008; Ruhe et al., 2011), and education (Billings & Kowalski, 2008; Clarke & Thornton, 2014; Dematteo & Reeves, 2011; Quaintance et al., 2010; Rubin et al., 2011). By examining the strengths and supports in an organization or situation, we focus on the positive "life giving properties" of an organization (Bushe, 2011, p. 2). The process requires four steps:

1. *Discovery:* Reflect on what is currently or has been the best experience in this situation.
2. *Dream:* Imagine the situation at the most ideal state.
3. *Design:* Plan and implement the change towards the ideal
4. *Destiny:* Take action to reach the goal in a positive manner.

The method of AI encompasses theories of discourse and narrative (Bushe, 2011) so the process is often done through storytelling. Telling the story about a time when everything came together and resulted in a positive outcome or when significant challenges were overcome to a positive victory energizes the participants for change. Sharing these stories with other team members increases everyone's understanding of shared values and goals, creates connections, reinforces use of positive word choices, and leads to constructive actions (Billings & Kowalski, 2008). See Tables 4-1 and 4-2 for more information about the process.

Strategies for Beginning

- *Start Small:* Design one case for one particular course, this allows for feasibility with your time and resources.
  - Finding SPs, persons to act as simulated patients, or one or two manikins to portray specific clinical needs is easier than trying to find simulated patients or manikins to demonstrate diverse needs in several case stories.
  - Consider conducting the high-fidelity simulation experience in a short time frame, such as having all of the experiences in one day instead of spreading the experiences over multiple days. This efficiency helps you manage your time with this program.
- *Scan Your Landscape:* What institutions or departments could be your collaborators? Is there anyone with experience on your campus? If not, is there a simulation center nearby? Interviewing someone from the center or a theater director or experienced artistic director (someone within the performing arts) can enhance the design aspects of your program.
- *Liability:* Discuss with your chair/program director any concerns about liability if you are bringing volunteer/paid SPs; this may influence the age range of your cast.
- *Rewards:* SPs may be rewarded in multiple ways. Think about rewards other than payment, such as sharing student feedback or thank you letters from students, providing food before and during the SP experience, or recognizing the SPs in a department newsletter or a letter to the Dean's Office.

Table 4-1. Appreciative Inquiry

Discovery	• Interview each other, tell stories of people when they are performing at their best • Determine what is positive, meaningful, successful, and effective • Identify shared values and goals	**Dream**	• Imagine the situation at the very best it can be • Identify common themes, qualities, and aspiration of this best of times • Envision a transformed future
Design	• Create a vision based on the themes that address success (from the stories) • Plan for and implement change	**Destiny**	• Take action to reach the goals identified in the vision • Evaluate progress • Sustain progress toward the goal

Table 4-2. Appreciative Inquiry Example

Example: You are faculty of an occupational therapist assistant program within a community college near a large city (less than 1 hour drive) with a large hospital and medical school. *Situation:* You want to add a simulation experience into your course that introduces basic clinical techniques (e.g., transfers, taking vitals).			
Discovery	• Interview each other, tell stories of people when they are performing at their best *See worksheet for questions; instructors describe their most valuable learning experiences with live patients* • Determine what is positive, meaningful, successful, and effective *Instructors agree that working with live patients is a valuable effective way to learn basic techniques* • Identify shared values and goals *All instructors agree that active learning and "hands on" with patients is a valuable learning method*	**Dream**	• Imagine the situation at the very best it can be *You imagine having live patients for students to work with in your lab* • Identify common themes, qualities, and aspiration of this best of times *Best experiences are with patients who are understanding when you are first learning basic techniques* • Envision a transformed future *You can offer this type of learning experience for your students*

(continued)

TABLE 4-2 (CONTINUED). APPRECIATIVE INQUIRY EXAMPLE

Design	• Create a vision based on the themes that address success (from the stories) *In discussion, one of the lab instructors shares a story about a positive experience they had with a theater group of older adults they volunteer with* • Plan for and implement change *Would this theater group be open to participating in your lab? You and the lab instructors develop a plan to reach out to the theatre group*	**Destiny**	• Take action to reach the goals identified in the vision *Reach out to the theater group and discuss possible collaboration* • Evaluate progress *Once collaboration begins, check in with the leader of the theater group and instructors. What's working? What needs to be changed?* • Sustain progress toward the goal *Continue supporting aspects that make the collaboration work; identify ways to meet challenges, move toward goal*

Worksheet 4-1

Appreciative Inquiry—Discovery

Purpose of This Activity

To provide an opportunity to experience an AI approach in order to build your simulation experiences. By going through the following process, you should have a deeper understanding of your institution's landscape and offerings.

Instructions

With a colleague, interview each other using the following questions. ***Be a generous listener. Do not dialogue.*** Allow your partner to speak freely. Ask additional follow-up questions if necessary. Use this sheet to record the notes from your interview.

Or, if you do not have a colleague, read the questions, reflect, and write down your answers.

- *Best Experience:* Tell me about one of the best times you have had at your organization/program/college/university/institution. When did you feel most alive? Involved? Connected? Excited? What made it so exciting? (Note: this does not have to be specifically related to simulation).

- *Values:* What are three things you value most about your organization/program/college/university/institution? What is the single most important thing that has contributed to your work as an educator in your situation?

- *Core Values:* What is a core value of your organization/program/college/university/institution? What is it, that if it did not exist, would make your situation very different than it currently is?

- *Three Wishes:* If you have three wishes for your organization/program/college/university/institution, what would they be?

Adapted from Appreciative Inquiry Guide for Organizations, Voyle and Voyle Consulting. http://www.appreciativeway.com/appreciative-inquiry-resources/AI-generic-ques-org.pdf. Used with permission.

Worksheet 4-2

Appreciative Inquiry—Dream, Design, and Destiny

When you finished reviewing your answers, ***Dream*** about your ideal future. What does it look like? Who is involved?

Next, ***Design*** the change. Generate a plan of action. What existing strengths and supports can you leverage? Who are the people you need to contact to bring on board? What resources are available?

Finally, move toward ***Destiny.*** Make a personal commitment to act. What is the first step? What do you need to do to make this happen?

Adapted from Appreciative Inquiry Guide for Organizations, Voyle and Voyle Consulting. http://www.appreciativeway.com/appreciative-inquiry-resources/appreciative-inquiry-resources.cfm. Used with permission.

References

Billings, D. M., & Kowalski, K. (2008). Appreciative inquiry. *The Journal of Continuing Education in Nursing, 39*(3), 104. https://doi.org/10.3928/00220124-20080301-11

Bushe, G. R. (1998). Five theories of change embedded in appreciative inquiry. In Cooperrider, D., Sorenson, P., Whitney, D., & Yeager, T. (eds.) *Appreciative inquiry: An emerging direction for organization development* (pp. 117-127). Stipes.

Bushe, G. R. (2011). Appreciative inquiry: Theory and critique. In Boje, D., Burnes, B., & Hassard, J. (Eds.) *The Routledge Companion to Organizational Change* (pp. 87-103). Routledge.

Carter, C. A., Ruhe, M. C., Weyer, S., Litaker, D., Fry, R. E., & Stange, K. C. (2007). An appreciative inquiry approach to practice improvement and transformative change in health care settings. *Quality Management in Health Care, 16*(3), 194-204. https://doi.org/10.1097/01.qmh.0000281055.15177.79

Clarke, M. & Thornton, J. (2014). Using appreciative inquiry to explore the potential of enhanced practice education opportunities. *British Journal of Occupational Therapy, 77*(9), 475-478. https://doi.org/10.4276/030802214x14098207541153

Cooperrider, D. L. & Srivastva, S. (1987). Appreciative inquiry in organizational life. *Research in Organizational Change and Development, 1,* 129-169. JAI Press, Inc. Retrieved from https://www.oio.nl/wp-content/uploads/APPRECIATIVE_INQUIRY_IN_Orgnizational_life.pdf

Dematteo, D., & Reeves, S. (2011). A critical examination of the role of appreciative inquiry within an interprofessional education initiative. *Journal of Interprofessional Care, 25*(3), 203-208. https://doi.org/10.3109/13561820.2010.504312

Lind, C., & Smith, D. (2008). Analyzing the state of community health nursing advancing from deficit to strengths-based practice using appreciative inquiry. *Advances in Nursing Science, 31*(1), 28-41. https://doi.org/10.1097/01.ans.0000311527.35446.4c

Quaintance, J. L., Arnold, L., & Thompson, G. S. (2010). What students learn about professionalism from faculty stories: An "appreciative inquiry" approach. *Academic Medicine, 85*(1), 118-123. https://doi.org/10.1097/acm.0b013e3181c42acd

Rubin, R., Kerrell, R., & Roberts, G. (2011). Appreciative inquiry in occupational therapy education. *British Journal of Occupational Therapy, 74*(5), 233-240. https://doi.org/10.4276/030802211x13046730116533

Ruhe, M. C., Bobiak, S. N., Litaker, D., Carter, C. A., Wu, L., Schroder, C., Zyzanski, S. J., Weyer, S. M., Werner, J. J., Fry, R. E., & Stange, K. C. (2001). Appreciative inquiry for quality improvement in primary care practices. *Quality Management in Health Care, 20*(1), 37-48. https://doi.org/10.1097/qmh.0b013e31820311be

References

Kern's Model Step 3
Goals and Objectives

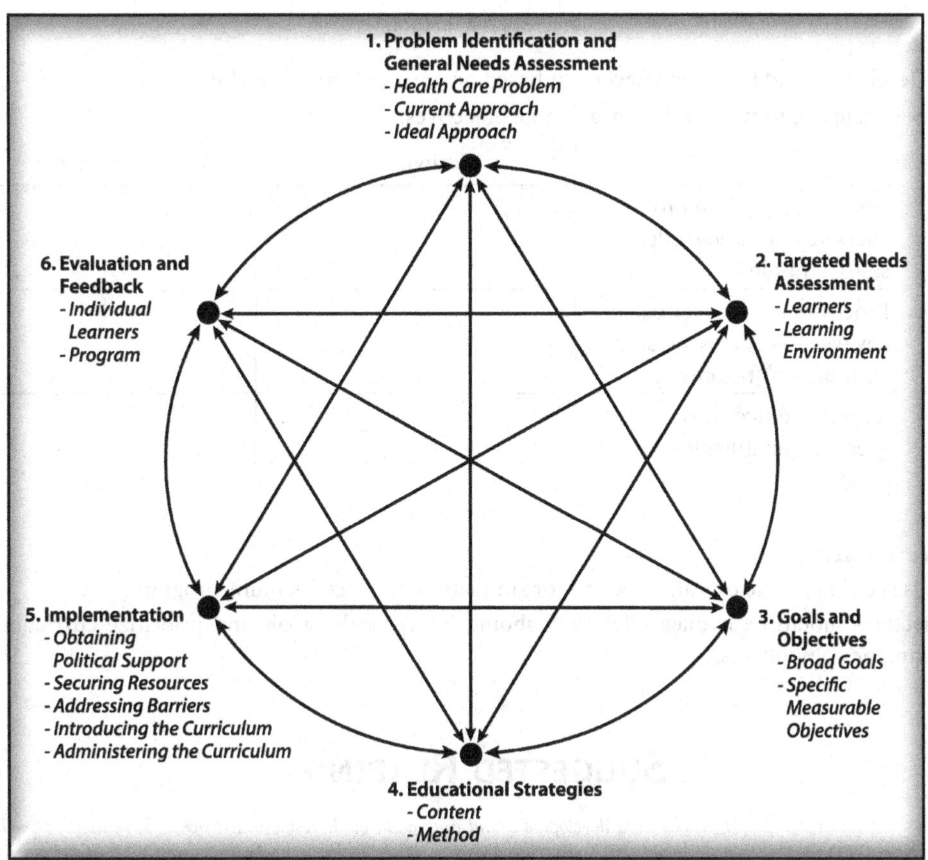

- The purpose of this step is to develop general goals and specific, measurable objectives to direct educational content, methods, and evaluation.
- This step defines the reason for teaching the content and communicates a curriculum/program vision.
- Goals are visionary, broad, and general and communicate the overall objective of the curriculum/program.
- Goals are typically not measurable and indicate where curricular/program efforts are directed.
- Objectives are precise, specific, and measurable and indicate what the learner should achieve.

- Objectives are focused on learning outcome measures and have specific quantifiable values or definitions.
- Objectives should include cognitive (knowledge), affective (attitude), and psychomotor (skills) components.
- Objectives direct content, identify learning methods, direct evaluation, support clear communication to the learner, and are often required by accrediting bodies.

- Goal:
  - Develop an overall, generalized objective for the curriculum/program.
    → Create one to two broad educational goals.

- Objectives:
  - Develop desired learner achievement based on current learner capabilities.
    → Create one to two specific measurable objectives.

	Individual	Program
Cognitive, psychomotor, affective (e.g., knowledge, skills, attitude)		
Process (i.e., consider use of key words/verbs associated with Bloom's taxonomy)		
Expected outcome (e.g., specific, quantifiable)		

After this step:

- Goals should provide overall direction for simulation in the curriculum/program.
- Objectives should be manageable: They should interpret the goals and prioritize curricular/programmatic components.

Suggested Readings

Farnan, J., & Schindler, N. (2013). *Curriculum development and evaluation guide resident as teacher: A mutually beneficial arrangement APPD/COMSEP pre course 2013.* Retrieved from: https://www.appd.org/meetings/2013SpringPresentations/PCWS1Handout.pdf

Kern, D. E. (2014). *Curriculum development: An essential educational skill, a public trust, a form of scholarship, an opportunity for organizational change.* Weill Cornell College of Medicine, Qatar. Retrieved from: https://dnnyqetna.blob.core.windows.net/portals/15/Six-Step%20Approach%20to%20Curriculum%20Development.pdf?sr=b&si=DNNFileManagerPolicy&sig=9sAOUX/lzfZQsN6QKLOpWJ46YLRuXmQwOghR7ptxnFw=

Khamis, N. N., Satava, R. M., Alnassar, S. A., & Kern, D. E. (2016). A stepwise model for simulation-based curriculum development for clinical skills, a modification of the six-step approach. *Surgical Endoscopy,* 279-287. https://doi.org/10.1007/s00464-015-4206x

5

How Does Learning Occur
Educational Theories to Support Simulation in Education and Training

Maureen M. Hoppe, EdD, MA, OTR/L, CPAM, CHSE
Tracy Van Oss, DHSc, MPH, OTR/L, FAOTA, CHSE

Learning Objectives

1. Describe educational theoretical frameworks to support clinical simulation use in health care education.
2. Analyze key constructs of constructivism, social cognitive learning, experiential learning, transformative learning, appreciative inquiry, and situated learning as foundational theories for clinical simulation instructional design.
3. Identify guiding pedagogical theories for development of clinical simulation within curriculum.

Kern's Model of Program Development

The content in this chapter articulates Step 3 of Kern's Model: Goals and Objectives. Information in this chapter contributes to the development of simulation goals and objectives that should articulate with, and identify, the teaching modality needed to meet curricular goals and objectives.

Zapletal, A. L., Baird, J. M., Van Oss, T., Hoppe, M. M., Prast, J. E., & Herge, E. A. *Clinical Simulation for Health Care Professionals* (pp. 47-56).

Educational Theoretical Frameworks

Educational theories are utilized to guide curricular design and instructional methodologies to facilitate learning in health care professions. When working on incorporating theory into clinical simulation development, a strengths-based approach based on appreciative inquiry should be considered (see Chapter 4 on Appreciative Inquiry; Cooperrider & Srivastva, 1987). Also, depending on unique curriculum design, it is important to examine how a theory will inform participant learning and provide support to change behavior and develop skill sets (Sabus & Macauley, 2016). In addition, when developing an interprofessional simulation, collaborating with other disciplines in choosing a theoretical framework is paramount to providing foundational understanding to guide simulation design and implementation process, thus improving the effectiveness of a simulation experience for the learner. Educational theories commonly utilized by simulation providers to guide, design, and implement a prelicensure curriculum are outlined in Table 5-1. Scientific theories relevant to simulation education researchers that may ground design including provision of pragmatic simulation use examples in Table 5-2.

Development of theory driven simulation experiences is guided by constructs from educational theories that emphasize how learning builds upon previous knowledge gained in curricula. Active experimentation and critical reflection by the learner based on experiential learning theory provides support for the use of clinical simulation. Figure 5-1 provides a conceptual representation of components of the clinical simulation process utilizing key constructs of experiential learning theory for theoretical support. Integration of active doing using simulation experience and reflective opportunities through debriefing facilitates learning in health care professions' students and practitioners allow for future application in clinical practice.

Table 5-1. Educational Learning Theory Constructs to Guide Clinical Simulation

Theory	Key Constructs	Learning Principles	Application to Clinical Simulation
Constructivism	Meaning is construed through experience. Knowledge builds upon existing knowledge (Brandon & All, 2010; Merriam et al., 2007).	Learning involves inquiry and active exploration to derive new meaning and deepen understanding of concepts (Fosnet, 1996).	Learners are actively involved in simulation experiences, with the expectation that knowledge builds on itself. Simulation providers can facilitate development through: • Learner reflection • Probing questions to help learners integrate new learning to past experiences • Scaffolding of simulation encounters throughout curriculum, based on learner educational level in program
Social Cognitive Learning	"Behavior is a function of the interaction of the person with the environment" (Merriam et al., 2007, p. 289). Learning impacted by observation of others, including the consequences of behaviors, not simply the direct imitation of behaviors. Cognitive processes and perceived self-efficacy contribute to learning (Bandura, 1989; 2005).	Learning facilitated through observational learning, contributing to intentional behavior change, and self-development (Bandura, 2005).	Role modeling of behavior by simulation provider or peer learners. May utilize small groups of learners with assigned roles within the simulation experience, allowing for learning to occur through observation of others. Video-recorded analysis of performance during simulated encounter to facilitate clinical reasoning of therapeutic process.
Experiential Learning	Learning is an ongoing process or continuous cycle depicted in four interactive stages: • Concrete experience • Reflective observation • Abstract conceptualization • Active experimentation (Kolb, 1984; Wenger, 2009)	"Knowledge is created through the transformation of experience" (Kolb, 1984, p. 38). Experiential learning involves application of didactic coursework with hands-on experience to improve critical thinking and clinical reasoning skills in an actual practice environment, as well as improvement of personal and professional attributes (Coker, 2010; Knecht-Sabres, 2010).	Learners actively participate in clinical simulation experience to apply and integrate knowledge in "real-time," including opportunities to respond to unforeseen circumstances consistent with clinical practice. Learners reflect during and after simulation encounter: what happened and what was response to situation. Debriefing occurs after the simulation encounter; this is not feedback but a guided teaching strategy. Learners can integrate key knowledge/skills gained into future simulated encounters, fieldwork, and clinical practice.

(continued)

Table 5-1 (continued). Educational Learning Theory Constructs to Guide Clinical Simulation

Theory	Key Constructs	Learning Principles	Application to Clinical Simulation
Situated Learning	Context provides a natural environment for knowledge. Knowledge "cannot be separated from the activity, context, and culture of the situation" (Gieselman et al., 2000, p. 264).	Learning occurs in the "real world" context or simulated environment (An, 2016; Lee & Wu, 2014). Situated learning environment referred to as a community of practice in which professional skills develop (Mann, 2011; Ebbers, 2015).	Learners may be immersed in a simulated environment that encompasses more experienced learners and provides an opportunity for "cognitive apprenticeship" to support learning of less experienced individuals involved in the simulation encounter (Gieselman et al., 2000). Situated learning provides students the opportunity to make real-time decisions about their interactions and response to them. Interprofessional simulation encounters foster collaboration, understanding of roles/responsibilities within the team, and allow for real-time decision making (Gieselman et al., 2000).
Transformative Learning	Critical reflection facilitates learning through changes in meaning, beliefs, or perspectives (Cranton, 1994; Hegge & Hallman, 2008; Merriam et al., 2007).	Transformative learning emerges from integration of "experience, critical reflection and development" of the learner (Merriam et al., 2007, p. 144).	Having learners critically reflect on simulated encounter. Video-recorded analysis can assist with critical reflection of performance, behaviors, and communication—providing insight that may not have been noticed by the learner during the actual encounter. Facilitated probing questions to consider beliefs and ways of thinking influencing interactions in simulated encounter. Simulation provider creates critical questions for learner self-reflection to create awareness of behaviors, skills, knowledge, and communication during simulated encounter (Cranton, 1994).
Appreciative Inquiry	Strengths-based approach to learning (Johnson & Leavitt, 2001).	Focus on the positive attributes and strengths of organization to manage or initiate change (Cooperrider & Srivastva, 1987)	5D cycle of appreciative inquiry. Simulation providers can use to guide simulation design with a focus on what resources, staff, space, budget is available vs. what is not available. Provides perspective to critically examine opportunities that may be available that had not previously been considered with a "glass half full" outlook (Johnson & Leavitt, 2001, p. 130).

Table 5-2. Scientific Theories Relevant to Simulation Education Researchers

Scientific Learning Theory	Main Tenets	Key Investigator	Evidence	Simulation Example
Learning Curve Theory	Learning consistently follows a logistic-shaped pattern across.	Thurstone	Studies in a wide range of contexts on individuals, groups, organizations, animals, and humans—all showing the learning curve pattern.	Operation times for laparoscopic surgery improve according to a learning curve.
Forgetting Curve Theory	Forgetting follows a nonlinear pattern with rapid initial decay.	Ebbinghaus	Studies in a wide range of contexts on individuals, groups, organizations, animals, and humans—all showing the forgetting curve pattern.	Clinicians lose CPR knowledge at an exponential rate.
Behaviorism	New behaviors can be developed using positive and negative reinforcement.	Skinner	Animal and human studies show skill learning according to lawful mechanisms.	Surgeons can learn a procedure to an "automaticity endpoint."
Constructivism	Knowledge of the world is constructed by every individual differently.	Piaget	Instructional designs that explicitly take into account the unique prior knowledge of the learner are more effective.	Inquiry-based learning in scenario-based simulation.
Social Constructivism	Knowledge of the world is constructed through social interaction and especially with "scaffolds."	Vygotsky, Bandura	The influence of social context on learning is seen when that context is varied.	The same virtual clinical cases are implemented across multiple medical schools with widely varying results.
Reflective Practice	Learning occurs best when organized according to a metacognitive framework that includes specific opportunities for reflection.	Schon	Any number of debriefing strategies that invoke reflection by simulation participants result in deeper and better retained learning.	Debriefing strategies that invoke self-monitoring or reflection are more effective.
Situated Learning	Learning is advantaged by "legitimate peripheral participation" in a community of practice.	Lave & Wenger	Simulation education that takes place in a community of practice (as opposed to separate from) is often more successful.	"See one-do one-teach one" progression is being replaced by more intentional and measured methods.

(continued)

Table 5-2 (continued). Scientific Theories Relevant to Simulation Education Researchers

Scientific Learning Theory	Main Tenets	Key Investigator	Evidence	Simulation Example
Activity Theory	De-emphasizes the measurement of knowledge states in favor of basing learning on the tools and social interactions necessary to accomplish relevant activities.	Engeström	Qualitative studies of real-life activities, with the researchers as active participants, have shown improved functional fidelity.	A simulation center can be considered as one activity system and the operating theater a second one. Each has its own instructional properties that interact.
Cognitive Load Theory	Human cognitive architecture includes specific bottlenecks that can be mitigated by instructional design.	Sweller	Several cognitive load effects have been enumerated, which can impair learning.	Clinical information can be deliberately apportioned to the learners' auditory and visual systems, allowing increased cognitive resources to be brought to bear on key concepts.

Reproduced with permission from Pusic, M. V., Boulis, K., & McGaghie, W. C. (2018). Role of scientific theory in simulation education research. *Simulation in Healthcare, 13*(35), S7-S14. https://doi.org/10.1097/sih.0000000000000282

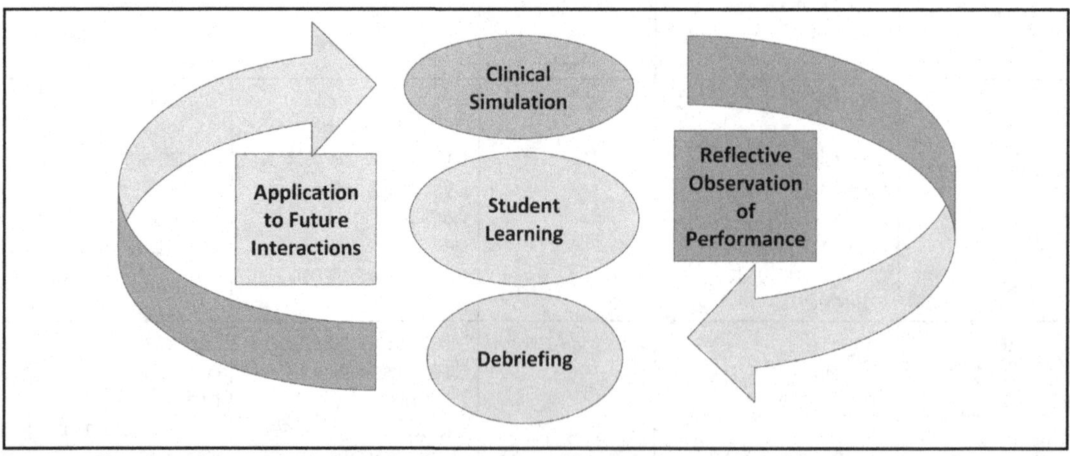

Figure 5-1. Clinical simulation conceptual model utilizing experiential learning theory. (Adapted from Dearmon et al., 2013 and Kolb, 1984.)

Worksheet 5-1
Theory in Simulation Design

Purpose of This Activity

Incorporation of the use of theory to guide simulation design.

Reflective Questions for Use of Clinical Simulation in Education and Training

- Identifying the gap or enhancement you are addressing in your curriculum (see Chapter 4).

- If your practice area is *academia:* ***What courses*** in your curriculum would be appropriate for clinical simulation?

- If your practice area is *academia:* ***How*** could clinical simulation be integrated and scaffolded through the curriculum to facilitate education and training of students?

- If your practice area is *clinical:* ***How*** could clinical simulation be integrated for educational/training purposes of *staff* at your site?

- If your practice area is *clinical:* ***How*** could clinical simulation be integrated for ***student*** learning opportunities at your site?

(continued)

Worksheet 5-1 (continued)
Theory in Simulation Design

Use the following table to analyze application of educational theories to guide instructional use of clinical simulation.

Educational Theory	*Key Constructs of Theory*	*Rationale for Use of Guiding Theory*	*Application to Clinical Simulation*	*Desired Student Learning Outcome From Participation in Clinical Simulation*

(continued)

Worksheet 5-1 (continued)
Theory in Simulation Design

Develop a goal for use of clinical simulation at your institution with supportive theoretical framework.

- Goal:

- Guiding educational theoretical framework:

- Rationale for theory use:

References

An, J. (2016). Learning to teach students with disabilities through situated learning experiences. *Research Quarterly for Exercise and Sport, 87,* A122-A123. Retrieved from https://search.proquest.com/docview/1817495194?accountid=34241

Bandura, A. (1989). Human agency in social cognitive theory. *American Psychologist, 44*(9), 1175-1184. https://doi.org/10.1037/0003-066X.44.9.1175

Bandura, A. (2005). Evolution of social cognitive theory. In K. G. Smith & M. A. Hitt (Eds.), *Great minds in management* (pp. 9-35). Oxford University Press.

Brandon, A. F., & All, A. C. (2010). Constructivism theory analysis and application to curricula. *Nursing Education Perspectives, 31*(2), 89-92. Retrieved from http://search.proquest.com/docview/219978672?accountid=58678

Coker, P. (2010). Effects of an experiential learning program on the clinical reasoning and critical thinking skills of occupational therapy students. *Journal of Allied Health, 39*(4), 280-286. Retrieved from http://search.proquest.com/docview/874211085?accountid=58678

Cooperrider, D. L., & Srivastva, S. (1987). Appreciative inquiry in organizational life. *Research in Organizational Change and Development, 1,* 129-169. JAI Press, Inc. Retrieved from https://www.oio.nl/wp-content/uploads/APPRECIATIVE_INQUIRY_IN_Orgnizational_life.pdf

Cranton, P. (1994). *Understanding and promoting transformative learning: A guide for educators of adults.* Jossey-Bass.

Dearmon, V., Graves, R. J., Hayden, S., Mulekar, M. S., Lawrence, S. M., Jones, L., & Farmer, J. E. (2013). Effectiveness of simulation-based orientation of baccalaureate nursing students preparing for their first clinical experience. *Journal of Nursing Education, 52*(1), 29-38. https://doi.org/10.3928/0148834-20121212-02

Ebbers, S. J. (2015). Situated learning. In J. M. Spector (Ed.), *The SAGE eEncyclopedia of educational technology* (pp. 650-651). https://doi.org/10.4135/9781483346397.n267

Fosnet, C. T. (Ed). (1996). *Constructivism: Theory, perspectives, and practice.* Teachers College Press.

Gieselman, J. A., Stark, N., & Farruggia, M. J. (2000). Implications of the situated learning model for teaching and learning nursing research. *The Journal of Continuing Education in Nursing, 31*(6), 263-8. https://doi.org/10.3928/0022-0124-20001101-07

Hegge, M. J., & Hallman, P. A. (2008). Changing nursing culture to welcome second-degree students: Herding and corralling sacred cows. *Journal of Nursing Education, 47*(12), 552-6. https://doi.org/10.3928/01484834-20081201-04

Johnson, G., & Leavitt, W. (2001). Building on success: Transforming organizations through an appreciative inquiry. *Public Personnel Management, 30*(1), 129-136. https://doi.org/10.1177/009102600103000111

Knecht-Sabres, L. J. (2010). The use of experiential learning in an occupational therapy program: Can it foster skills for clinical practice? *Occupational Therapy in Health Care 24*(4), 320-334. https://doi.org/10.3109/07380577.2010.514382

Kolb, D. A. (1984). *Experiential learning: Experience as the source of learning and development.* Prentice Hall.

Lee, Y., & Wu, W. (2014). The effects of situated learning and health knowledge involvement on health communications. *Reproductive Health, 11*(93), 1-7. https://doi.org/10.1186/1742-4755-11-93

Mann, K. V. (2011). Theoretical perspectives in medical education: Past experience and future possibilities. *Medical Education, 45,* 60–68. https://doi.org/10.1111/j.1365-2923.2010.03757.x

Merriam, S., Caffarella, R. S., & Baumgartner, L. M. (2007). *Learning in adulthood: A comprehensive guide* (3rd ed.). Jossey-Bass.

Pusic, M. V., Boulis, K., & McGaghie, W. C. (2018). Role of scientific theory in simulation education research. *Simulation in Healthcare, 13*(35), S7-S14. https://doi.org/10.1097/sih.0000000000000282

Sabus, C., & Macauley, K. (2016). Simulation in physical therapy education and practice opportunities and evidence-based instruction to achieve meaningful learning outcomes. *Journal of Physical Therapy Education, 30*(1), 3-13. https://doi.org/10.1097/00001416-201630010-00002

Wenger, E. A. (2009). Social theory of learning. In K. Illeris (Ed.), *Contemporary theories of learning: Learning theorists in their own words* (pp. 147-158). Routledge.

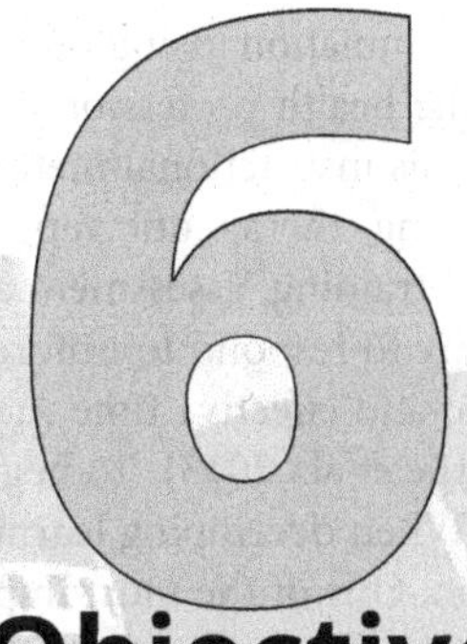

Developing Learning Objectives

Jean E. Prast, OTD, MSOT, OTRL, CHSE
Tracy Van Oss, DHSc, MPH, OTR/L, FAOTA, CHSE

Learning Objectives

1. Describe key components of behavioral learning objectives used in clinical simulation necessary to facilitate learning.
2. Discuss the knowledge and skills that students will acquire from participating in the simulation.
3. Develop clearly defined, measurable learning objectives to support the achievement of desired simulation outcomes.

Kern's Model of Program Development

The content in this chapter articulates Step 3 of Kern's Model: Goals and Objectives. Information in this chapter explains how to develop specific learning objectives that are the building blocks of a rigorous simulation. This information articulates the measurable objectives necessary to develop a sound curriculum.

Zapletal, A. L., Baird, J. M., Van Oss, T., Hoppe, M. M., Prast, J. E., & Herge, E. A. *Clinical Simulation for Health Care Professionals* (pp. 57-64).

Clinical simulation using standardized patients and high-fidelity simulators can be integrated throughout the health profession curriculum and adapted based on the student level to facilitate skill acquisition. This instructional method can prepare students in the following areas: functional transfer/mobility training, therapeutic rapport, professional communication appropriate for client education, technical skill training, assessment administration, clinical reasoning and problem solving in real time with the ability to respond to unforeseen circumstances that arise in clinical practice, interprofessional collaboration, and effective time management skills with patient care delivery (Castillo, 2011; Giles et al., 2014; Herge et al., 2013). To begin the process for the learner, learning objectives are used to guide the process. When developing learning objectives think about the what, where, when, how, and why of the simulation. One of the most important steps of creating the objectives is to know what you want or expect as an overall outcome from the learning experience itself. Whether you are an experienced health care professional or educator, outcomes are an essential component of instruction and education (client or student). Regardless of the setting, health care or academia, we use outcome measures to determine the impact of learning in academia activities and, in this case, simulation-based experiences.

In the academic setting, simulation should be integrated into your program and tied to the curricula (INACLS, 2016a, 2016b; Khamis et al., 2016). Consider the courses and content taught along with the course objectives, assignments, and learning activities. Think about the following:

1. Why do you want to integrate simulation?
2. How does it fit and why?
3. Where does it fit and who should be involved in planning?
4. Overall, what are your desired outcomes?

To have achievable outcomes, clearly defined, measurable objectives are necessary. These objectives can be either broad or specific. Reflect on the following: What do you want them to learn and how will you get there? Answering this question with a clear connection to your course or clinical objectives is a great first step in developing the learning objectives.

Learning Objectives

A learning objective is a statement that describes what the learner will be able to do or achieve upon completion of an educational activity. This can include areas such as knowledge, skills, behaviors, and/or attitudes to be acquired by the learner from participation in the lesson or, in this case, simulation. These objectives are guiding tools to facilitate the achievement of learning outcomes and should be central when designing educational activities. Learning objectives need to be determined early to use as a guide in selecting the instructional method (e.g., simulation), choosing the appropriate instructional materials (e.g., type of simulation modality, tools, resources), developing the educational content (e.g., simulation scenario), and establishing tests or evaluation tools to measure learning outcomes. In some health professions, when designing simulation there may only be one learning objective or measurable goal. Following are examples of two methods to help create measurable learning objectives.

The ABCDs

When developing learning objectives, consider the basics of ABCDs to get you started. Identify the following:

- *A*udience: Identify your learners, who are they?
- *B*ehavior/Performance: What do you want the learning to be able to do?
- *C*ondition: Under what circumstances or in what situation will they perform?
- *D*egree: How will the learner's performance be measured?

SMART Goal Acronym

When developing the learning objectives of your simulation, it is important to reference the acronym SMART (Specific, Measurable, Achievable, Realistic, Timely). This acronym was created to use as a framework to write meaningful, measurable objectives that focus on the desired knowledge, skills, and attitudes that learners should demonstrate upon completion of a simulation (Doran, 1981). According to the International Nursing Association for Clinical Simulation and Learning (INACSL, 2016a), the following are required elements to construct SMART learning objectives based on expected outcomes:

- *S*pecific:
  - Identify the learners, scenario, fidelity, facilitation, debriefing, assessment, and evaluation methods.
  - Include the three categories of Bloom's taxonomy with varying levels.
  - Keep in mind that being specific enhances the ability to measure outcomes.
  - Consider what will change from the simulation (to who and how).
- *M*easurable:
  - Make sure they are useful for evaluation.
  - Determine a baseline to measure changes you expect to occur.
  - Use a reliable and valid method of measurement to assess outcomes.
- *A*chievable:
  - Ensure they are created at the learners' level of knowledge, experience, and skill level.
  - Make sure they are attainable within a realistic time frame.
  - Ensure that adequate resources are available to achieve the desired outcomes.
- *R*ealistic:
  - Have links to your programs design, mission, vision, and outcomes.
  - Make sure they are linked to expected outcomes.
  - Make sure they are appropriate to the learners' knowledge, skills, and attitudes.
  - Ensure they are aligned with current evidence, standards, and guidelines.
- *T*ime-Phased Objectives:
  - Establish a desired time frame to meet the objectives.
  - Create a specific time frame to plan, implement, and evaluate outcomes.

According to the Centers for Disease Control and Prevention (CDC, 2009), potential consequences of not following this standard can lead to ambiguity, unintended outcomes, and failure to meet simulation objectives.

Learning Taxonomies

When developing your learning objectives, it's important to reference a learning taxonomy to ensure a variety of learning occurs. Learning taxonomies were created to describe various learning behaviors and characteristics that we want our learners to develop. These taxonomies are often used to identify different stages of learning development and classify behavioral objectives (Krathwohl, 2002). The use of a learning taxonomy to write learning objectives that describe the skills and abilities that you desire learners to master and demonstrate can be extremely beneficial. One of the most commonly used in education is Bloom's Taxonomy, which is divided into three broad categories or domains (i.e., cognitive, affective, and psychomotor) that are hierarchical with a general rule that an earlier level must be mastered before the next level (Anderson & Krathwohl, 2001). The following includes a brief overview of each category:

- *Cognitive (knowledge):* The thinking domain; this is where information is acquired with the ability to process what is obtained.
- *Affective (attitudes):* The feeling domain; learners make an internal commitment to the experience and demonstrate emotional responses to tasks learned.
- *Psychomotor (skills)*: The skills domain; learners recognize the value of the experience and acquire the abilities to carry out the skills obtained.

A general rule when writing learning objectives is to have at least one objective for each category; however, it ultimately depends on the desired outcomes (e.g., mastery of a specific skill may result in only one learning objective). Another general rule is to start with an action verb to help provide structure and communicate the knowledge, skills, and/or attitudes the learner is supposed to achieve because of participating in the simulation. There are numerous resources that you can find online that provide action verbs (e.g., identify, explain, demonstrate), especially those linked to Bloom's. As you create the learning objectives of your simulation, keep in mind that higher levels of the learning taxonomy can lead to deeper learning and transfer of knowledge and skills to a greater variety of tasks and contexts (Adams, 2015).

Depending on the "simulation" that you develop, learners may not reach the level of mastery. Some simulations may include remembering and understanding vs. evaluating and creating (Bloom's taxonomy), it really depends on the desired outcomes and learning objectives developed and the level of the learner. Some examples include:

- *Interprofessional Team Case Review:* The objective is to identify the roles of other health care providers in order to make a referral.
- *Safe Patient Handling With Transfers:* The objective is to list the steps of a safe patient transfer vs. demonstrating one.

Writing Learning Objectives

When developing learning objectives, it is important to keep your focus on the learner—not the educator performance. To do this, think about the following question: "What is it that you want or expect the learner to achieve from the learning activity?" As you begin to answer this question make sure you keep the emphasis on the behavior that can be observed during or following the activity, not the content or subject matter itself (Tables 6-1 and 6-2).

Avoiding Pitfalls for Writing Objectives

Keep in mind the following when developing learning objectives:

- Make sure learning objectives are linked to program goals
- Review the curriculum design to strategically embed simulation for optimal student learning
- Know what you want from the simulation (e.g., learning expectations/outcomes) before you get started creating learning objectives
- Make sure the learning objectives are specific and measurable
- Focus on the learner to create valuable learning experiences
- Use an action verb and the ABCD rule to be SMART
- Make revisions based on evaluation measures
- Make sure the learner's level of knowledge and skill can meet the learning objective

Table 6-1. Checklist for Writing Learning Objectives

Writing learning objectives can be challenging; however, once you master the skill of creating them you will appreciate how much they can support measuring the outcomes of your simulation. To help you create learning objectives for your simulation, make sure that each statement:

- ☐ Is learner oriented, not educator oriented
- ☐ Meets the components necessary for a measurable learning objective (e.g., ABCD: identified audience, observable behavior, performance conditions, and degree for measurement)
- ☐ Has a clear description of the learning outcome that you want the learner to achieve
- ☐ Starts with an action verb that specifies the desired observable behavior
- ☐ Is clearly observable (e.g., written, verbal, and/or visual demonstration)
- ☐ Is measurable
- ☐ Has a range of complexity based on learning taxonomies (e.g., application, problem solving)
- ☐ Includes written documentation from each domain (e.g., cognitive, affective, psychomotor); consider writing objectives in all domains
- ☐ Does not include ambiguity verbs such as know, understand, and learn
- ☐ Includes only one general learning outcome in each objective

Table 6-2. Learning Objectives for the Simulation Encounter

1. Demonstrate administration of a standardized assessment with a patient in an acute care setting.
2. Recognize the impact of early patient mobilization interventions to enhance occupation-based performance.
3. Identify proper standard precautions prior to start of each simulation scenario.
4. Discuss various forms of communication necessary to provide quality service working with an interprofessional team in a home care setting.
5. Assess vital signs to determine appropriate responses during an intervention session.
6. Develop goals and discharge recommendations based on treatment interventions.
7. Design a patient-centered plan for early mobilization with nursing and respiratory care.

Worksheet 6-1
Developing Learning Objectives

Purpose of This Activity

This worksheet is designed to guide the process of developing learning objectives for your simulation.

Date: ____

Goal of the simulation: ______________________________________

Title of the simulation: ______________________________________

Brief description of the simulation encounter (one to two sentences): ______________________

____

____

Setting: ____

____

1. Begin with defining the philosophy and/or mission of your program.

2. Next, identify curricular or program design including threads.

3. Restate the educational theory that is guiding your simulation.

4. Identify course(s) and why it is appropriate for simulation.

5. Identify what you expect the learners to learn and the rationale. (What in your needs assessment led you to this focus?)

(continued)

Worksheet 6-1 (continued)
Developing Learning Objectives

6. Using a learning taxonomy (Bloom's is referenced here), identify an action verb that you would like to include in your learning objectives.
   - ☐ Cognitive (knowledge): ______________________________
   - ☐ Affective (attitudes): ______________________________
   - ☐ Psychomotor (skills): ______________________________

7. Using the ABCDs, fill out the following:
   - ☐ A (audience):______________________________
   - ☐ B (behavior): ______________________________
   - ☐ C (condition): ______________________________
   - ☐ D (degree): ______________________________

8. Using your course objectives and curricular aims, create one to three learning objectives for your simulation.
   - ☐ Learning objective 1:______________________________
   - ☐ Learning objective 2:______________________________
   - ☐ Learning objective 3:______________________________

9. Review the learning objective(s) to check that they meet the SMART guidelines.
   - ☐ S: specific
   - ☐ M: measurable
   - ☐ A: achievable
   - ☐ R: realistic
   - ☐ T: timely

10. Keep in mind your learning objectives for the case.
    - ☐ What do the learners need to know to get ready (e.g., SIM prior to SP, labs to practice)?

    - ☐ What do you have for the learners to review or learn prior to coming into the scenario (e.g., readings, videos, resources, practice labs)?

References

Adams, N. (2015). Bloom's taxonomy of cognitive learning objectives. *Journal of the Medical Library Association, 103*(3), 152-153. Retrieved from: https://www.ncbi.nlm.nih.gov/pmc/articles/PMC4511057/

Anderson, L. W., & Krathwohl, D. R., (Eds.). (2001). *A taxonomy for learning, teaching, and assessing: A revision of Bloom's taxonomy of educational objectives.* Allyn & Bacon.

Castillo, D. C. (2011). Experiences in a simulated hospital: Virtual training in occupational therapy. *OT Practice, 16*(22), 21-23. Retrieved from http://search.proquest.com/docview/912764952?accountid=58678

Centers for Disease Control and Prevention. (2009). *Evaluation briefs: Writing SMART objectives.* Retrieved from http://www.cdc.gov/healthyyouth/evaluation/pdf/breif3b.pdf

Doran, G. T. (1981). There's a S.M.A.R.T. way to write management's goals and objectives. *Management Review, 70*(11), 35-36. Retrieved from: https://community.mis.temple.edu/mis0855002fall2015/files/2015/10/S.M.A.R.T-Way-Management-Review.pdf

Giles, A. K., Carson, N. E., Breland, H. L., Coker-Bolt, P., & Bowman, P. J. (2014). Use of simulated patients and reflective video analysis to assess occupational therapy students' preparedness for fieldwork. *American Journal of Occupational Therapy, 68*(2), S57-S66. https://doi.org/10.5014/ajot.2014.685s03

Herge, E. A., Lorch, A., DeAngelis, T., Vause-Earland, T., Mollo, K., & Zapletal, A. (2013). The standardized patient encounter: A dynamic educational approach to enhance students' clinical healthcare skills. *Journal of Allied Health, 42*(4), 229-235. Retrieved from http://search.proquest.com/docview/1493991946?accountid=58678

Khamis, N. N., Satava, R. M., Alnassar, S. A., & Kern, D. E. (2016). A stepwise model for simulation-based curriculum developmental approach for clinical skills, a modification of the six-step approach. *Surgical Endoscopy, 30*(1), 279-287. https://doi.org/10.1007/s00464-015-4206-x

Krathwohl, D. (2002). A revision of Bloom's taxonomy: An overview. *Theory Into Practice, 41*(4). 212-218. https://doi.org/ 10.1207/s15430421tip4104_2

INACSL Standards Committee (2016a). INACSL Standards of Best Practice: Simulation^{SM} Outcomes and Objectives. *Clinical Simulation in Nursing, 12*(S), S13-S15. https://doi.org/10.1016/j.ecns.2016.09.006

INACSL Standards Committee (2016b). INACSL Standards of Best Practice: Simulation^{SM} Design. *Clinical Simulation in Nursing, 12*(S), S5-S12. https://doi.org/10.1016/j.ecns.2016.09.005

7

Art and Science of Measurement

Assessment Development for Simulation

Tracy Van Oss, DHSc, MPH, OTR/L, FAOTA, CHSE
E. Adel Herge, OTD, OTR/L, FAOTA

Learning Objectives

1. Understand the different types of assessments available for use with a variety of simulation encounters.
2. Evaluate available assessments to determine the best option for your simulation encounter.
3. Apply assessment tool to individualized clinical simulation encounters.

Kern's Model of Program Development

The content in this chapter articulates Step 3 of Kern's Model: Goals and Objectives. Information in this chapter explains how to assess student learning. This articulates with the curricular objectives that direct student evaluation and can often be further associated with accreditation.

Zapletal, A. L., Baird, J. M., Van Oss, T., Hoppe, M. M., Prast, J. E., & Herge, E. A. *Clinical Simulation for Health Care Professionals* (pp. 65-77).

Assessing Student Performance

There are many ways student learning can be assessed when using simulation. One way to get started is to decide whether the assessment is formative or summative or both. *Formative assessment* is performed in the process of learning and provides information to adjust teaching/learning in real time. *Summative assessment* is performed periodically and determines what learners do/do not know at a particular point in time (Garrison & Ehrlinghaus, 2010). Both are advantageous and should be considered when planning the simulation experiences.

Assessing With Simulation

Experiential learning is one way for learners to practice skills needed to work in a health care system. Simulation allows for repeated practice to sharpen the skills needed to be an effective and safe health care practitioner. Allowing learners to work with a multitude of persons with various conditions can help to increase confidence and competence in selected skills (Bambini et al., 2009; Duffy & Harding, 2004; Greenwood et al., 2014; Hall et al. 2011; Schirmer et al., 2005). This type of learning also allows learners to improve clinical judgment and clinical reasoning (Guhde, 2010; Lasater, 2007). Learners may make a mistake; however, the simulation encounter should provide a safe environment with support to reflect and make changes prior to entry into the fast-paced health care system. Learners also can assess satisfaction with the simulation experience itself (Leonard et al., 2010; Shoemaker et al., 2009). By allowing learners to provide input on the type of learning it will create memorable experiences to reflect on when working with patients in the future as clinicians.

The following stakeholders can participate assessing a simulation:

- *Faculty:* Faculty observe the simulation and assess student performance. This may be through observing a two-way mirror, watching a videotape of the simulation, or actually being part of the simulation. Faculty can use checklists or other structured assessments to evaluate student performance.
- *Peer Observer:* Grouping students together allows peer support, as well as the opportunity for at least one student to have the role of the observer. This allows the student to be intimately involved in the simulation even if they are not performing the hands-on skills. This is a valuable role to learn what to do and sometimes what not to do.
- *Standardized Patient:* SPs can assess student performance. To do this effectively SP training needs to include specific areas of student performance (i.e., where to place hands during a transfer). SPs can also assess "soft skills" such as communication, professionalism, or empathy. SPs can use checklists and open-ended questions to rate student performance.
- *Student (Self-Rating):* Simulation sessions can be videotaped for students to self-rate, and/or provide a reflection on a particular skill set or the entire session. Quantitative questions may be used, but there should also be open-ended questions to allow the student to elaborate on why they felt the simulation went well or how they can improve for next time.

When choosing an assessment tool faculty should consider the following:

1. Learning objectives of the simulation should parallel the assessment tool measures
2. Utility of the assessment tool in the simulation including:
    - Skill set of the person administering the tool—take into consideration inter-reliability if there are multiple assessors
    - How the results of the assessment will be used; is this a *formative* assessment (i.e., to provide feedback to the student re: their performance during or immediately following the simulation) or *summative* (i.e., to determine whether a student has mastered a specific skill or is ready to move to the next level of training)

3. Psychometrics of the tool, including reliability and validity
4. Process to train other observers (e.g., lab instructors, SPs, peer observers) to use the assessment tool correctly and effectively

Format of Assessments

There are a variety of methods including:

- Observation is commonly used and incorporated as the use of clinical judgment (Duffy & Harding, 2004; Hall et al., 2011; Lasater, 2007; Guhde, 2010; Shoemaker et al., 2009)
- Checklist survey/scale provide specific areas to address (Bambini et al., 2009; Duffy & Harding, 2004; Greenwood et al., 2014; Guhde, 2010; Heinerichs et al., 2013; Henry et al., 2007; Leonard et al., 2010; Merryman, 2010; Silberman et al., 2013; Titzer et al., 2012)
- Focus groups and questionnaires can include open ended questions to allow for more in-depth responses (Lasater, 2007)
- Standardized measures can provide objective information with consistency in the delivery (Greenwood et al., 2014; Hall et al., 2011; Henry et al., 2007; Jones & Sheppard, 2011; Schirmer et al., 2005)

Which assessment used will depend on the objectives for your simulation experience. A variety of pre-established assessment tools are available. These are listed in Table 7-1.

Table 7-1. Simulation Assessment Tools

Name	Citation	What it Measures	Psychometrics
17-Item Standardized Patient Checklist	Cohen, D. S., Colliver, J. A., Marcy, M. S., Fried, E. D., & Swartz, M. H. (1996). Psychometric properties of a standardized-patient checklist and rating-scale form used to assess interpersonal and communication skills. *Academic Medicine, 71*(1). Retrieved from http://journals.lww.com/academicmedicine/pages/default.aspx?desktopMode=true	Interpersonal and communication skills	Reliability: • Inter-case reliability of 0.65 Validity: • No information
Actions, Communication, and Teaching in Simulation (ACTS) Tool	Sanko, J. S., Shekhter, I., Gattamorta, K. A., & Birnbach, D. J. (2016). Development and psychometric analysis of a tool to evaluate confederates. *Clinical Simulation in Nursing, 12*(11), 475-481. https://doi.org/10.1016/j.ecns.2016.07.006	Acting, verbal, and nonverbal characterization; flexibility and adaptability; use of props and attire; and interactions with participants	Reliability: • Inter-rater reliability of 0.91 • Parallel reliability of 0.963 • Internal consistency: Cronbach's alpha of 0.93 • All item total correlations between 0.52 to 0.96 Validity: • Content and face validity used to review each version of the measure until it was felt that the included items correctly measured the construct
Acute Care Confidence Survey	Greenwood, K., Nicoloro, D., & Iversen, M. (2014). Reliability and validity of the acute care confidence survey: An objective measure to assess students' self-confidence and predict student performance for inpatient clinical experiences. *Journal of Acute Care Physical Therapy, 5*(1). Retrieved from http://journals.lww.com/jacpt/Pages/default.aspx	Self-confidence and predictor for student performance for inpatient clinical experiences	Reliability: • Sufficient homogeneity was found for the full scale (α=0.91) and 3 subscales (α=0.75, instruct; α=0.86, judgment; and α=0.83, mobility) but not for the manual subscale (α=0.22) • Test-retest reliability was excellent (intraclass correlation coefficient, 0.78 to 0.91) Validity: • A low-to-moderate correlation was found between midterm Clinical Performance Instrument scores and overall ACCS scores (r=0.5; p=.02)

(continued)

Table 7-1. Simulation Assessment Tools (continued)

Name	Citation	What it Measures	Psychometrics
Common Ground Instrument	Lang, F. L., McCord, R., Harvill, L., & Anderson, D. S. (2004). Communication assessment using the common ground instrument: Psychometric properties. *Family Medicine, 36*(3). Retrieved from http://www.stfm.org/NewsJournals/FamilyMedicine	Core communication skills	Reliability: • Inter-rater reliability was 0.85 for overall global ratings and 0.92 for the overall checklist assessment • Generalizability coefficient was 0.80 for 50 minutes of testing Validity: • The correlation between the ratings of trainer raters and a panel of communication experts was 0.84
DARE[2] Patient Safety Rubric	Walshe, N., O'Brien, S., Murphy, S., & Graham, R. (2014). Simulation performance evaluation: Inter-rater reliability of the DARE[2] Patient Safety Rubric. *Clinical Simulation in Nursing, 10*(9). https://doi.org/10.1016/j.ecns.2014.06.005	Systematic patient assessment, clinical response, clinical-psychomotor skills, and communication proficiency	Reliability: • Intraclass correlation coefficients were greater than 0.7 for three of the four domains of practice and 0.58 for the fourth • Intraclass correlation coefficient for overall rubric score was 0.75 • Percentage agreement for the overall rubric was 59% Validity: • All correlations were significant at $p<.01$ and indicate that the individual domains are supporting constructs within the rubric • A content validity index of 97% indicates that almost 100% of indicators were considered relevant by 100% of participants

(continued)

Table 7-1. Simulation Assessment Tools (continued)

Name	Citation	What it Measures	Psychometrics
Debriefing Assessment for Simulation in Healthcare (DASH)	Simon, R., Raemer, D. B., & Rudolph, J. W. (2010). *Debriefing assessment for simulation in healthcare (DASH) rater's handbook*. Center for Medical Simulation. https://harvardmedsim.org/wp-content/uploads/2017/01/DASH.handbook.2010.Final.Rev.2.pdf.	Instructor behaviors that facilitate learning during the introduction to the simulation course and the postsimulation debriefing	Reliability: • Intraclass correlation coefficient for the combined elements was 0.74 • Intraclass correlation coefficients for the individual elements were predominantly greater than 0.60 • Cronbach's alpha=0.89 across the webinar raters Validity: • There were significant differences among the ratings for the three standardized debriefings (p<.001). Brett-Fleegler, M., Rudolph, J., Eppich, W., Monuteaux, M., Fleegler, E., Cheng, A., & Simon, R. (2012). Debriefing assessment for simulation in healthcare: Development and psychometric properties. *Simulation in Healthcare, 7*(5), 288-294. https://doi.org/ 10.1097/SIH.0b013e3182620228
Debriefing for Meaningful Learning Evaluation Scale	Bradley, C. S., & Dreifuerst, K. T. (2016). Pilot testing the debriefing for meaningful learning evaluation scale. *Clinical Simulation in Nursing, 12*(7), 277-280. https://doi.org/10.1016/j.ecns.2016.01.008	Debriefer's ability to implement the Debriefing for Meaningful Learning Evaluation Scale	Reliability: • Internal consistency: Cronbach's alpha of 0.88 • Inter-rater reliability of 0.86, total scale ICC [p<0.01] Validity: • Content validity: (scale-level CVI 0.92) • Face validity established
Educational Practices Questionnaire	National League for Nursing, 2005. Retrieved from http://www.nln.org/docs/default-source/default-document-library/instrument-1_educational-practices-questionnaire.pdf?sfvrsn=0	Perceptions of the importance of educational best practices in simulation	Reliability: • Discrimination scores ranged from 75% to 95% • Cronbach's alpha of 0.95 Validity: • Correlations among the conceptual factors were from 0.77 and 0.86 Franklin, A. E., Burns, P., & Lee, C. S. (2014). Psychometric testing on the NLN student satisfaction and self-confidence in learning, simulation design scale, and educational practices questionnaire using a sample of prelicensure novice nurses. *Nurse Education Today, 34*(10). https://doi.org/10.1016/j.nedt.2014.06.011

(continued)

Table 7-1. Simulation Assessment Tools (continued)

Name	Citation	What it Measures	Psychometrics
Healthcare Provider Priority Survey	Titzer, J., Swenty, C., & Hoehn, G. (2012). An interprofessional simulation promoting collaboration and problem solving among nursing and allied health professional students. *Clinical Simulation in Nursing, 8*(8). http://dx.doi.org.proxy1.lib.tju.edu/10.1016/j.ecns.2011.01.001	Interprofessional simulation focused on collaboration and problem solving	• Qualitative survey • No psychometrics available
Lasater Clinical Judgment Rubric (LCJR)	Lasater, K. (2007). Clinical judgment development: Using simulation to create an assessment rubric. *Journal of Nursing Education, 46*(11). Retrieved from www.routledge.com/9781630917357	Focused observation, recognizing deviations from expected patterns, information seeking, prioritizing data, making sense of data, confidence, communication, skillfulness, self-analysis, commitment to improvement	Reliability: • Study #1: Inter-rater reliability of 0.889 • Study #2: Inter-rater reliability of 92% to 96% • Study #3: Used level of agreement for reliability analyses—results ranged from 57% to 100% Validity: • Findings from each of these studies provided evidence supporting the validity of the LCJR for assessing clinical judgment during simulated patient care scenarios Adamson, K. A., Gubrud, P., Sideras, S., & Lasater, K. (2012). Assessing the reliability, validity, and use of the Lasater clinical judgment rubric: Three approaches. *Journal of Nursing Education, 51*(2), 66-73. https://doi.org/10.3928/01484834-20111130-03
McMaster-Ottawa Team Observed Structured Clinical Encounter	Hall, P., Marshall, D., Weaver, L., Boyle, A., & Taniguchi, A. (2011). A method to enhance student teams in palliative care: Piloting the McMaster-Ottawa team observed structured clinical encounter. *Journal of Palliative Medicine, 14*(6). https://doi.org/10.1089/jpm.2010.0295	Interprofessional team competencies in primary care	Reliability: • Inter-rater reliability of 0.916 • Internal consistency for the IPE scales (checklists) for three stations ranged from 0.725 to 0.865—two observers Validity: • Correlation between the two observers for the teams' global scores for all three stations combined was 0.844

(continued)

Table 7-1. Simulation Assessment Tools (continued)

Name	Citation	What it Measures	Psychometrics
Objective Structured Clinical Assessment (OSCA)	Najjar, R. H., Docherty, A., & Miehl, N. (2016). Psychometric properties of an objective structured clinical assessment tool. *Clinical Simulation in Nursing, 12*(3), 88-95. https://doi.org/10.1016/j.ecns.2016.01.003	Communication, medication administration, client education, performance and behavioral outcomes	Reliability: • Inter-rater reliability: The single measure and average measure for consistency ranged from 0.63 to 0.94 and 0.77 to 0.97, respectively. Validity: • Expert panel agreed that content of the scenario (M = 3.43, standard deviation [SD] = 0.53), constructs being measured in the OSCA (M = 3.57, SD = 0.53), and the skills being tested aligned well with the course outcomes (M = 3.71, SD = 0.49).
Quint Leveled Clinical Competency Tool	Prion, S. K., Gilbert, G. E., Adamson, K. A., Kardong-Edgren, S., & Quint, S. (2017). Development and testing of Quint Leveled Clinical Competency Tool. *Clinical Simulation in Nursing, 13*(3), 106-115. https://doi.org/10.1016/j.ecns.2016.10.008	Clinical judgment with prelicensure nursing students	Reliability: • Inter-rater reliability of 0.87 • Coefficient α of 0.83 Validity: • Limited face validity • Content validity index of 0.72
Rochester Communi-cations Rating Scale	Epstein, R. M., Dannefer, E. F., Nofziger, A. C., Hansen, J. T., Schultz, S.H., Jospe, N., Connard, L. W., Meldrum, S. C., & Henson, L. C. (2010). Comprehensive assessment of pro-fessional competence: The Rochester Experiment. *Teaching and Learning in Medicine, 16*(2). https://doi.org/10.1207/s15328015tlm1602_12	Physician's interest in patient as a person, understanding patient's experience of illness, attention to context, participation in care	Reliability: • Inter-rater reliability of 0.59 • Internal consistency: Cronbach's alpha of 0.91 Validity: • No information on validity
Seattle College of Nursing Simulation Evaluation	Mikasa, A. W., Cicero, T. F., & Adamson, K. A. (2013). Outcome-based evaluation tool to evaluate student performance in high-fidelity simulation. *Clinical Simulation in Nursing, 9*(9), e361- e367. http://dx.doi.org/10.1016/j.ecns.2012.06.001	Assessment, intervention, evaluation, critical thinking, direct patient care, communication, collaboration, and professional behaviors	Reliability: • Internal consistency: Cronbach's alpha of 0.97 • Inter-rater reliability of 0.858 • Intra-rater reliability of 0.907 Validity: • Descriptive analyses of the data provided evidence supporting the validity of the tool. • No additional information

(continued)

Table 7-1. Simulation Assessment Tools (continued)

Name	Citation	What it Measures	Psychometrics
Simulation Design Scale	National League for Nursing. (2005). Retrieved from: http://www.nln.org/docs/default-source/professional-development-programs/nln-instrument_simulation-design-scale.pdf?sfvrsn=0	Perceptions of objectives, information support, problem solving, feedback, and fidelity in simulation	Reliability: • Items had similar standard deviations and inter-item correlations • Discrimination scores ranged from 79% to 93% • Cronbach's alpha of 0.96 Validity: • Correlations among theoretical factors were 0.67 to 0.89. Franklin, A. E., Burns, P., & Lee, C. S. (2014). Psychometric testing on the NLN student satisfaction and self-confidence in learning, simulation design scale, and educational practices questionnaire using a sample of prelicensure novice nurses. *Nurse Education Today, 34*(10). http://dx.doi.org/10.1016/j.nedt.2014.06.011
Student Satisfaction and Self-Confidence in Learning	National League for Nursing. (2005). Retrieved from: http://www.nln.org/docs/default-source/default-document-library/instrument-2_satisfaction-and-self-confidence-in-learning.pdf?sfvrsn=0	Attitudes toward satisfaction with instruction and self-confidence in learning in simulation	Reliability: • Discrimination scores ranged from 67% to 94% • Cronbach's alpha of 0.92 Validity: • Correlation between satisfaction and self-confidence factors of 0.78 • Concordant validity of 0.78 • Discordant validity of SCLS and SDS of 0.66 Franklin, A. E., Burns, P., & Lee, C. S. (2014). Psychometric testing on the NLN student satisfaction and self-confidence in learning, simulation design scale, and educational practices questionnaire using a sample of prelicensure novice nurses. *Nurse Education Today, 34*(10). http://dx.doi.org/10.1016/j.nedt.2014.06.011

(continued)

Table 7-1. Simulation Assessment Tools (continued)

Name	Citation	What it Measures	Psychometrics
Van Gelderen Family-Care Rubric (VGFCR)	Van Gelderen, S., Krumwiede, N., & Christian, A. (2016). Teaching family nursing through simulation: Family-care rubric development. *Clinical Simulation in Nursing, 12*(5), 159-170. https://doi.org/10.1016/j.ecns.2016.01.002	Three-phase design: (a) literature review, (b) refinement of family constructs, and (c) psychometric testing of the VGFCR	Reliability: • Overall intraclass correlation coefficient of 0.928 • Cronbach's alpha of 0.956 • All constructs significant at the p=.05 level Validity: • Face validity demonstrated • Content validity demonstrated

Worksheet 7-1
Assessments

Purpose of This Activity

To create the assessment plan.

Complete this worksheet as you gather more information related to your simulation.

Date: ______________________________

Title of the simulation: ______________________________

Brief description of the simulation encounter (one to two sentences): ______________________________

____

____

Setting: ______________________________

____

Simulation modality/ies (SP, task trainers, manikin, other): ______________________________

____

Start by rewriting the learning objectives for this simulation.

1. What types of assessment will be utilized in this scenario?
   - ☐ Formative ______________________________
   - ☐ Summative ______________________________
   - ☐ Both ______________________________

   Notes:

2. Who will assess the clinical simulation encounters?
   - ☐ Faculty ______________________________
   - ☐ Observer ______________________________
   - ☐ Standardized patient ______________________________
   - ☐ Student peers ______________________________
   - ☐ Student (self-rating) ______________________________

   Notes:

(continued)

Worksheet 7-1 (continued)

Assessments

3. What format of assessment will be utilized?
   - ☐ Observation____________________
   - ☐ Checklist survey/scale____________________
   - ☐ Focus groups____________________
   - ☐ Questionnaires ____________________
   - ☐ Standardized measures ____________________

   Notes:

4. How will you assess the simulation experience before/after the simulation encounter for the learner?
   - ☐ Prebriefing____________________
   - ☐ Debriefing____________________
   - ☐ Reflection ____________________
   - ☐ Completing assessments (pre-established or individually created)____________________

   Notes:

5. When planning a research project, list the tasks you must complete prior to the start of the simulation experience:

References

Bambini, D., Washburn, J., & Perkins, R. (2009). Outcomes of clinical simulation for novice nursing students: Communication, confidence, clinical judgment. *Nursing Education Perspectives, 30*(2), 79-82. Retrieved from: https://www.ncbi.nlm.nih.gov/pubmed/19476069

Duffy, D. M., & Harding, J. H. (2004). Simulation of organic monolayers as templates for the nucleation of calcite crystals. *Langmuir, 20*(18), 7630-7636. https://doi.org/10.1021/la049552b

Garrison, C., & Ehrlinghaus, M. (2010). *Formative and summative assessments.* Retrieved from http://standardslearning.pbworks.com/f/Formative+and+Summative+Assessments+in+the+Classroom.pdf

Greenwood, K., Nicoloro, D., & Iversen, M. (2014). Reliability and validity of the acute care confidence survey: An objective measure to assess students' self-confidence and predict student performance for inpatient clinical experiences. *Journal of Acute Care Physical Therapy, 5*(1). https://doi.org/10.1097/01.jat.0000446087.82782.f5

Guhde, J. (2010). Using online exercises and patient simulation to improve students' clinical decision-making. *Nursing Education Perspectives, 31*(6), 387-9. Retrieved from: https://www.ncbi.nlm.nih.gov/pubmed/21280447

Hall, P., Marshall, D., Weaver, L., Boyle, A., & Taniguchi, A. (2011). A method to enhance student teams in palliative care: Piloting the McMaster-Ottawa team observed structured clinical encounter. *Journal of Palliative Medicine, 14*(6). https://doi.org/10.1089/jpm.2010.0295

Heinerichs, S., Cattano, N. M., & Morrison, K. E. (2013). Assessing nonverbal communication skills through video recordings and debriefings of clinical simulation exams. *Athletic Training Education Journal, 8*(1), 17-22. https://doi.org/10.4085/08010217

Henry, B. W., Douglass, C., & Kostiwa, I. M. (2007). Effects of participation in an aging game simulation activity on the attitudes of allied health students toward older adults. *Internet Journal of Allied Health Sciences and Practice, 5*(4), 5. Retrieved from: https://nsuworks.nova.edu/ijahsp/vol5/iss4/5/

Jones, A., & Sheppard, L. (2011). Use of a human patient simulator to improve physiotherapy cardiorespiratory clinical skills in undergraduate physiotherapy students: A randomised controlled trial. *Internet Journal of Allied Health Sciences and Practice*, 9, 1-11. Retrieved from: https://nsuworks.nova.edu/ijahsp/vol9/iss1/12/

Lasater, K. (2007). Clinical judgment development: Using simulation to create an assessment rubric. *Journal of Nursing Education, 46*(11). Retrieved from www.routledge.com/9781630917357

Leonard, B., Shuhaibar, E. L., & Chen, R. (2010). Nursing student perceptions of intraprofessional team education using high-fidelity simulation. *Journal of Nursing Education, 49*(11), 628-631. https://doi.org/10.3928/01484834-20100730-06

Merryman, M. B. (2010). Effects of simulated learning and facilitated debriefing on student understanding of mental illness. *Occupational Therapy in Mental Health, 26*(1), 18-31. https://doi.org/10.1080/01642120903513933

Schirmer, J. M., Mauksch, L., Lang, F., Marvel, M. K., Zoppi, K., Epstein, R. M., & Pryzbylski, M. (2005). Assessing communication competence: A review of current tools. *Fam Med, 37*(3), 184-192.

Shoemaker, M. J., Riemersma, L., & Perkins, R. (2009). Use of high fidelity human simulation to teach physical therapist decision-making skills for intensive care setting. *Cardiopulmonary Physical Therapy Journal, 20*(1), 13-18. Retrieved from: https://www.ncbi.nlm.nih.gov/pubmed/15739134

Silberman, N. J., Panzarella, K. J., & Melzer, B. A. (2013). Using human simulation to prepare physical therapy students for acute care practice. *Journal of Allied Health, 42*(1), 25-32. Retrieved from: https://www.ncbi.nlm.nih.gov/pubmed/23471282

Titzer, J., Swenty, C. & Hoehn, G. (2012). An interprofessional simulation promoting collaboration and problem solving among nursing and allied health professional students. *Clinical Simulation in Nursing, 8*(8). http://dx.doi.org.proxy1.lib.tju.edu/10.1016/j.ecns.2011.01.001

References

Kern's Model Step 4
Educational Strategies

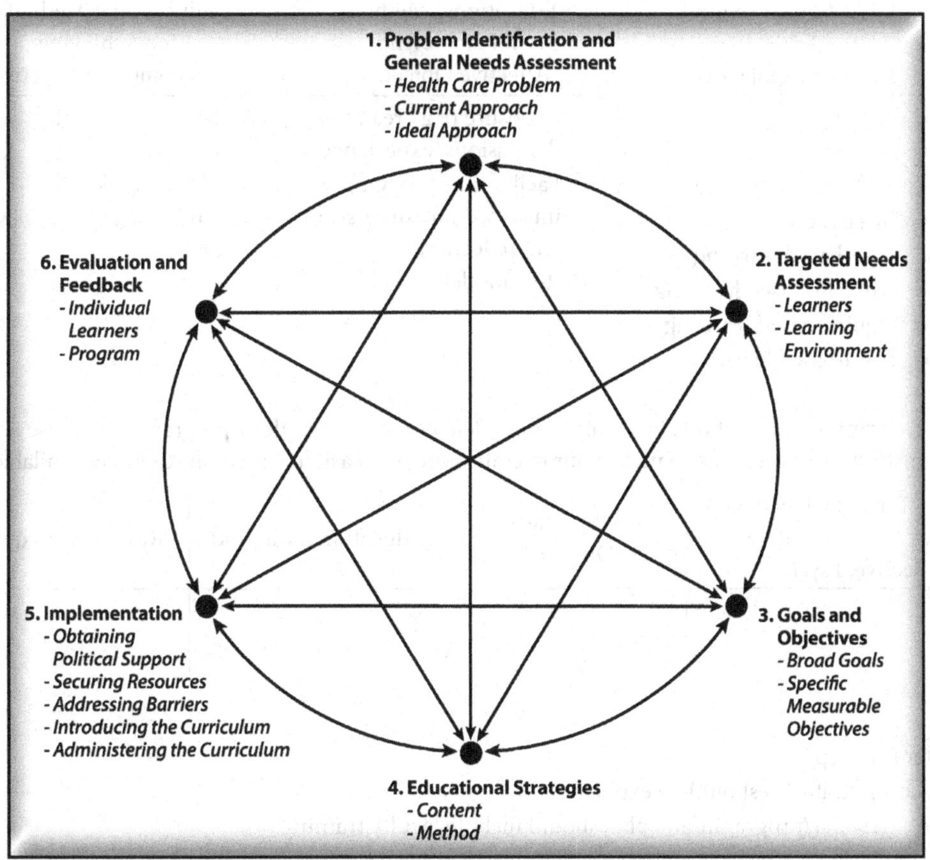

- The purpose of this step is to develop specific content and methods that will accomplish the educational objectives established.
- This step is especially important in simulation because errors are very the focus of simulation experiences so that learners can identify and avoid them; and when errors are made, remediation can be taught.
- Simulation curricula is resource intensive; thus, attention to content validity, establishment of benchmarks, and a varying complexity of tasks is important.

- Educational content preparation should include deconstructing the skills/procedure into key components; this helps in establishing criteria for expected levels of proficiency and input from literature and clinical expert practitioners.
- Educational method preparation should include using multiple educational methods, choosing the most appropriate simulation method, a plan to increase simulation complexity, opportunities for practice, and a review of performance.
- Attention should be given to faculty/staff development to ensure expertise in simulation methods, feedback, and debriefing.

- Educational strategies:
  - Methods used to achieve cognitive, affective, and psychomotor objectives:

Educational Methods for Achieving Cognitive Objectives	Educational Methods for Achieving Affective Objectives	Educational Methods for Achieving Psychomotor Objectives
• Reading • Lecture • Audiovisual materials • Discussion • Case-based learning • Problem-based learning • Inquiry-based learning • Team-based learning	• Exposure (e.g., readings, discussions, experiences) • Facilitation of openness, introspection, discussion, and reflection • Role models	• Supervised clinical experience • Simulations • Audio or visual review of skills

  - Determine two methods (at minimum) to deliver your curriculum/program. Try to use multiple instructional methods to make your overall strategies feasible, based on resources available.

Type of Objective (e.g., Cognitive, Affective, Psychomotor)	Specific Learning Objective	Educational Method	Resources Required

After this step:

- Teaching strategies should be explicit.
- The curricular/programmatic plan should include faculty training.

Suggested Readings

Farnan, J., & Schindler, N. (2013). *Curriculum development and evaluation guide resident as teacher: A mutually beneficial arrangement APPD/COMSEP pre course 2013.* Retrieved from: https://www.appd.org/meetings/2013SpringPresentations/PCWS1Handout.pdf

Kern, D. E. (2014). *Curriculum development: An essential educational skill, a public trust, a form of scholarship, an opportunity for organizational change.* Weill Cornell College of Medicine, Qatar. Retrieved from: https://dnnyqetna.blob.core.windows.net/portals/15/Six-Step%20Approach%20to%20Curriculum%20Development.pdf?sr=b&si=DNNFileManagerPolicy&sig=9sAOUX/lzfZQsN6QKLOpWJ46YLRuXmQwOghR7ptxnFw=

Khamis, N. N., Satava, R. M., Alnassar, S. A., & Kern, D. E. (2016). A stepwise model for simulation-based curriculum development for clinical skills, a modification of the six-step approach. *Surgical Endoscopy,* 279-287. https://doi.org/10.1007/s00464-015-4206x

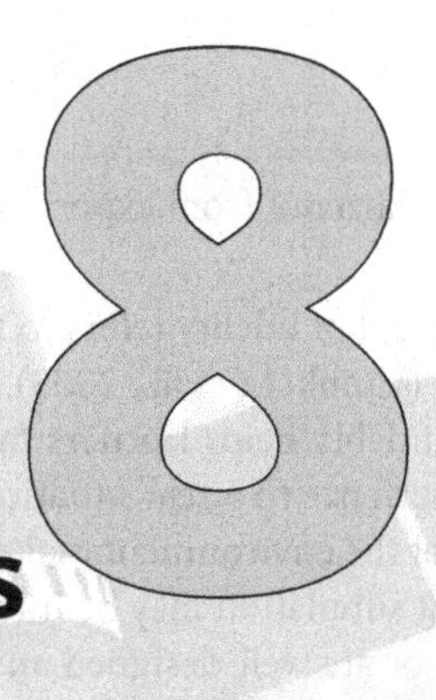

Simulation Modalities and Fidelity

Joanne M. Baird, PhD, OTR/L, CHSE, FAOTA
Maureen M. Hoppe, EdD, MA, OTR/L, CPAM, CHSE

Learning Objectives

1. Define and describe the role of fidelity in simulation education.
2. Recognize the advantages and challenges of fidelity with different types of simulation.
3. Discuss strategies to promote fidelity when creating simulation experiences.

Kern's Model of Program Development

The content in this chapter articulates Step 4 of Kern's Model: Educational Strategies. Information in this chapter contributes to the development of simulations that promote learning in a safe and believable environment. This articulates with the focus on content validity and establishment of benchmarks.

Zapletal, A. L., Baird, J. M., Van Oss, T., Hoppe, M. M., Prast, J. E., & Herge, E. A. *Clinical Simulation for Health Care Professionals* (pp. 81-90).

Fidelity: What Is It?

"People learn not from experience, but in it...." (Hoffman & Donaldson, 2004, p. 449)

The concept of fidelity refers to the match between the realism of the simulation and an actual clinical situation (Issenberg et al., 2005). An important consideration when developing a simulation experience is that fidelity helps learners take an active role in simulation, which increases the likeness of the learning experience to a real situation (Dieckmann et al., 2007). Fidelity is valuable for learners because the realism of the environment makes the experience believable for learners (Giles et al., 2014). Research indicates that simulation may be integrated in a prelicensure health care curriculum with positive results if the scenarios are well-designed and realistic (Wotton et al., 2010).

The amount, or level of, fidelity associated with a simulation is directly related to the simulation environment (Issenberg et al., 2005; Kneebone et al., 2005; Resnick & Sanchez, 2009). Fidelity is often described as a binary concept, with simulation experiences referred to as high fidelity or low fidelity. Because fidelity is created by the environment and because the type of simulator is a major environmental factor, this binary classification is based largely on the type of simulator used (Cunningham, 2010; Munshi et al., 2015; Tosterud et al., 2013). Table 8-1 outlines simulation types with associated levels of fidelity.

Paper and video-based simulations reflect ***Miller's levels*** of *knows and knows how,* and thus have lower levels of fidelity (refer to Chapter 1 for information about Miller's Pyramid). Simulations using manikins or simulated patients reflect learner performance at the Miller's level of *shows how* level, while performance in an actual health care practice reflects Miller's level of *does* (Munishi et al., 2015). No single simulation encounter will assess an entire range of skills, knowledge, or competency (Epstein & Hundert, 2002).

Aspects of Fidelity

While the binary classification of simulation activities as either high fidelity or low fidelity is simple, it has shortcomings. In simulation, the learning environment is really a spectrum, rather than a set menu, of situations. Fidelity is not truly a binary concept, because the environment is comprised of much more than the type of simulator used. Thus, there are several ways to consider fidelity more closely. An examination reveals that simulation encompasses the environment (physical fidelity), the scenario (conceptual fidelity), and the learner's experience (emotional fidelity). All of these factors are thought to contribute to the overall fidelity of the simulation (Dieckmann et al., 2007; Nanji et al., 2013; Rudolph et al., 2007). Each type of fidelity influences the realism of the simulation for the learner (Table 8-2). If learners experience the scenario as reality, they will act spontaneously and obtain the true benefit of simulation (Aliner, 2011).

- *Physical Fidelity:* Represents the degree to which the environment and supplies used in the simulation reflect the appearance and function of actual equipment that the learner would be using in a real-life scenario. Physical fidelity represents the visual, tactile, auditory, olfactory, and other sensory cues that the learner would experience in real life. This category can also include subcategories of fidelity such as equipment fidelity (Beaubien & Baker, 2004). The use of moulage, which is defined as "the art of applying mock injuries for the purpose of training," further contributes to this aspect of fidelity (Cornelle, 2015).
- *Conceptual Fidelity:* Represents the degree to which the simulation progresses in a plausible manner. Conceptual fidelity includes the realism of each aspect of the scenario, individually and taken as a whole. The scenario must unfold in a realistic manner. Conceptual fidelity is integral to a positive learning experience. While the physical (e.g., environmental or equipment) fidelity of a simulation can improve learner experiences, it cannot compensate for simulation experiences that have poor conceptual fidelity (Beaubien & Baker, 2004).

Table 8-1. Simulation Types and Associated Fidelity

Low Fidelity	High Fidelity
Role playing Paper-based case studies	Manikin
Video-based simulations Task trainers	Standardized patients
Adapted from Cunningham, 2010 and Tosterud et al., 2013.	

Table 8-2. Phases of the Simulation Experience

Terms	*Prebriefing* "An *information or orientation session held prior to the start of* a simulation activity in which instructions or preparatory information is given to the participants" (Lopreiato et al., 2016, p. 28).	*Briefing* "An *activity immediately preceding the start of a simulation* where the participants receive essential information about the simulation scenario" (Lopreiato et al., 2016, p. 6).	*Simulation Experience* The *simulated encounter itself is designed* for learner participation. (Lopreiato et al., 2016).	*Debriefing* Debriefing is a teaching method *utilized to enhance student learning after the simulation experience occurs,* consisting of student reflective analysis of performance for future application (Dreifuerst, 2012).
Examples	A few weeks before the simulation, discuss/share the encounter and explain expectations. Discuss during lectures the laboratory and learning experiences and how they relate to the simulation.	During the week of the simulation, the class preceding the simulation, or on the day of the simulation, discuss where participants will go: what room or area, where important equipment is located within that area, where the instructor will be/can be reached, etc. Information can be provided in writing on a handout for reference.	This is the actual simulation itself, which may include a manikin, an SP, or another simulation modality.	After the simulation students meet with the instructors, SPs, and colleagues and discuss their experiences with the goal of reflective learning.

- *Psychological Fidelity:* This represents what the learner experiences during the simulation, whether it be relief, pressure, frustration, or satisfaction (Lopreiato et al., 2016). Psychological fidelity represents the "buy-in" that the learner experiences during the scenario; it is also defined as how well the learner's performance during the simulation would match what would be expected during a real-life scenario (Beaubien & Baker, 2004).

Psychological Fidelity or Suspending Disbelief

While all aspects of fidelity are important, psychological fidelity is thought to be the most essential (Rudolph et al., 2014). An important aspect of psychological fidelity is the role that the learner plays. A learner must consider the scenario and simulation as real so that treatment occurs as it would in reality (Issenberg & Scalese, 2007). It is important that the learner accepts the simulation as reality to gain the most from the experience. Psychological fidelity can be influenced by all aspects of the simulation, ranging from the accuracy and function of the equipment or manikin (equipment fidelity) to the level of acting portrayed by standardized patient (SP), or the accuracy of the age, size, and gender represented in the scenario (physical fidelity; Rudolph et al., 2014).

One method to promote psychological fidelity is through the use of a fiction contract, an agreement between the instructor and the learner that explicitly acknowledges the limitations and expectations of the simulation and those involved. A fiction contract helps the learner suspend disbelief and fully engage in the simulation by outlining the roles and responsibilities of each party. Whether this contract is verbal, through a discussion with the learner, and/or in writing, it is done prior to the simulation in the prebriefing or briefing phase of the simulation experience, as depicted in Table 8-2.

The fiction contract asks the learner to temporarily suspend judgment of realism during the simulation learning experience and to engage in the simulation, even if the situation isn't entirely representative of a real-life event. The educator is responsible to support the learner through striving for realism, properly preparing the learner, and offering a safe educational environment (Dieckmann et al., 2007). The educator acknowledges the limitations of the simulation and requests a voluntary commitment from the learner to act as if the simulation is real. The contract also conveys that the quality of the experience for the learner depends, in large part, on the learner's genuine participation (Rudolph et al., 2014).

The Role of Fidelity in Simulation Education

The learning environment must be considered, no matter what type of simulation is used (Issenberg et al., 2005; Kneebone et al., 2005; Resnick & Sanchez, 2009). The learning environment directly contributes to fidelity or the level of realism present during the simulation (Alinier, 2011). Students prefer realism during simulations, thus the learning environment should be of significant concern (Rudolph et al., 2014). However, a simulation does not have to be high fidelity to promote transfer of skills to the clinical environment (Maran & Glavin, 2003; Munshi, et al., 2015; Salas & Burke, 2002). In fact, research indicates that high-fidelity simulation does not promote skill carryover when used to train novice learners, and that low-fidelity simulation can be used effectively to train complex skills (Salas & Burke, 2002). The most important consideration when developing a simulation is that the type of task, method of simulation, and level of the learner are all aligned. Indeed, the learning objectives should dictate the type of fidelity used. Table 8-3 provides an overview of how fidelity can be managed within the design of a simulation. In general, it appears that the level of fidelity should equate to the level of the learner and the complexity of the task. Thus, a high level of fidelity is not necessary if novice learners are to demonstrate basic skills (Maran & Glavin, 2003; Munshi et al., 2015; Salas & Burke, 2002). If advanced learners are performing complex skills; however, high-fidelity simulation may result in better transfer of skills.

Table 8-3. Methods to Address Fidelity Considerations With Simulation Design

Type of Fidelity	Definition	Examples

Physical/ environmental	Where the simulation will take place; ensure environment is set up and mirrors the actual setting as closely as possible (hospital room, ICU, home situation, etc.):
	• Incorporate medical equipment, moulage, props to increase realism of simulated encounter
	• Replicate body fluids/wounds
	• Sensory experiences are important, include as appropriate:
	  ◦ Alarms with equipment
	  ◦ Odors associated with wounds, body fluids
	• Age, gender, and clinical condition of the client are replicated as close as possible
		SP only interacts with student(s) in one room with a hospital bed, monitor, bedside table, sink, overbed table meant to replicate an acute care environment
		• Use of IV pole and line, oxygen cannula
		• Foley catheter bag with colored water or apple juice to simulate urine
		• Set monitors or pumps to alarm as appropriate for simulation
		• If a case is written for an older adult, make sure the SP's age is 55 or older, rather than a younger adult

Conceptual fidelity	Set the stage for an accurate representation of what the learner would experience in "real life" Ensure scenario progresses in realistic manner SPs are trained on procedures and scripted for learning to accurately depict clinical conditions/behaviors Temporal considerations appropriate to expectations in clinical practice Time parameters for evaluation/ intervention/ documentation of client session	Simulation should be realistic, thus if a student calls for help in an acute care simulation without using the call bell and the door to the room is closed, this may be an opportunity to review safety and communication Consideration should be given to patient responses when a specific objective is key (the student's response to a friendly disruption rather than the student's response to a rude or mean disruption) and also when a specific motor behavior is desired (a gait deviation, limitation in range of motion, or speech limitation) Students are actively learning and often perform assessments and interventions more slowly than typical clinical norms; scenarios can address this by setting task timelines or introducing patient fatigue or impatience

(continued)

Table 8-3 (continued). Methods to Address Fidelity Considerations With Simulation Design

Type of Fidelity	Definition	Examples
Psychological fidelity	Consider the use of a fiction contract with learners Have learners dress the part and wear what would be expected of them in clinical practice Design consideration with physical and conceptual fidelity will contribute substantially to psychological fidelity of the learner The more realistic the preparation and actual simulation design, the more likely the learner will buy into the simulated encounter	This is a verbal (or it can be written) contract that addresses that simulation is not the same as actual practice and that in order for all to benefit, belief must be temporarily suspended so that the student can treat the simulation as reality Consider street clothes instead of hospital gowns, night/bath wear; obtain permission in advance from the SP if alternate clothing would benefit the simulation All aspects of the simulation should be compatible; if the scenario occurs in the early morning, lighting should be overly bright. If the scenario occurs at home, everyday objects should be evident. Consider the use of confederates—others within the simulation that are not the focus but may have a role secondary to the SP, such as someone portraying a family member or member of the health care or educational team.

Strategies to Use When Creating Simulations

Consider these aspects of your simulation as you begin planning.

Setting

Can the simulation mimic key aspects of the desired setting?

One measure of skill mastery is technical performance in a realistic clinical environment. Tasks mastered easily in a classroom may not be directly applicable as learned if they need to be completed in a clinical care environment, such as at the bedside, on an intensive care unit, in a busy rehabilitation clinic, or in a client's home.

Environment

Simulations are strongly influenced by all aspects of the environment. Typically there are several environmental aspects to consider. What *physical* environment is available and would be the best match for the task and level of the learner?

- Classroom
- Classroom laboratory
- Simulation center

- Simulation space (room or area designed to be realistic to a particular setting; e.g., an apartment with working appliances and plumbing, a bed area mimicking an acute setting, a conference room)
- Hospital/clinic
- Clinical fieldwork setting
- Community area

What *temporal* environment is available and would be the best match for the task and level of the learner?

- Will this simulation be time-limited? If so, will the learner need to use a maximum amount of time (i.e., provide a 30-minute intervention) or complete a task within a maximum amount of time (i.e., finish an evaluation within 30 minutes)?
- Will this simulation be trial-limited? For example, will the student have three trials to correctly demonstrate a skill or complete a task no matter how long it takes?

What *behavioral* environment is available and would be the best match for the task/skill and level of the learner?

- Does the simulation lend itself to a behavioral if/then manipulation? For example, if the student takes a certain course of action, do you want the SP or manikin to respond in a specific way?
  - If a student does not introduce themself, do you want the SP to ask for the student's name or provide feedback later about not having the student's name?
  - If a student forgets to lock the brakes of a wheelchair before a transfer, does the SP provide a cue or allow the wheelchair to move, requiring the student to problem solve how to safely manage the situation. What if the student misses the wheelchair movement and proceeds? Does the SP provide a cue at this time or do you?
- Do you want to consider using an SP or another individual who plays a non-patient role in a scenario, such as a family member or member of the health care team? This individual plays a role in the simulation, whether to add a challenge, provide support or information to the learner or contribute to the realism of the scenario. This individual is known as a *confederate.**
  - Consider a simulation of an older adult with cognitive impairment and a confederate who plays the role of a caregiver.
  - A confederate can also be used to play the role of a peer professional from another discipline. (*A request to remove this term has been sent to the Society for Simulation in Healthcare, the authors of the *Simulation in Healthcare Dictionary.*)

Worksheet 8-1
Fidelity Considerations With Simulation Design

Purpose of This Activity

Explore fidelity considerations with simulation design.

Date: ____

Title of the simulation: ____

Brief description of the simulation encounter (one to two sentences): ______________________
____
____

Setting: ____
____

Learning objectives: ____
____

Simulation modality/ies (SP, task trainers, manikin, other): ______________________________
____

Reflective Questions to Consider With Regard to Fidelity and Use of Clinical Simulation

- What strategies can be used to improve the psychological fidelity of the clinical simulation for the learner?

- Utilizing an appreciative inquiry approach, what resources are available to improve fidelity of simulated learning environment?

- How can fidelity be enhanced in simulation design to maximize learning related to educational objectives?

(continued)

Worksheet 8-1 (continued)

Fidelity Considerations With Simulation Design

Use the following bulleted points to guide fidelity considerations with simulation design.

- Type of clinical simulation:
- Rationale for use of selected simulation type (relate to educational objectives):
- Methods/strategies to address psychological fidelity of the learner:
- Methods/strategies to address environmental fidelity of the simulated encounter:
- Methods/strategies to address equipment fidelity in simulation design:

References

Aliner, G. (2011). Developing high-fidelity health care simulation scenarios: A guide for educators and professionals. *Simulation & Gaming, 42,* 9-26. https://doi.org/10.1177/1046878109355683

Beaubien, J. M., & Baker, D. P. (2004). The use of simulation for training teamwork skills in health care: How low can you go? *BMJ Quality & Safety, 13*(Suppl. 1), i51-i-56. https://doi.org/10.1136/qhc.13.suppl1.i51

Cornelle, J. T. (2015). Moulage in simulation. In Wilson, L. & Wittmann, R. A. (Eds.), *Review manual for the certified healthcare simulation educator exam.* Springer Publishing Company.

Cunningham, D. D. (2010). Incorporating medium fidelity simulation in a practical nurse education program. *Journal of Practical Nursing, 60*(1), 2-5. Retrieved from https://libraryproxy.csm.edu:2069/docview/878223590?accountid=58678

Dieckmann, P., Gaba, D., & Rall, M. (2007). Deepening the theoretical foundations of patient simulationion as social practice. *Simulation in Healthcare, 2,* 183-193.

Dreifuerst, K. (2012). Using debriefing for meaningful learning to foster development of clinical reasoning in simulation. *Journal of Nursing Education, 51,* 326-333. http://dx.doi.org/10.3928/01484834-20120409-02

Epstein, R. M., & Hundert, E. M. (2002). Defining and assessing professional competence. *Journal of American Medical Association, 287*(2), 226-235.

Giles, A. K., Carson, N. E., Breland, H. L., Coker-Bolt, P., & Bowman, P. J. (2014). Use of simulated patients and reflective video analysis to assess occupational therapy students' preparedness for fieldwork. *The American Journal of Occupational Therapy, 68*(Suppl. 2), S57-S66. https://doi.org/10.5014/ajot.2014.685S03.

Gore, T. (2017). The relationship between levels of fidelity in simulation, traditional clinical experiences and objectives. *International Journal of Nursing Education Scholarship, 14*(1), 337-344. http://libraryproxy.csm.edu:2156/10.1515/ijnes-2017-0012

Hoffman, K. G. & Donaldson, J. F. (2004) Contextual tensions of the clinical environment and their influence on teaching and learning. *Medical Education, 38,* 448-454. https://doi.org/10.1046/j.1365-2923.2004.01799.x

Issenberg, S. B., McGaghie, W. C., Petrusa, E. R., Gordon, D. L., & Scalese, R. J. (2005). Features and uses of high-fidelity medical simulations that lead to effective learning: A BEME systematic review. *Medical Teacher, 27,* 10–28. https://doi.org/10.1080/01421590500046924

Issenberg, B., & Scalese, R. (2007). Best evidence on high-fidelity simulation: What clinical teachers need to know. *Clinical Teacher,* 4(2), 73-77. https://doi.org/10.1111/j.1743-498X.2007.00161.x

Kneebone, R. L., Kidd, J., Nestel, D., Barnet, A., Lo, B., King, R., Yang, G. Z. & Brown, R. (2005). Blurring the boundaries: Scenario-based simulation in a clinical setting. *Medical Education, 39,* 580-587.

Lopreiato, J. O. (Ed.), Downing, D., Gammon, W., Lioce, L., Sittner, B., Slot, V., Spain, A. E. (Associate Eds.), and the Terminology & Concepts Working Group. (2016). *Healthcare simulation dictionary.* Retrieved from http://www.ssih.org/dictionary.

Maran, N. J. & Glavin, R. J. (2003). Low- to high-fidelity simulation—A continuum of medical education? *Medical Education, 37,* S1-S9. https://doi.org/10.1046/j.1365-2923.37.s1.9.x

Munshi, F., Lababidi, H., & Alyousef, S. (2015). Low-versus high-fidelity simulations in teaching and assessing clinical skills. *Journal of Taibah University Medical Sciences, 10,* 12-15. http://dx.doi.org/10.1016/j.jtumed.2015.01.008

Nanji, K. C., Baca, K. & Raemer, D. B (2013). The effect of an olfactory and visual cue on realism and engagement in a healthcare simulation experience. *Simulation in Healthcare: The Journal of the Society of Medical Simulation 8,* 143-147.

Resnick, M. L. & Sanchez, R. (2009). Reducing patient handling injuries through contextual training. *Journal of Emergency Nursing, 35,* 504-508. https://doi.org/10.1016/j.jen.2008.10.017.

Rudolph, J. W., Raemer, D. B. & Simon, R. (2014). Establishing a safe container for learning in simulation: The role of the pre simulation briefing, *Simulation in Healthcare, 9,* 339-349.

Rudolph, J. W., Simon, R., & Raemer, D. B. (2007). Which reality matters? Questions on the road to high engagement in healthcare simulation. *Simulation in Healthcare: The Journal of the Society of Medical Simulation 2*(3), 161-163.

Salas, E., & Burke, C. (2002). Simulation for training is effective when … *BMJ Quality & Safety, 11,* 119-120. https://doi.org/10.1136/qhc.11.2.119

Tosterud, R., Hedelin, B., & Hall-Lord, M. (2013). Nursing students' perceptions of high- and low-fidelity simulation used as learning methods. *Nurse Education in Practice, 13*(4), 262-270. http://dx.doi.org/10.1016/j.nepr.2013.02.002

Wotton, K., Davis, J., Button, D., & Kelton, M. (2010). Third-year undergraduate nursing students' perceptions of high-fidelity simulation. *Journal of Nursing Education, 49*(11), 632-639. http://dx.doi.org/10.3928/01484834-20100831-01

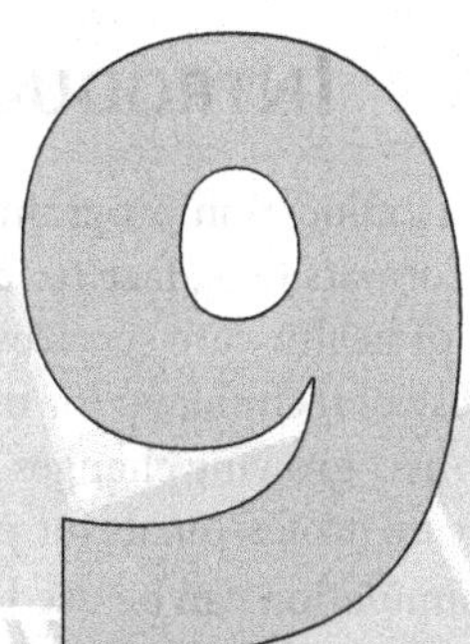

Virtual Learning in Simulation

Jean E. Prast, OTD, MSOT, OTRL, CHSE
Maureen M. Hoppe, EdD, MA, OTR/L, CPAM, CHSE

Learning Objectives

1. Discuss effective use of virtual simulation methods to address educational objectives.
2. Establish technological and resource needs to effectively implement a virtual simulation.
3. Design a virtual clinical simulation in health professional curricula to facilitate student learning while utilizing best practices.

Kern's Model of Program Development

The content in this chapter articulates Step 4 of Kern's Model: Educational Strategies. Information in this chapter discusses the types and uses of virtual simulation modalities. This articulates with choosing the most appropriate simulation method.

Zapletal, A. L., Baird, J. M., Van Oss, T., Hoppe, M. M., Prast, J. E., & Herge, E. A. *Clinical Simulation for Health Care Professionals* (pp. 91-99).

Introduction to Virtual Learning

Health care education programs have changed over time with variations in teaching and learning methods and formats (e.g., face to face, hybrid, online). Similarly, changes and trends have been seen in the provision of health care services based on consumer needs and accessibility (e.g., office visits, telehealth visits, use of technology for medical reporting). Innovative strategies can provide valuable opportunities to connect growing changes in health care technology and population needs as programs prepare future health care professionals for practice.

Clinical simulation can be used as an effective instructional methodology in health professions curricula to enhance student learning and preparation for successful transitions to future practice. Virtual simulation experiences can provide opportunities to practice critical and clinical reasoning, as well as technical and professional skills in a safe, low risk environment, allowing students to adjust their responses to complex scenarios consistent with clinical practice (Herge et al., 2013). Through online debriefing and feedback from peers, standardized patients (SPs), and/or faculty instructors, students can reflect on their experiences, assess strengths, and recognize areas for growth. Current evidence demonstrates an increase in students' comfort and confidence with specific skills and techniques after a high-fidelity clinical simulation experience in a face-to-face environment; however, there is limited research related to effectiveness of remote virtual simulation learning in health profession education (Herge et al., 2013). Some evidence has shown that the use of virtual patients can improve clinical reasoning, procedural skills, and team skills when compared to traditional educational methodologies (Kononowicz et al., 2019). The International Nursing Association for Clinical Simulation and Learning provides an evidence-based framework of best practice for use of simulation, which can serve as a model for education (INACSL, 2016).

Creating an effective clinical simulation program and embedding it into a health profession curriculum is normally challenging but can be heightened with a transition from face to face to online or hybrid format delivery. There are many components to this teaching/learning experience that need to be considered, such as identifying learning objectives, designing the virtual environment, selecting appropriate assessment measures, and determining which courses are optimal for this learner-centered instructional method. Use of exclusive virtual simulation can pose unique challenges related to the availability of resources, transformation of existing pedagogical methods, student volume, technology needs, and funding for simulation programs. Faculty need to be creative with implementation of virtual simulations while being cognizant of best practice guidelines. This may be especially challenging for 'hands-on' manual techniques (psychomotor skills) traditionally taught and assessed during in-person simulation sessions.

However, virtual simulations with the use of SPs can be a valuable method to allow students to practice establishing rapport with appropriate communication skills, obtaining a medical or occupational history, administration of cognitive screens, as well as clinical observation skill sets. In addition, the use of virtual platforms, including multiple breakout rooms proctored by medical faculty has been used for a web-based OSCE (Objective Structured Clinical Examination) with students reporting favorable learning despite the inability to complete a physical examination in a virtual world (Major et al., 2020). With clear written and verbal communication, simulation guidelines, preparation, as well as training of individuals in simulation roles including SP roles and faculty, virtual simulations can be designed to mimic a telehealth visit consistent with clinical practice.

Telehealth has been effectively used in health care practice to provide improved access to services, but as a result of COVID-19 there was a rapid shift to virtual platforms to provide telehealth services across disciplines. Thus, students in health care programs may need additional learning experiences and exposure to online virtual technologies to best prepare for the changing health care environments, as well as future work in clinical and community settings. Use of virtual SPs, video case scenarios, and simulated clients may be effective methods to assist with the transition to future practice and provide an adjunct for clinical experiences to supplement learning opportunities.

Virtual Simulation Planning, Design, and Implementation Considerations

Planning and designing a virtual simulation, requires different considerations and resources than an in-person simulation experience. The following unique components should be addressed with the development and implementation of a virtual simulation:

Netiquette

Professionalism in a virtual environment should mimic expectations of those in a health care environment. Be clear and descriptive with student expectations working in a virtual context. Things to consider:

- Participants should have clear identification of professional name for entrance to virtual simulated environment
- Appropriate background should be captured with webcam (e.g., virtual or natural background choice)
- Recommend distractors minimized in and around the physical work environment (e.g., people, animals, noise)
- Ensure participants are able to listen and communicate effectively (e.g., headset, microphone, speakers)
- Written permission for recording is obtained from all participants
- Privacy considerations should be outlined for all participants (i.e., policies restricting unauthorized individuals in virtual learning environment and unauthorized screen shots/recordings of simulated experience)
- Netiquette training should be provided to both the learner and SP.

Standardized Patient Preparation

Screening, hiring, and training is essential in planning for the use of an SP, regardless of the simulation format. Some core areas to consider with training and preparation of an SP in a virtual environment include the following:

- Identifying the purpose and learning objectives of the simulation
- Provision of a script inclusive of key statements as well as clear guidelines and expectations essential for student learning
- Provide a specific schedule with an algorithm of events as they are expected to occur
- Make sure to provide training on the use of selected tools or evaluation instruments being used
- Educate the SP on equipment or resources needed to carry out the simulation (e.g., modalities, household items, environmental set-up)

Student Preparation

Intentional student preparation is imperative throughout the various stages of simulation particularly in a virtual learning environment. Much of the preparation and education will occur during the prebriefing phase of the simulation. This will vary greatly depending on the simulation. Some considerations include:

- Video of a hand off or patient report from another professional with detailed, step-by-step instructions with visual images on use of the virtual learning platform (e.g., chat feature, muting, recording, share screen, share video); protocols or parameters involved in the scenario; and a schedule with expectations and assigned roles.
- During the briefing phase, students should be reminded of learning objectives and expectations. If they are completing the simulation in collaboration with a peer, time should be allocated to develop a plan and set everything up before implementation (e.g., enter platform, identify role, navigate features, hit record). When the virtual simulation is completed, debriefing and feedback should occur based on the selected model and timeframe allocated (e.g., immediate, delayed; or faculty-led, peer-led, SP-led).

Resources

Similar to planning for any type of simulation, human and material resources need to be considered for virtual simulation including ensuring that all participants have the necessary resources/tools to successfully engage in the simulation before the day of event. A component of simulation preparation may include the provision of a checklist to all participants that consists of equipment, resource, and materials needed for use during the simulation experience at least 2 weeks prior to the simulation. Educators are responsible for following up and supplying any necessary resources that participants report that they do not have readily accessible. In a virtual simulation, there are additional considerations with simulation design and implementation such as:

- Who will be responsible for monitoring the virtual simulation?
- Who will be available for troubleshooting with any technology issues?
- Who will prepare materials and ensure all involved parties are trained or educated on all components of the simulation?
- What evaluation tools will be used?
    - Who will be responsible for conducting the evaluations?
- Who will facilitate and observe the simulation sessions?
- Who will manage the students and any needs associated with the virtual simulation?

Technology

The selection of a virtual platform or app should be made based on cost, availability, ease of use, and ease of access for all involved parties (e.g., SPs, students, faculty, staff). Consider platforms or apps that are readily available and supported by the facility (this is helpful with training, troubleshooting, and support needs). Depending on the structure of the simulation, security and recording features should be considered.

Learner Evaluation

Learner evaluation is an important aspect of simulation with the method aligning to the educational objectives and type of assessment (formative or summative). Educators need to:

- Consider how and when the learner or simulation itself will be evaluated.
- Are there tools that were previously developed for an on-site simulation that can be used for the virtual simulation?
- Is a summative or formative evaluation preferred? Is there training involved in administration of the tools (Web-OSCE, CAT-M)?

Assessment Tools

Choosing the appropriate assessment tools is important to gather and collect data to inform future curriculum design, programmatic needs, and learner outcomes. Depending on the type of assessment, these may be completed by the educator, observer, SP, or learner. The simulationist needs to contemplate the following:

- If standardized or nonstandardized instruments are preferred for the virtual simulation, take into consideration the use of realistic and appropriate tools that can be used based on observation skills and resources needed and available for administration.
- Will they be readily available for the student and SP?
- Are the results easy to interpret in a virtual environment?
- Are screen shares needed to accurately assess outcomes?

Documentation

Depending on the purpose, expectation, and learning objectives of the virtual simulation, documentation of the event may be considered. Educators need to determine whether the purpose of the simulation documentation is for clinical preparation, professional growth consistent with reflective practice, or guided clinical reasoning development. For example, there are various encounters in clinical practice that require documentation (e.g., initial evaluation, meetings, SOAP or narrative note, interview, patient intake, assessment data). In addition, there are various platforms that can be used (e.g., EHRgo, Microsoft Excel, academic learning management systems, electronic health record systems). In some cases, a timer may be set to practice time management with patient reporting and documentation consistent with clinical practice expectations.

Debriefing

Debriefing is an integral part of the experience, if not the most important aspect. It consists of a semi-structured conversation or questions to facilitate guided reflection and enhance learning from the simulation experience. There are many formats and models to guide the process. The following includes examples of models to structure the debriefing process: PEARLS, 4D Model, +/Δ, GAS (Gather, Analyze, Summarize), Good Judgment Method.

In addition, a number of formats can be used to facilitate the debriefing process in a virtual environment.

- Educator-provided focused questions for peer-led online discussion
- Guided debriefing by trained SP
- Reflective discussion threads developed by the educator
- Synchronous small group virtual debrief with educator in breakout rooms or designated time slots

Course/Program Integration

A review of the purpose and desired outcomes of using virtual simulation as a teaching method should be considered before development and integration.

- Are there curriculum, accreditation, or program standards that need to be considered?
- Is there a set place or better fit for the virtual learning to occur within the program to best meet learner needs?
- Collaboration with colleagues with planning and design is critical to enhance continuity and progression of learner skill development/growth, as well as to ensure adequate foundational learner knowledge is present prior to simulation participation to maximize success.

Table 9-1. Schedule Templates

Appointment Times (Patient Enter/Exit)	8:30 to 9:00 a.m.	9:15 to 9:45 a.m.	10:00 to 10:30 a.m.
Breakout Room #l	Faculty/Staff A	SP/Role Player A	Moderator A
Student(s)	1, 2, 3	4, 5, 6	7, 8, 9
Breakout Room #2	Faculty/Staff B	SP/Role Player B	Moderator B
Student(s)	10, 11, 12	13, 14, 15	16, 17, 18

Include time built into schedule for students to brief (i.e., 10 minute prep/record) and debrief (i.e., 15 minute predetermined questions to guide). These built-in times will occur before arrival and after departure of the client who is receiving the health care service.

Institutional/Programmatic Policies

Policies and procedures for the virtual simulation should be established (e.g., similar to that of a face-to-face encounter). Content such as student and SP safety (e.g., physical and emotional), liability insurance and coverage, privacy policies (e.g., HIPAA, FERPA), and permissions to participate (e.g., recording, personal information gathered) should be considered. At some facilities, a compliance officer or administrator will be available to support the development of policies and procedures to ensure that health and safety are considered as part of the virtual simulation event.

Table 9-1 provides examples of scheduling templates.

Worksheet 9-1
Brainstorming Innovative Strategies for Creating a Virtual Simulation

Planning the Virtual Simulation	*Resources (e.g., Human, Materials, Technology)*	*Needs/ Considerations*
Where does it fit best in the program/ curriculum? • Identify the best or most appropriate fit in terms of program needs, threads, and content delivery (e.g., class, workshop, clinical)		
What type of virtual simulation is preferred? • Identify the program needs, curricular threads, learning objectives, and desired outcomes • Examples: use of an avatar, SP, role playing, case scenarios, video-based		
What type of technology is preferred and available? • Identify the preferred tools with consideration of devices, internet access (e.g., broadband width), and privacy		
What is the preferred platform? • Consider the ease of access across devices and troubleshooting support (e.g., Zoom, MS Teams, Google Meet, FaceTime, Telehealth Apps)		
What are the expectations of students? • Consider professional behaviors (netiquette), how they will be informed of the expectations, and how they will inform others as displayed virtually (i.e., looking at screen vs. webcam will impact eye contact)		
How will SPs or those fulfilling simulation roles be prepared? • Consider when and where virtual training will occur and what it will entail (e.g., simulation schedule, expectations, tools and resources needed, use of evaluation methods)		

(continued)

Worksheet 9-1 (continued)
Brainstorming Innovative Strategies for Creating a Virtual Simulation

Planning the Virtual Simulation	*Resources (e.g., Human, Materials, Technology)*	*Needs/ Considerations*
How will students be prepared? • Consider prebriefing, briefing, and debriefing materials and detailed instructions (simulation schedule, expectations, navigation, tools and resources needed, environmental set-up)		
What evaluation tools will be used to measure simulation outcomes? • Identify the method (e.g., formative, summative), instruments or resources that will be used (e.g., Web-OSCE, CAT-M, SET-M), who is responsible for administration/completion (e.g., student, peer, SP, faculty/staff), and the timeframes for implementation		
What standardized or nonstandardized health care assessment tools are preferred? • Identify tools that are appropriate to implement and realistic to interpret in a virtual learning platform to assess the SP or person fulfilling a role (e.g., developmental, cognition, auditory, physical function)		
Will the virtual simulation encounter include a documentation component? • Identify the need for written communication to capture the encounter • Consider note-taking, filling out discipline-specific documentation forms, charting, use of an electronic health record		
What institutional or programmatic policies are needed? • Consider student and SP safety, liability, ethical issues that may arise, privacy (FERPA), and permissions (recording)		

REFERENCES

Herge, A., Lorch, A., DeAngelis, T., Vause-Earland, T., Mollo, K., & Zapletal, A. (2013.) The standardized patient encounter: A dynamic educational approach to enhance students' clinical healthcare skills. *Journal of Allied Health, 42*(4), 229-235.

INACSL Standards Committee (2016). INACSL standards of best practice: Simulation SM simulation design. *Clinical Simulation in Nursing, 12*(S), S5-S12. http://dx.doi.org/10.1016/j.ecns.2016.09.005

Kononowicz, A. A., Woodham, L. A., Edelbring, S., Stathakarou, N., Davies, D., Saxena, N., Tudor Car, L., Carlstedt-Duke, J., Car, J., & Zary, N. (2019). Virtual patient simulations in health professions education: Systematic review and meta-analysis by the digital health education collaboration. *Journal of Medical Internet Research, 21*(7), e14676. https://doi.org/10.2196/14676

Major, S., Sawan, L., Vognsen, J. & Jabre, M. (2020). Covid-19 pandemic prompts the development of web-OSCE Zoom teleconferencing to resume medical students' clinical skills training at Weill Cornell Medicine-Qatar. *BMJ Simulation & Technology Enhanced Learning, 6*:376-377. https://doi.org/10.1136/bmjstel-2020-000629

10

Gamification and Gameful Simulation

Victoria L. B. Grieve, PharmD

Learning Objectives

1. Define and describe gamification, gameful design, and the difference between them.
2. Recognize the benefit to engagement that comes with applying gameful concepts by way of self-determinism theory.
3. Identify potential opportunities for applying gamification or gameful design to educational simulations.

Kern's Model of Program Development

The content in this chapter articulates Step 4 of Kern's Model: Educational Strategies. Information in this chapter contributes to the development of simulation that involves gaming and learner motivation. This articulates with selecting the most appropriate simulation methods and strategies for a successful delivery.

Zapletal, A. L., Baird, J. M., Van Oss, T., Hoppe, M. M., Prast, J. E., & Herge, E. A. *Clinical Simulation for Health Care Professionals* (pp. 101-108).

Games and Motivations

Playing games has become one of the most ubiquitous activities engaged in by a large portion of the population. 2.7 billion people play games regularly (Wijman, 2020). Each one of those gamers spends about 7 hours a week playing games (Anderton, 2019). As of 2020, the projected market for video games alone is $159 billion (Wijman, 2020). In an attempt to explain the wide-spread engagement with video games, researchers have turned to link it with Self-Determination Theory. This theory tries to explain why humans engage in certain activities and splits motivation into two camps: extrinsic motivation and intrinsic motivation. Extrinsic motivational concepts are very similar to those of operant conditioning: also known as rewards and punishments. The act of awarding points or grades in a class is an example of extrinsic reward, just as the act of delivering negative reviews or requiring additional work are examples of extrinsic punishment. Humans are motivated to seek out rewards and avoid punishments (Ryan et al., 2006). However, these simple concepts have been found to be limiting in driving long-term engagement, which leads to the other side of self-determination: intrinsic motivation. These motivations are separated into three main drives: autonomy, competence, and relatedness. Humans desire autonomy and are more motivated to participate in an activity where they can approach the situation at their own pace and in their own way. The drive for competence revolves around how much a person can see themselves get better at an activity over time. Relatedness is the drive for a person to interact with other participants during the activity, whether in a competitive fashion or a cooperative one. These three intrinsically motivating categories are shown to increase long-term motivation with a given task (Deci & Ryan, 1985). Additionally, there is another category of intrinsic motivation that could be added to this list specific to game activities: that of immersion (Tondello et al., 2017). The motivation of immersion is the drive for novel experiences that can take a person away from their norm and can include mental immersion in a story or physical immersion through the act of gameplay.

Games are extremely good at delivering experiences that cover extrinsic motivations and intrinsic motivations. Many online games and mobile games utilize extrinsic motivators to keep players coming back each day. Classic scoring systems seen in many arcade games are also extrinsically motivating. Intrinsic motivations are usually covered via the interaction that a player has with a game. The act of maneuvering in a game world and responding to challenges enhances a player's sense of autonomy. The challenges of a game increasing as a player gets better at overcoming them enhances the sense of competence, especially when a player re-engages with old challenges and finds them easier the second time. The act of cooperating with or competing with other players and nonplayer entities in the game world enhance a player's connectedness. The act of becoming invested in the moment-to-moment gameplay or the story being told enhances a player's immersion. Take, for instance, a massively successful video game like From Software's *Dark Souls. Dark Souls* is a large, third person action adventure game set in a mysterious world. The main aspects of the game involve combating challenging monsters and exploring the world around you. Within the game, overcoming enemies gives you currency to upgrade your equipment and avatar's strength (i.e., extrinsic motivation rewarding combat). Additionally, exploring the world and engaging with the plot rewards you with unique items or stories (i.e., extrinsic motivation rewarding exploration). The player can set off in a variety of directions to meet their goals and every combat can be tackled in different ways (e.g., autonomy). The enemies you fight become increasingly difficult to face and you are encouraged to engage with early enemies later in the game after you have mastered fighting them (e.g., competence). There is a system to directly combat other players via invading their game or joining with fellow players to overcome challenges together (e.g., connectedness). The world building and backstory of the game is complex and well-conceived, and the controls translate player agency into avatar action fluidly (e.g., immersion). There is little wonder why games are so massively popular, given how many ways they can incorporate self-determination theory motivations.

Not all motivations are equally useful for all participants, however. Everyone who experiences your simulation/game will engage with extrinsic and intrinsic motivations differently. Some learners may be encouraged by competing with their fellows, while others will disengage completely. Some participants may become immersed in your designed experience, while others will never quite be able to suspend

TABLE 10-1. MOTIVATION TYPES AND EXAMPLES

Type	Name	Example	Extent
Extrinsic	Reward	Traditional grade systems, scoring systems used for feedback, food provided upon completion	Short-term
	Punishment	Requiring extra homework due to poor performance, open verbal reprimand, failing a class	
Intrinsic	Autonomy	Open-ended activities allowing the learners to dictate the actions in a simulation, task trainers that a student can access when they want to	Long-term
	Competence	Performing a simulation multiple times with a focus on improving performance; targeted, positive feedback highlighting learner performance; increasing the challenge of activities over time and iteration	
	Relatedness	Allowing the learners to compare metrics of their performance to breed competition, roundtable-style discussions where learners are encouraged to critique each other's performance, cooperative group scenarios	
	Immersion	Educators playing characters appropriate for the scenario, providing a website and a means to interact with a scenario outside of simulation hours, establishing a scene by engaging learner's senses	

disbelief. This means that, if you plan to incorporate concepts of self-determination theory into your simulations, you should make sure to either provide a wide range of motivations or cater your simulations to your learners' preferred motivations. The choice between these two approaches is ultimately up to the simulation educator, but will likely vary based on how familiar you are with the students' personalities and preferences. The more you understand your learner, the better you can design the experience to engage. See Table 10-1 for more information.

Educational simulations are not inherently built to be games, but simulation specialists can learn much from the way games engage their players. The rest of this chapter will be discussing the two ways in which game design concepts can be incorporated into simulation education, the kinds of motivations that can be leveraged by these strategies, as well as tips for designing your own game simulations.

GAMIFICATION

Gamification is the act of applying elements of games to non-game experiences (Deterding et al., 2011). The concept of gamification may have started earlier, but 2008 was when it started to become prevalent in software development and adjacent tech fields (Walz & Deterding, 2015). Since then, gamification has been applied to many fields, including education and simulation.

Some common elements taken from games are scoring systems, leaderboards, and achievements. Scoring systems are seen in a variety of places, from task trainer simulation programs to modifications of traditional grading schemes. Some success has been found in converting traditional grading structures into "experience point" systems and "leveling structures," which are elaborations of the scoring concept (Sheldon, 2020). The benefit to scoring systems is that it is a form of feedback that the learner can receive relatively quickly and can improve over time, but the downsides include a lack of specificity in the feedback and some confusion as to how certain scores are generated. Leaderboards tend to be related to scoring systems in that many scoring systems can be converted into leaderboards, but also quantifiable statistics like time to finish simulation or number of simulations completed would also make reasonable leaderboards. The primary theory of using leaderboards is to take an explicit motivation like scoring and add in a social competition element to drive more intrinsic motivation. However, this has found mixed success, since some participants were actually discouraged from participating and competing once their score fell too low (Mekler et al., 2013). Also, there is some concern as to the ethical ramifications of including potentially embarrassing metrics in a form that all participants can see.

Achievement systems, also known as "badging" systems or "microcredentials," are a way to reward certain milestones of learning. In many video games, achievements unlock for your account under three broadly defined scenarios. From least difficult to design to most difficult to design, they are: milestone progress for the main activity, extra recognition for performing a nonvital activity, or performing an action that shows a deeper understanding of the activity/scenario. As a quick example of these three achievement types, consider the application to a standardized patient scenario where the learner is speaking to a patient who is coming down with a novel respiratory infection. Milestone progress would be motivational interviewing to assess the patient's infection risk, nonvital activity might be checking if the patient has asthma or some other kind of chronic illness that would make the situation worse, deeper understanding would be to consider the patient's partner's risk of infection and look into contact tracing for other possible infected people. These could all be anticipated and awarded to a learner during the debriefing in the form of achievements.

This is not an exhaustive list of elements of games that could be applied to nongame activities, but it should provide a reasonable starting point and serve as a useful explanation of gamification. The important thing to remember is that gamification is the addition of game elements to an activity that is otherwise not considered to be a game in an effort to enhance engagement in the participant through extrinsic and/or intrinsic motivations.

Strategies for Implementing Gamification

Gamification has been considered a relatively simple way to add value to existing simulations. However, to get the most benefit out of gamification strategies, you must be very deliberate in what kind of elements you employ and in what way. It should be mostly used to enhance intrinsic motivations, since often extrinsically motivating factors are already present (e.g., rewards for completion of the simulation task or avoidance of reprisal for not performing the task) and do little to meaningfully increase learner engagement.

If possible, a great starting point is to survey your learners so that you can better target the innate motivations they respond to. If you end up with many students who are motivated from competing with each other, consider leaning more into elements that encourage ways for the participants to compare themselves. If learners are more interested in immersive elements, you should consider small ways to make your scenarios come alive by engaging more senses. Nearly all students tend to respond well to elements related to autonomy and competence, so be mindful of ways you can enhance these areas.

Here are some more targeted strategies and examples to help get you thinking about how to gamify your simulations:

- *Autonomy:* Simulations that allow learners to solve problems organically allow greater autonomy than simulations that are more procedural. Even if the simulation objective is related to following an established procedure (i.e., CPR training or Code Blue simulations), the designer can make it so that the nature of the simulation is not obvious and allows the participants to figure out the best way to help the patient. Also consider that when and where to deploy a simulation can enhance autonomy. Allowing students the choice of scenario or even the schedule of when the learning will occur can help them feel more personally involved with their learning and enhance autonomy. The main takeaway is that the more open the simulation is (or appears to be), the more learners can solve on their own and the greater the level of autonomy you will incorporate.

- *Competence:* Most simulation learning already touches on competence as an inherent part of the process of learning. After all, the main objective of learning in any form is to enhance the learner's competence in the task. However, there are still ways that a simulation designer can deliberately enhance the feeling of competence. Providing some means of incremental feedback throughout an experience can help with this, such as through a scoring system. Points and scores awarded throughout a scenario become a kind of microfeedback, reinforcing good behavior while also giving the student a numerical value that demonstrates their increasing competence. Usually, the bulk of feedback is reserved for debriefing, and this can also generate a great feeling of competence at the conclusion of the simulation. Another great opportunity for instilling competence is through repetition of scenarios. Learners who encounter similar scenarios get better at engaging with those scenarios in a way that is obvious and internalized, enhancing their feelings of competence with each new case. This allows the educator to scaffold the student through more challenging variants of similar scenarios, with the student witnessing their own growth organically.
- *Relatedness/Competition:* Competition tends to be more divisive than the other motivations on this list. Some people respond well and thrive under a competitive atmosphere, while others find the comparisons of work to be stressful or demotivating. To really leverage this motivation, you as the designer must know your participants and get a feel for how they might respond to this. A simple way to introduce competition has been mentioned previously: leaderboards. Publicly displaying metrics related to your participants' performance can lead some learners to strive to be at the top of that list. Another reasonable way to have participants compete would be to have multiple learning groups go through the simulation simultaneously. Some groups will inevitably try to perform better than their fellows to impress the instructors. Another way that you might include competition while not alienating some participants is creating a fictional third party for the learners to compete against in the scenario. This could be a standardized colleague-actor that the participants are supposed to argue with on the best way to proceed, or even including fictional participants into the leaderboard structure. That way participants can strive to overcome a conflicting party without the social dynamic of it being a real person they interact with outside of the scenario.
- *Relatedness/Cooperation:* Cooperation tends to be a more universal motivation than competition and many educational simulations involve teams of learners working together to achieve their goals. There can be problems with group cohesion and intergroup conflict, and a simulation educator should be on the lookout for individuals who are feeling forced out of the group dynamic. Efforts should be made to introduce group mates to each other if they are unfamiliar, and a reasonable way to do this is through simple icebreaker games before the simulation starts. This kind of short cooperative activity can help group cohesion during the simulation. Even having the learners name their groups can help with cooperation and provides the educator with an easy shorthand when referring to them. Additionally, consider how cooperation and competition can be connected through having groups of learners working together against other groups of learners. This has the added benefit of group social dynamics motivating high-functional group members to assist low-functional group members in order to uplift the team as a whole. It also shields the egos of participants from the shame of poor performance, reducing the potential of individuals becoming demotivated from the competition.
- *Immersion:* There are countless ways to enhance the immersion of a simulation, and the methods always should focus on engaging the learner's senses. Highly advanced simulations using virtual reality equipment are highly immersive, cognitively transporting the learner into the simulation space. However, virtual reality simulations are extremely expensive to produce and fundamentally tend to be solitary experiences, which may conflict with your objectives. Much simpler ways of enhancing immersion might involve playing a background loop of sounds to match the environment the simulation is supposed to be taking place in (such as ambient noises recorded from an ICU, the realistic beeping of a machine, or outdoor sounds if the scenario takes place outside). Also consider the use of scents in simulation. Smells tend to be closely tied to memory and can be a very subtle way to increase immersion. Burning a scented candle that smells like pine for a scenario in the woods or wiping down the simulated ICU with the same cleaner used in the functional ICUs can go a long way towards helping the learners suspend their disbelief.

Gameful Design

Whereas gamification is the consideration of including game-like elements to already existing educational simulations, gameful design is the process of designing the simulation to be a game from the beginning. This allows the educator to incorporate intrinsic, gameful motivations more holistically and pervasively. The cornerstone of this design philosophy is that simulations already contain all the core qualities of games and it just takes a different perspective to design. The core elements of what makes a game to be a game can be summed up by the following four concepts: goals, rules, feedback systems, and voluntary participation (McGonigal, 2011). The goal of a game can be somewhat like the objectives set forth in the creation of a simulation, but it's more than just what you want the learner to get out of the experience—it is also where you what them to end up in the scenario. The rules of a game create the boundary of the experience, dictating what is allowable and what is not. In simulation education, some rules could be how the manikin functions, what kinds of procedures you can perform given the room and equipment that is part of the scenario, or even the ability to "time out" and ask some questions. Some rules are explicit, while others are attended to during the set-up of the simulation. Feedback is a critical component of both games and simulations, but games tend to give more regular and varied feedback than the average simulation. Traditional simulations hold back the bulk of feedback until the debriefing, but that doesn't have to be the case. Finally, voluntary participation really relates to the invitation to the participants to suspend disbelief and agree to play by the rules to reach the goal while using the feedback. In games, this is called the "magic circle" and represents the artificial space that the game takes up, allowing players to experience something outside their normal world (Fairfield, 2008).

After establishing that simulations contain all the elements of a game, a designer can consider the process along different lines entirely: that of creating a game. All of the comments above about gamification can be relevant when designing gameful simulations: all the same motivations are coming into play and many of the suggestions can be incorporated into the design. A major difference is that the motivational elements can be included in the baseline creation of the simulation rather than being added in later. For example, instead of having points earned by the students being abstract and disconnected, perhaps they now earn money that is accrued to their group's "account" that can be utilized in future simulations to buy hints or gain access to equipment that is unnecessary but more efficient. This way the students still see a gain in a metric that is a direct result of their actions (e.g., competence), can spend that metric at their own discretion (e.g., autonomy), and can feel more connected to the greater narrative connecting the simulation experiences (e.g., immersion). It also could allow for groups to collaborate in new ways, lending fake money to each other to all manage the simulations ahead of them.

Furthermore, one very important design philosophy of games can be leaned on in educational simulations: learning from failure. If the designer can distance the penalties for failure from the learners, or abstract them in some way, the learners may feel more comfortable experimenting and less stress around failing. This is especially true if the simulations are part of a series wherein the learners can approach similar tasks repetitively until achieving success. In many simulations, the learners are prevented from failing, either from a facilitator stepping in to correct something or the design of the scenario itself preventing it. When a designer realizes that they can pull those safety nets back a little, they find that there is much more space to design in and for participants to learn from. Failure shouldn't be trivial, but it should be penalizing either. One way that has achieved this in some gameful simulations is through the creation of a scenario-specific metric (e.g., arbitrary score, fake money, percent out of 100 representing public approval) that can be penalized that does not impact the learner's grade or educational well-being. The student will feel the sting of the loss in that metric, but will not be penalized outside the scenario, allowing them to be more circumspect and reapproach the experience with drive and fervor.

Strategies of Designing Gameful Simulations

Since this book is not a primer on how to design games, a list of books related to game design is included at the end of this chapter. A simulation educator can learn a surprising amount from the work of entertainment and educational game designers.

However, some concepts can be covered here to get you thinking gamefully about designing simulation education:

- Consider the space around the use of the simulations you already have. Is there some way you can link the experiences naturally? Is there a metaphor or story that can wrap and shape the experience? For instance, if you perform several simulated patient cases as part of a classroom setting, you could frame the experience as a fake hospital with student groups serving in different wings of said hospital. The cases could be tweaked to allow longitudinal care, with patients coming back for follow-ups. Those follow-ups could be tweaked to react to the recommendations that individual groups enacted in previous visits. The feedback from individual cases could be presented as postvisit surveys that reflect the recommendations, but also reflect bedside manner or whatever other elements you wish to assess them on.
- Consider metrics you can gather or calculate that are part of the game-space created from your metaphor. These metrics and scores have more meaning than simple point values, can be controlled by the learners, and are removed from potential grade point assessments. To continue the previous example, you could use the postvisit survey assessments to determine star ratings for the different teams, with breakdowns of the specific components that make up that rank. The star ratings could be used to drive conversations about the learner's performance, change the attitude of future simulated patients, and could allow changes to nonessential resources during the simulations as an abstraction of financial incentives usually tied to star ratings in hospitals.
- Consider ways to increase the immersion of the story you create. Something as simple as making separate email accounts for fictional characters the learners interact with can go a long way towards the suspension of disbelief. You could also make an email account or use an online texting service to have ways for the simulated patients to contact the learners prior to or following a visit. This could allow opportunities for microlessons about telephonic communication, managing medical errors, or responding to contact over new symptoms.

An important thing to keep in mind is to be very clear to your learners when you are acting "in character" and when you are the instructor. Given more complex scenarios, students can become confused with the information they receive and become frustrated. Be sure to check in with your learners frequently and be considerate of their concerns. Designing a game is an iterative process and gameful simulations should be no exception.

References

Anderton, K. (2019). Research report shows how much time we spend gaming. *Forbes,* March 21.

Deci, E. L., & Ryan, R. (1985). *Intrinsic motivation and self-determination in human behavior.* Plenum.

Deterding, S., Dixon, D., Khaled, R., & Nacke, L. (2011). From game design elements to gamefulness: defining" gamification". Paper presented at the Proceedings of the 15th international academic MindTrek conference: Envisioning future media environments.

Fairfield, J. A. (2008). The magic circle. *Vanderbilt Journal of Entertainment and Technology, 11,* 823.

McGonigal, J. (2011). *Reality is broken: Why games make us better and how they can change the world.* Penguin.

Mekler, E. D., Brühlmann, F., Opwis, K., & Tuch, A. N. (2013). *Do points, levels and leaderboards harm intrinsic motivation? An empirical analysis of common gamification elements.* Paper presented at the Proceedings of the First International Conference on Gameful Design, Research, and Applications.

Ryan, R. M., Rigby, C. S., & Przybylski, A. (2006). The motivational pull of video games: A self-determination theory approach. *Motivation and Emotion, 30*(4), 344-360.

Sheldon, L. (2020). *The multiplayer classroom: Designing coursework as a game.* CRC Press.

Tondello, G. F., Mora, A., & Nacke, L. E. (2017). *Elements of gameful design emerging from user preferences.* Paper presented at the Proceedings of the Annual Symposium on Computer-Human Interaction in Play.

Walz, S. P., & Deterding, S. (2015). *The gameful world: Approaches, issues, applications.* MIT Press.

Wijman, T. (2020). The world's 2.7 billion gamers will spend $159.3 billion on games in 2020; The market will surpass $200 billion by 2023. *New Zoo.* Retrieved from https://newzoo.com/insights/articles/newzoo-games-market-numbers-revenues-and-audience-2020-2023/

Suggested Readings

Carnes, M. C., & Carnes, M. C. (2014). *Minds on fire: How role-immersion games transform college.* Harvard University Press.

Culyba, S. (2018). *The Transformational Framework: A process tool for the development of transformational games.* Carnegie Mellon University.

Fullerton, T. (2014). *Game design workshop: A playcentric approach to creating innovative games.* CRC press.

Juul, J. (2013). *The art of failure: An essay on the pain of playing video games.* MIT press.

McGonigal, J. (2011). *Reality is broken: Why games make us better and how they can change the world.* Penguin.

Schell, J. (2008). *The Art of Game Design: A book of lenses.* CRC press.

Weston, A. (2018). *Teaching as the art of staging: A scenario-based college pedagogy in action.* Stylus Publishing, LLC.

11

Simulation Design and the Impact on Student Stress

Jennifer A. Merz, OTD, OTR/L
Pari Kumar, OTD, OTR/L
Audrey L. Zapletal, OTD, OTR/L, CLA

Learning Objectives

1. Discuss how the design of the simulation experience can impact the student experience.
2. Describe how students perceive the simulation encounter before and after the experience (e.g., physiological, positives, and negatives).
3. Formulate strategies that enhance workflow and decrease student stress during the simulation encounter.

Kern's Model of Program Development

The content in this chapter articulates Step 4 of Kern's Model: Educational Strategies. Information in this chapter addresses how to develop simulations with an emphasis on student preparation. This method contributes to accomplishing established educational objectives.

Zapletal, A. L., Baird, J. M., Van Oss, T., Hoppe, M. M., Prast, J. E., & Herge, E. A. *Clinical Simulation for Health Care Professionals* (pp. 109-115).

Stress, Learning, and Simulation

Evidence has shown that learners across health professions engaged in high-fidelity simulations feel stressed and have increased anxiety (Beischel, 2013; Gibbs et al., 2017; Nielsen & Harder, 2013; Ohtake et al., 2013; Yockey & Henry, 2019). Simulationists and team members should be aware of how stress behaviors impact learning as well as the learner's physiological state.

Learners naturally perceive any simulation encounter as a stressful event. Some learners are excited about the experience, while others tremble at the thought of interacting with a patient. It's important that you, as the simulation coordinator/simulationist, are aware of the range of emotions that learners could experience before, during, and after the event. Most adult learners will use this learning experience as an opportunity to assess their current knowledge and skill; while others fear that the patient could be too challenging or they do not have the self-confidence to complete particular skills, such as helping a patient move from one surface to another. A few learners may freeze when they knock on the door (indicating the beginning of the simulation). Other learners will have difficulty suspending reality and discussing the event as "fake" and not helpful.

Faculty and staff need to be available during the simulation to support students. Having faculty/staff stationed in the halls and watching simulations in a video room allows faculty/staff to respond quickly to an unplanned situation with a learner (or standardized patient [SP] or manikin, which can make a learner anxious). In most cases, once the learner enters the room, introduces themselves, and begins the encounter—the perceived stress begins to dissipate. The learner's endorphins and enkephalins increase and cortisol, the stress hormone, decreases (Bong et al., 2010; Judd et al., 2016). Even if the learner's experience is not ideal, they are able to function within the room as the therapist because they are forced to meet the demands of the situation or, if built into the encounter, they can ask their peers for help. Because simulation experiences require quick problem solving, demand a high cognitive load, and operate in a complex multi-dimensional environment (e.g., the SP, equipment, supplies, lighting, cues from the environment), these elements enhance the learner's coping skills. Even when learners think they have performed poorly, the learner (and anyone observing) can find some strengths to the performance (i.e., no one got hurt during a poorly performed transfer). Simulation encounters provide everyone the opportunity to assess their strengths and determine their areas of growth.

When designing the simulation, it's important to think about elements that can induce more stress than intended. Elements to consider include:

- Is the simulation experience graded (the actual performance)?
- Do the learners know prior to the experience of their role in a specific case (if multiple cases are part of the preparation; Yockey & Henry, 2019)?
- Are there any observers in the room: peers, faculty, etc.? And everyone understands how their role supports the learner (Harder et al., 2013)?
- Have learners practiced technical skills with enough instructor guidance and feedback to perform independently in a safe learning environment?
- Is there a plan to remediate students in private (Yockey & Henry, 2019)?
- How will learners access their personal videos, and can this be done in private (Cato, 2013)?
- How has faculty been trained to facilitate a safe debriefing learning experience where learners can express their challenges (INACSL, 2016)?

Simulation encounters provide faculty with insight into how learners may perform in the clinical setting. Learning is a process; students benefit from deliberate practice coupled with simulation or real-life supervised experience. The clinical fieldwork/internship provides an additional opportunity to further develop their skills. Simulation experiences embedded into the entry level curriculum are not the only solution to train learners to be entry level clinicians prior to their clinical internships (i.e., Level II fieldwork, clinical rotations). Simulation experiences are a learning modality that enhances the training cycle and, for example, cannot prepare a learner to operate independently in the intensive care unit during the first week of a clinical internship.

How Simulation Design Impacts the Student Experience

Simulation design impacts the learner's perceived stress level. In the sections following, the learner's physiological state during the learning experience is shared. The sections also describe the benefits and unfavorable aspects of simulation, according to the existing literature.

Physiological Responses During Simulation, Clinical, and Other Learning Experiences

Physiological responses, such as elevation in heart rate and cortisol levels, are expected to occur during both simulation experiences and clinical training (Judd et al., 2016). Increasing the number of peers observing a learner during a simulation experience can also increase anxiety and heart rate secondary to social evaluation anxiety (Mills et al., 2016). This phenomenon, however, occurs only in the first minute of the simulation experience; it then reduces to levels comparable to having no peers observing (Mills et al., 2016). The experience of stress is most common when the ability to respond to a situation is underdeveloped and experience is novel, intense, or unpredictable (McGraw et al., 2013). Because learners have often not mastered the skills that are being targeted during a simulation experience, they are expected to experience some level of stress. Mills et al. (2016) states it is also normal for learners to experience anticipation anxiety prior to a simulation experience. Evain et al. (2017) found that having a high quality debriefing after a simulation experience can reduce residual anxiety; however, this is not as common among individuals with higher trait anxiety who may require additional attention during debriefing (refer to Chapter 15 for information about debriefing).

Benefits of Stress Incorporated Simulation

Although simulations are often viewed by students as stressful events, this stress can allow learners to develop coping skills for high-stress clinical situations (Selye, 1985). A study by DeMaria et al. (2010) found that students who experienced a simulation with the addition of a stressful event retained knowledge at a higher level and were better able to apply the practical skills learned. Additionally, this heightened anxiety correlated with increased performance 6 months following the study intervention (DeMaria et al., 2010). It is hypothesized that this increase in performance and skill retention following anxiety provoking events occurs via activation of the amygdala (Cahill et al., 1996; Sandi & Pinelo-Nava, 2007).

Viewing video recordings has been determined to be a valuable component of learning, with 86% of students rating that it was useful in improving their abilities to respond to clinical emergencies (Gordon & Buckley, 2009). Giles and colleagues (2014) also incorporated video analysis of self-performance to help students determine areas of strength and growth. This post-performance video analysis and reflection allows the learner an opportunity to self-debrief and analyze the successes and challenges experienced in the event and develop a personalized learning plan. This type of planning provides the learner an opportunity to be proactive and control their educational experience.

Challenges of Simulation

When compared to clinical training, a simulation experience may be perceived as more psychologically stressful despite exhibiting a similar physiological response (Judd et al., 2016). Paskins & Peile (2010) found that learners reflected on past simulation experiences with strong words such as "terror," "humiliation," and "panic." Biernacki and Dziuda (2012) also suggested that learners mimicked symptoms of posttraumatic stress disorder following a simulation experience that they labeled as "simulator sickness." Fear of making mistakes may cause a student to lose focus, reducing their effectiveness and overall sense of direction with a patient (White, 2003). Mills et al. (2016) suggests that stress could be caused by fear of being reprimanded or embarrassing oneself in front of peers and professors, ultimately causing inhibitory stress as opposed to motivational stress. This could also occur when receiving feedback from an SP or faculty member in front of peers after the simulation experience (INACSL, 2016, 2020; Turner & Harder, 2018; Yockey & Henry, 2019).

Adding distractions within a simulation experience can take away from what is supposed to be the core focus and make it more stressful for a learner (DeMaria et al., 2010; LeBlanc, 2009). For example, Nielsen and Harder (2013) found that learners experienced greater anxiety when observed or video recorded during a simulation experience. In addition, unfamiliar surroundings in a simulation room may cause stress, unnatural speech and behavior, and poor skill learning (Li et al., 2015). By creating more potential for stress, a learner's cortisol levels may continue to increase, which has been associated with impaired clinical reasoning (Bong et al., 2010; Judd et al., 2016; Yockey & Henry, 2019).

Strategies to Mitigate Stress of Simulation

Creating a psychologically safe environment for students to perform is critical. The more information students know about the structure and expectations of the encounter, the more likely they will be successful. Table 11-1 provides strategies for the faculty/simulation team to consider when designing the encounter.

Avoiding Pitfalls and Strategies to Decrease Stress During Simulation

- Prior to a simulation experience, learners should get sufficient sleep, eat well, and anticipate a good grade (Beischel, 2013).
- Residual anxiety, anxiety that remains following the debriefing process for a simulation, can be reduced by providing high quality debriefing sessions (Evain et al., 2017; INACSL, 2016, 2020).
- Reducing the number of peers watching in the room can decrease the anxiety experienced by a student (Mills et al., 2016; Yockey & Henry, 2019).
- Create simulation environments that are as realistic as possible in order to create an environment that is high fidelity and feels "real" to the learner (DeMaria et al., 2010).
- Promote students' familiarity with the simulation environment and objects that may be encountered in order to increase comfort with simulation-related tasks (Li et al., 2016).
- Providing students with the tools to practice and prepare for simulations at their own pace can help ease anxiety (Blazeck & Zewe, 2013). Learning bundles contain materials, such as videos and the necessary items needed to complete the tasks, that allow students to practice the necessary skills ahead of time and in a self-paced manner (Blazeck & Zewe, 2013).
- Introducing video recording early in the curriculum can make the process of video recording feel less daunting (Henneman & Cunningham, 2005).
- Confidentiality agreements should accompany video recordings, with disclosing methods that the video may be used, if applicable (Arafeh et al., 2010; Cato, 2013).
- Anticipating unexpected events during a simulation may increase the experience of anxiety; learners should be encouraged to work with what is in front of them at the moment (Lasater, 2007).
- Consider progressing from low to high-fidelity simulations to improve practice performance (Mills et al., 2016).

Table 11-1. Methods to Promote Learning Through Psychological Safety

Learners are explicitly made aware of (through written materials, discussions, electronic resources, demonstrations, and explanations):	
Expectations	• Set clear course objectives • Describe simulation goals • Discuss anticipated learning outcomes • Emphasize professional behaviors • Review confidentiality agreement • Outline the assessment method and/or instrument of student performance • Describe how simulation performance will influence progress in program/course (high stakes?) • Discuss the value of their perspective
"Fiction Contract"	• Review the importance of engaging like it is a real experience • Understand the role of the instructor is to create an engaging environment and promote learning • Emphasize limitations of the type of simulation used (manikin, task trainer, SP, etc.)
Details of Simulation	• Describe the properties of equipment • Review the length of the simulation experience • Discuss if/when break times are scheduled • Share pre- and postsimulation activities • Inform whether there will be observers • Disclose if simulation will be recorded or reviewed at a later time • Discuss the use of electronic devices during the simulation experience

Adapted from Rudolph et al., 2014.

- Consider implementing stress training programming to teach stress management techniques and applications prior to simulation. Individuals who underwent the training felt the skills learned were valuable and could be utilized during real situations (Goldberg et al., 2017).
- In order to reduce anxiety, ensure that learners are aware that no one can be harmed during a simulation (Lasater, 2007; Rhodes & Curran, 2005).
- Encouraging group planning sessions can decrease anxiety. When practicing in a group, unexpected situations or commentary will be present and the learner will be used to these experiences. Therefore, the learner feels a decreased sense of being "put on the spot" during the actual simulation (Elfrink et al., 2009).
- All faculty, lab instructors, simulation staff, etc. should be familiar with safety policies and procedures, including access to first aid and mental health counselors, at the home institution, and the location of the simulation encounter (if different from home institution).

Conclusion

Simulation experiences can be stressful since learners are held accountable for their actions; faculty/simulationists are responsible for systematically creating an simulation encounter that attempts to reduce stress and help the learner focus on their training. Not all stress can be alleviated; a good design will have proactive measures to mitigate the effects.

References

Arafeh, J. M., Hansen, S. S., & Nichols, A. (2010). Debriefing in simulation-based learning: Facilitating a reflective discussion. *The Journal of Perinatal and & Neonatal Nursing, 24*(4), 302-309. https://doi.org/10.1097/JPN.0b013e3181f6b5ec

Beischel, K. P. (2013). Variables affecting learning in a simulation experience: A mixed methods study. *Western Journal of Nursing Research, 35*(2), 226–247. https://doi.org/10.1177/0193945911408444

Biernacki, M., & Dziuda, L. (2012). Simulator sickness as a valid issue of simulator-based research. *Medycyna Pracy, 63*(3), 377-388. Retrieved from https://www.ncbi.nlm.nih.gov/pubmed/22880458

Blazeck, A., & Zewe, G. (2013). Simulating simulation: Promoting perfect practice with learning bundle-supported videos in an applied, learner-driven curriculum design. *Clinical Simulation in Nursing, 9*(1), 21-24. https://doi.org/10.1016/j.ecns.2011.07.002

Bong, C., Lightdale, J., Fredette, M., & Weinstock, P. (2010). Effects of simulation versus traditional tutorial-based training on physiologic stress levels among clinicians: A pilot study simulation in healthcare. *Simulation in Healthcare, 5*(5), 272-278. https://doi.org/10.1097/SIH.0b013e3181e98b29

Cahill, L., Haier, R. J., Fallon, J., Alkire, M. T., Tang, C., Keator, D., Wu, J., Mcgaugh, J. L. (1996). Amygdala activity at encoding correlated with long-term, free recall of emotional information. *Proceedings of the National Academy of Sciences, 93*(15), 8016-8021. https://doi.org/10.1073/pnas.93.15.8016

Cato, M. L. (2013). *Nursing student anxiety in simulation settings: A mixed methods study.* Retrieved from https://pdxscholar.library.pdx.edu/cgi/viewcontent.cgi?article=2034&context=open_access_etds

DeMaria, S., Bryson, E. O., Mooney, T. J., Silverstein, J. H., Reich, D. L., Bodian, C., & Levine, A. I. (2010). Adding emotional stressors to training in simulated cardiopulmonary arrest enhances participant performance. *Medical Education, 44,* 1006-1015. https://doi.org/10.1111/j.1365-2923.2010.03775.x

Elfrink, V. L., Nininger, J., Rohig, L., & Lee, J. (2009). The case for group planning in human patient simulation. *Nursing Education Perspectives, 30*(2), 83-86. Retrieved from https://www.ncbi.nlm.nih.gov/pubmed/19476070

Evain, J., Zoric, L., Mattatia, L., Picard, O., Ripart, J., & Cuvillon, P. (2017). Residual anxiety after high fidelity simulation in anaesthesiology: An observational, prospective, pilot study. *Anaesthesia Critical Care & Pain Medicine, 36*(4), 205-212. https://doi.org/10.1016/j.accpm.2016.09.008

Gibbs, D. M. & Dietrich, M. (2017). Using high fidelity simulation to impact occupational therapy student knowledge, comfort, and confidence in acute care. *The Open Journal of Occupational Therapy, 5*(1), 10. https://doi.org/10.15453/2168-6408.1225

Giles, A. K., Carson, N. E., Breland, H. L., Coker-Bolt, P., & Bowman, P. (2014). Use of simulated patients and reflective video analysis to assess occupational therapy students' preparedness for fieldwork. *American Journal of Occupational Therapy, 68,* 57-66. https://doi.org/10.5014/ajot.2014.685S03

Goldberg, M. B., Mazzei, M., Maher, Z., Fish, J. H., Milner, R., Yu, D., & Goldberg, A. J. (2017). Optimizing performance through stress training: An educational strategy for surgical residents. *American Journal of Surgery, 10*(17). https://doi.org/10.1016/j.amjsurg.2017.11.040

Gordon, C. J., & Buckley, T. (2009). The effect of high-fidelity simulation training on medical-surgical graduate nurses' perceived ability to respond to patient clinical emergencies. *Journal of Continuing Education in Nursing, 40*(11), 499-500. https://doi.org/10.3928/00220124-20091023-06

Harder, N., Ross, C. J. M., & Paul, P. (2013). Student perspective of roles assignment in high-fidelity simulation: An ethnographic study. *Clinical Simulation in Nursing, 9*(9), e329-e334. https://doi.org/10.1016/j.ecns.2012.09.003

Henneman, E. A., & Cunningham, H. (2005). Using clinical simulation to teach patient safety in an acute/critical care nursing course. *Nurse Educator, 30*(4), 172-177. https://doi.org/10.1097/00006223-200507000-00010

INACSL Standards Committee, Decker, S., Alinier, G., Crawford, S. B., Gordon, R. M., Jenkins, D., & Wilson, C. (2021). Healthcare simulation standards of best practice: The debriefing process. *Clinical Simulation in Nursing, 58*(27-32). https://doi.org/10.1016/j.ecns.2021.08.011

Judd, B., Alison, J., Waters, D., & Gordon, C. (2016). Comparison of psychophysiological stress in physiotherapy students undertaking simulation and hospital-based clinical education. *Simulation in Healthcare, 11*(4), 271–277. https://doi.org/10.1097/SIH.0000000000000155

Lasater, K. (2007). High-fidelity simulation and the development of clinical judgment: Students' experiences. *The Journal of Nursing Education, 46*(6), 269-276. https://doi.org/10.3928/01484834-20070601-06

LeBlanc, V. R. (2009). The effects of acute stress on performance: Implications for health professions education. *Academic Medicine: Journal of the Association of American Medical Colleges, 84*(10), 25-33. https://doi.org/10.1097/ACM.0b013e3181b37b8f

Li, H., Jin, D., Qiao, F., Chen, J., & Gong, J. (2015). Relationship between the Self-Rating Anxiety Scale score and the success rate of 64-slice computed tomography coronary angiography. *The International Journal of Psychiatry in Medicine, 51*(1), 47-55. https://doi.org/10.1177/0091217415621265

McGraw, L. K., Out, D., Hammermeister, J. J., Ohlson, C. J., Pickering, M. A., & Granger, D. A. (2013). Nature, correlates, and consequences of stress-related biological reactivity and regulation in Army nurses during combat casualty simulation. *Psychoneuroendocrinology, 38*(1), 135-144. https://doi.org/10.1016/j.psyneuen.2012.05.009

Mills, B., Carter, O., Rudd, C., Claxton, L., & O'Brien, R. (2016). An experimental investigation into the extent social evaluation anxiety impairs performance in simulation-based learning environments amongst final-year undergraduate nursing students. *Nurse Education Today, 45,* 9-15. https://doi.org/10.1016/j.nedt.2016.06.006

Nielsen, B., & Harder, N. (2013). Causes of student anxiety during simulation: What the literature says. *Clinical Simulation in Nursing, 9*(11), e507-e512. https://doi.org/10.1016/j.ecns.2013.03.003

Ohtake, P. J., Lazarus, M., Schillo, R., & Rosen, M. (2013). Simulation experience enhances physical therapist student confidence in managing a patient in the critical care environment. *Critical Illness Special Series, 93*(2), 216-228. https://doi.org/10.2522/ptj.20110463

Paskins, Z., & Peile, E. (2010). Final year medical students' views on simulation-based teaching: A comparison with the Best Evidence Medical Education Systematic Review. *Medical Teacher, 32*(7), 569-577. https://doi.org/10.3109/01421590903544710

Rhodes, M. L., & Curran, C. (2005). Use of the human patient simulator to teach clinical judgment skills in a baccalaureate nursing program. *Computers, Informatics, Nursing: CIN, 23*(5), 256-262. https://doi.org/10.1097/00024665-200509000-00009

Rudolph, J. W., Raemer, D. B., & Simon, R. (2014). Establishing a safe container for learning in simulation: The role of the pre-simulation briefing. *Simulation in Healthcare, 9,* 339-349. https://doi.org/10.1097/SIH.0000000000000047

Sandi, C., & Pinelo-Nava, M. T. (2007). Stress and memory: Behavioral effects and neurobiological mechanisms. *Neural Plasticity, 78970.* https://doi.org/10.1155/2007/78970

Selye, H. (1985). *Stress without distress.* J. B. Lippincott.

Turner, S., & Harder, N. (2018). Psychological safe environment: A concept analysis. *Clinical Simulation in Nursing,18,* 47-55. https://doi.org/10.1016/j.ecns.2018.02.004

White, A. H. (2003). Clinical decision making among fourth-year nursing students: An interpretive study. *Journal of Nursing Education, 42*(3), 113-120. Retrieved from https://www.ncbi.nlm.nih.gov/pubmed/12661711

Yockey, J., & Henry, M. (2019). Simulation anxiety across the curriculum. *Clinical Simulation in Nursing, 29,* 29-37. https://doi.org/10.1016/j.ecns.2018.12.004

Kern's Model Step 5
Implementation

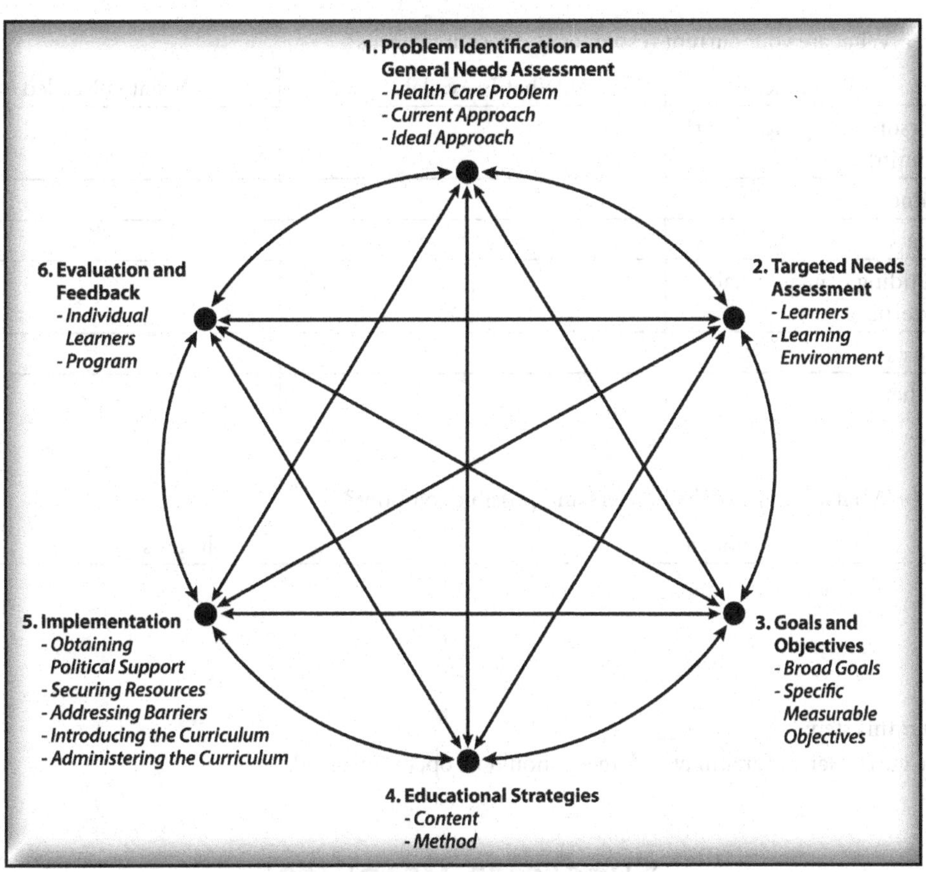

- The purpose of this step is to accomplish the plan by making the simulation a reality and turning it into an achievement.
- Ensure support for the curricular program: whose buy-in is needed before implementation?
- Identify and obtain resources (i.e., those existing, those needed in addition to).
- Consider various sources of support (e.g., funding, political, administrative).
- Anticipate, identify, and address any internal or external barriers that may impact implementation.
- Have a plan for introducing the curricular changes into the program, as well as for maintenance and enhancement.

- Consider how and when the curriculum will be administered, establishing a timeline for a pilot phase, a phase-in period, and then full implementation.

- Identify resources:
    - Determine resources, supports, and barriers for your simulation.
        → What are some possible sources of support?

Internal	External

→ What are your current resources and resource needs?

Resource	What Is Available	What Is Needed
Personnel (e.g., teaching/ admin)		
Time		
Space		
Funding (e.g., internal/ external)		
Costs		
Other		

→ What are some of the barriers and possible solutions?

Barriers	Solutions

After this step:

- The curricular/programmatic changes should be operationalized.

Suggested Readings

Farnan, J., & Schindler, N. (2013). *Curriculum development and evaluation guide resident as teacher: A mutually beneficial arrangement APPD/COMSEP pre course 2013.* Retrieved from: https://www.appd.org/meetings/2013SpringPresentations/PCWS1Handout.pdf

Kern, D. E. (2014). *Curriculum development: An essential educational skill, a public trust, a form of scholarship, an opportunity for organizational change.* Weill Cornell College of Medicine, Qatar. Retrieved from: https://dnnyqetna.blob.core.windows.net/portals/15/Six-Step%20Approach%20to%20Curriculum%20Development.pdf?sr=b&si=DNNFileManagerPolicy&sig=9sAOUX/lzfZQsN6QKLOpWJ46YLRuXmQwOghR7ptxnFw=

Khamis, N. N., Satava, R. M., Alnassar, S. A., & Kern, D. E. (2016). A stepwise model for simulation-based curriculum development for clinical skills, a modification of the six-step approach. *Surgical Endoscopy,* 279-287. https://doi.org/10.1007/s00464-015-4206x

12

Simulation on a Budget
Creative Solutions

Jean E. Prast, OTD, MSOT, OTRL, CHSE
Maureen M. Hoppe, EdD, MA, OTR/L, CPAM, CHSE

Learning Objectives

1. Identify resources necessary to successfully carry out a clinical simulation based on the scenario and desired outcomes.
2. Describe innovative strategies to facilitate learning with limited funding and resources to deliver an effective clinical simulation.
3. Formulate creative solutions in an effort to reach the desired learning outcomes that best support implementation of a high-fidelity clinical simulation.

Kern's Model of Program Development

The content in this chapter articulates Step 5 of Kern's Model: Implementation. Information in this chapter contributes to implementation of the simulation program by identifying innovative options to address limited budgets. This type of planning ensures funding support by addressing potential barriers proactively.

Zapletal, A. L., Baird, J. M., Van Oss, T., Hoppe, M. M., Prast, J. E., & Herge, E. A. *Clinical Simulation for Health Care Professionals* (pp. 119-127).

Simulation Use to Support Education

In health care professions, accreditation and practice standards are being revised to meet educational needs for learners as they prepare for clinical practice. Research shows that the use of simulation can prepare students for clinical practice, if done correctly. Although the methods and rigor vary, research focusing on the use of simulation in comparison to traditional classroom teaching in discrete knowledge and skill areas has demonstrated they are equal, and in some cases more beneficial, learning outcomes. In a national simulation study conducted by the National Council of State Boards of Nursing (2014), "substituting high-quality simulation experiences for up to half of traditional clinical hours produces comparable end-of-program educational outcomes and new graduates that are ready for clinical practice" (p. S3). There is also evidence that high-fidelity simulations are an effective teaching method to prepare learners for clinical practice and can be used in place of 50% of traditional clinical experiences for student education (Curl et al., 2016).

One challenge in health care education is finding an adequate number of clinical placements with skilled educators who have a sufficient amount of time allocated for student education (National Council of State Boards of Nursing, 2014). One specific example is in the field of occupational therapy. To assist with the shortage of clinical or fieldwork placements, simulation is an alternative option to provide students with an opportunity to apply learned skills in a safe and controlled environment (Accreditation Council for Occupational Therapy Education, 2018).

Balancing Resource Needs for Success

If a facility has simulation staff, it is recommended to connect with those who have extensive training and experience to help facilitate learning and implementation. It is important to note that often facilities do not have designated, skilled staff to support the design and implementation efforts necessitating developers to assume multiple roles in simulation. Using simulation as an educational tool or teaching method does have its challenges but it can be done. The most difficult thing is finding a balance, but how does one do it without taking on too much? First, consider identifying others who have a similar interest (e.g., colleagues, clinicians, students, other professions) or those who have experience using simulation as a teaching tool. Next, schedule a time to meet to set a timeline along with goals and assigned tasks. Be sure to set a realistic time frame and start out with something small, so losing momentum can be avoided. Some examples could include: 15-minute mock interviews, standardized cognitive screen (e.g., MOCA [Montreal Cognitive Assessment], SLUM [Saint Louis University Mental Status Examination], MMSE [Mini-Mental Status Examination]), or specific technical skills (e.g., client transfer, administration of meds, assessment of extremity, strength). These examples are just a few ideas to get a large group of learners through a simulation in a limited amount of time with few resources. Developing, implementing, and assessing a simulation can be time and labor intensive, but the experience provides valuable educational benefits to the learner (Giles et al., 2014; Ohtake et al., 2013).

Simulation Design and Implementation: Workforce Considerations

During the planning phase of a simulation, human resources need to be determined. This can be a challenging task, especially when working with a limited budget. The following are creative solutions to best support these needs:

- *Simulation Staff:* Does the facility have experts (trained simulation staff) available to support the simulation endeavors? If so, contact them for assistance with planning, equipment, and simulation technology. Keep in mind these experts may not be aware of the specific profession, curriculum, program, or learning objectives—so working together is essential for your success.
- *Service/Volunteer Work:* Is there anyone at the facility who is required to fulfill a certain amount of service to an organization? At some colleges and universities, faculty are required to partake in service projects. Some programs also require students to fulfill hours for community service. Capturing those in need of serving can help, regardless of budget needs.
- *Adjunct Faculty/Lab Staff/Alumni:* Does the facility allow contract work? If so, are there professionals from the clinic that can be hired via contract? This can help during the planning as well as the implementation phase.
- *Interprofessional Collaboration:* Are there established relationships with other faculty/staff outside the department/program? If so, is there a way to help and support each other? One suggestion would be to share resources and have an interprofessional education simulation. Another suggestion (which may be easier at the beginning) is to help each other with program specific simulations. For example, a physical therapy professional can fulfill the role of a standardized patient (SP) for respiratory therapy students during a simulation encounter, and vice versa.
- *Students/Graduate Assistants:* Are there varying levels of students at the institution or in the program? If so, consider requesting their services. Many times, senior or higher-level students want to give back to help peers prepare for clinical practice. Training students to role play or fulfill the role of an SP may be beneficial. Also, they can help with set-up or provide technology support throughout the simulation process as needed.
- *Partnerships:* Consider developing a partnership with other departments (outside of health care). Does the facility have a performing arts program? Are there programs in the area? If so, contact a faculty or staff member to discuss collaborative projects. A performing arts club, theater course, or drama club may have students or community members interested in assisting with the experience.
- *Continuing Education:* If payment is not an option, consider offering continuing education to professionals. Depending on the professional organization's requirements, this can be a valuable opportunity for professional development while educating future health care professionals. Professionals can bring much expertise to the experience, especially if they fulfill an SP role and help with debriefing of the simulation.
- *Community Agencies:* Partners from the community can add value to a simulation, especially if they have expertise working with the targeted population. Is there an organization that has an established relationship with the facility? A staff member from a shelter, school, support group, or resource agency may be interested in assisting with the experience (especially if their population would benefit from services in the future).
- *Personal Volunteers:* Are there colleagues who have family members or close friends who would like to donate their time to help with the simulation (e.g., training, implementation)? If so, get them into the facility and train them to get started.
- *Administration/Administrators:* Do not underestimate the value of having someone in an administrative position involved in the simulation. It's a great way to get them to support future simulation endeavors, as well as get to know what is being done for student learning in the professional programs.
- *Ongoing Support:* Consider building a team that will be committed to the simulation process from start to finish. Having members collaborate in the development, implementation, and outcome measurement phase may help with continuity and consistency for improved outcomes.
- *Continuity of Grading:* Once assessment tools are determined, the tool should be reviewed, so members of the simulation team are looking at the same thing (maybe even discuss the same rubric over lunch and provide a checklist of things to look for under each assessment area). This will help with inter-rater reliability and consistency.

Clinical Simulation Space Considerations

When planning and designing clinical simulations, it is important to consider space needs to best mirror desired practice locations for simulation scenarios. Table 12-1 provides an overview of questions to guide this process and facilitate creative thinking and solutions to address unique program needs.

Table 12-1. Clinical Simulation Space Considerations

Planning Questions to Consider	Response	Additional Comments/ Considerations
What type of space will you need to carry out desired simulation? • It is important to consider fidelity and realism to stage simulation (e.g., outpatient treatment room, hospital room)		
Do you have partnerships with any health care facilities or community organizations in your area? If yes: • What kind of space do they have available that may work for clinical simulation? • Is there an expert on simulation who can help mentor you with design and implementation? If no: • Can you identify a few facilities that you would like to contact? • Consider other local colleges/universities that may provide collaboration opportunities?	Yes or No	
Are there other health care programs at your facility? If yes: • Do they have similar desires or goals? • Is there an expert on simulation that can mentor you throughout the process? If no: • Can you identify other programs or professions that you would like to collaborate with? • Does your institution offer other health care professional programs that may be able to share space/resources?	Yes or No	

Creative Solutions for Simulation Use on a Budget

- *Fees:* Depending on the setting, the addition of fees may be considered. Some academic institutions can build in associated fees to student learning (e.g., lab fees, technology fees). Students can also purchase supply kits or required materials (e.g., stethoscope, gait belt, assessment tools) to partake in a simulation or threaded simulations throughout the program.
- *Grants:* Look at the availability of grants that could support the clinical simulation. Whether the simulation is conducted in an academic or clinical setting, there should be specific grants related to education (e.g., innovative teaching awards, research grants) at the facility, community, state, and/or national levels. An additional opinion could be contacting an academic institution to identify opportunities and resources that may be available (e.g., student research, collaborative awards).
- *Donations:* Identify the resources (e.g., equipment, tools) needed to implement the clinical simulation and make it known to others (i.e., market a donation drive or reach out to health care vendors). Designate a location to collect the desired resources and keep a list of those who donate time to gather and deliver these items (e.g., in-kind donations). Keep in mind that the more realistic the simulation the higher the fidelity, which can impact learning outcomes and ability for learners to transfer skills into the clinic. Keep a detailed record of those who donated and make sure to send a thank you note.
- *Consignment Shops:* Consider visiting local consignment shops to collect resources to support the simulation. Keep in mind that products are donated daily and depending on the items needed, the shops should be visited more than once (e.g., make-up for moulage after Halloween, winter attire after the season ends, spring and fall cleaning).
- *Technology:* Consider the use of technology, especially the tools used daily, as a resource to better support the simulation endeavor. There are various apps and creative ways to use technology (e.g., smartphones, laptops, camcorders). It really depends on the simulation developed and how the outcomes will be measured (e.g., recording for debriefing, translate language, app for treatment or resource).
- *Recruitment:* Consider various cost-effective ways to recruit human or physical resources and market the simulation. Ask around or create a social media post for local volunteers or equipment needs. Some ideas include add to community webpage, email blasts, letters to alumni. Fostering collaborative relationships can lead to partnerships, which will assist with cost containment.
- *Training:* As learned from previous chapters, there are a lot of components to simulation that will require training for those supporting the event (e.g., SPs, debriefers, facilitators). Identifying alternative ways to train can help with costs as well as scheduling. Accessing or creating online, web-based, training to prepare those supporting the event may be a cost-effective, viable option. Some ideas to include are an overview of the scenario and learning objectives; a visual of the setting, simulation environment, and resources; expectations of various roles a person will fulfill; tools used to assess outcome measures (e.g., grading, scoring, and evaluating); selected debriefing format and questions developed to guide the learning process; how to provide feedback (and how it differs from debriefing); or a description of resources and tools that will be used.
- *Scheduling Flexibility:* Consider adjusting the time that the course is being offered based on space and resource availability. A local clinic may be closed in the evening or on a weekend, but may be willing to support the simulation endeavors during the off hours.
- *Community Outreach:* Reach out to community organizations and clinical partners to share the simulation plan and any unmet needs. Consider requesting old resources that are being updated or replaced at their facilities (e.g., wheelchair, mats, pumps, beds).
- *Shared Space:* Consider the vast array of space that may be available (internal or external) to implement the simulation. When doing so, keep in mind what the learning outcomes are and what space will allow the highest fidelity for learning. In other words, utilize the actual setting and space most realistic to clinical practice (e.g., hospital room, outpatient treatment room, inpatient rehab gym, or

office). What can be offered to the facility in exchange for their resources? Can staff be offered continuing education or professional development opportunities for involvement (which can be costly for some)? Can space be offered for the collaborative partner to use in return (i.e., an outpatient treatment room in exchange for a classroom with a guest speaker or lab space to demonstrate annual competencies)?

- *Interprofessional:* Collaborating with other disciplines or professionals can help with the financial hardships that may be encountered with costs associated with simulation-based education. Regardless of the setting, many accreditation standards include or are considering the inclusion of interprofessional education and practice components. Consider connecting with other departments, programs, and schools within the organization or in the community to share space, resources, and costs. Some ideas include an academic setting (i.e., theater department for SPs or utilization of space) or a clinical setting (i.e., a designated patient room [hospital] or classroom [school] during times not in use).

Worksheet 12-1

Brainstorming Creative Solutions for Clinical Simulation Use on a Budget

Purpose of This Activity

Brainstorm resource needs and creative solutions for simulation design and implementation. Use this worksheet to guide creative thinking with simulation design and implementation with consideration of fiscal constraints.

Planning the Simulation	*Response*	*Anticipated Simulation Cost*	*Additional Comments or Creative Options to Address Need*
What is your current budget? • Identify funds allocated or available			
Where will your funding come from? • List possible funding options that may be available (consider grants, in-kind donations, etc.)			
What type(s) are available? • Identify your preferred simulation method (e.g., task trainer, standardized patient, manikin, role play)			
What is the desired setting or environment you would like to simulate? • Consider the practice setting (e.g., skilled nursing facility, hospital, rehab, home) or space to carry out desired tasks (e.g., emergency room, kitchen, operating room, therapy gym)			

(continued)

Worksheet 12-1 (continued)

Brainstorming Creative Solutions for Clinical Simulation Use on a Budget

Planning the Simulation	*Response*	*Anticipated Simulation Cost*	*Additional Comments or Creative Options to Address Need*
Describe the location/space that would best simulate the actual environment. • Consider physical fidelity			
What resources do you currently have available? • Consider human and physical resources			
What resources will you need? • Consider space, tools, materials, supplies, equipment, and staff			
How much time will you need to carry out the simulation? • Identify the length of time for each encounter and how many encounters based on number of learners			
What type of training will need to be provided? • Consider staff, standardized patients, educators, and support help			
What are your fidelity considerations? • Consider physical, conceptual, and psychological			

References

Accreditation Council for Occupational Therapy Education. (2018). *2018 Accreditation Council for Occupational Therapy Education standards and interpretive guide.* Retrieved from https://www.aota.org/~/media/Corporate/Files/EducationCareers/Accredit/StandardsReview/2018-ACOTE-Standards-Interpretive-Guide.pdf

Curl, E., Smith, S., Chisholm, L., McGee, L., & Das, K. (2016). Effectiveness of integrated simulation and clinical experiences compared to traditional clinical experiences for nursing students. *Nursing Education Perspectives, 37*(2), 72-77. https://doi.org/10.5480/15-1647

Giles, A. K., Carson, N. E., Breland, H. L., Coker-Bolt, P., & Bowman, P. J. (2014). Use of simulated patients and reflective video analysis to assess occupational therapy students' preparedness for fieldwork. *American Journal of Occupational Therapy, 68*(2), S57-S66. https://doi.org/10.5014/ajot.2014.685S03

National Council of State Boards of Nursing. (2014). The NCSBN national simulation study: A longitudinal, randomized, controlled study replacing clinical hours with simulation in prelicensure nursing education. *Journal of Nursing Regulation, 5*(2), S3-S50. https://doi.org/10.1016/s2155-8256(15)30062-4

Ohtake, P. J., Lazarus, M., Schillo, R., & Rosen, M. (2013). Simulation experience enhances physical therapist student confidence in managing a patient in the critical care environment. *Physical Therapy, 93*(2), 216-228. https://doi.org/10.1016/s2155-8256(15)30062-4

REFERENCES

13

Designing the Simulation Encounter

Audrey L. Zapletal, OTD, OTR/L, CLA
Joanne M. Baird, PhD, OTR/L, CHSE, FAOTA
E. Adel Herge, OTD, OTR/L, FAOTA
Maureen M. Hoppe, EdD, MA, OTR/L, CPAM, CHSE

Learning Objectives

1. Describe multiple clinical simulation methods and supporting pedagogical theoretical frameworks.
2. Identify key components of best practice clinical simulation used to facilitate learning.
3. Formulate strategies to address challenges associated with clinical simulation used in occupational therapy curricula.
4. Integrate formative and summative assessment measures of clinical simulation processes for quality improvement.

Kern's Model of Program Development

The content in this chapter articulates Step 5 of Kern's Model: Implementation. Information in this chapter discusses the development and preparation for implementation of planned simulations. This articulates with accomplishing the plan by making the simulation a reality and achieving successful outcomes.

Zapletal, A. L., Baird, J. M., Van Oss, T., Hoppe, M. M., Prast, J. E., & Herge, E. A. *Clinical Simulation for Health Care Professionals* (pp. 129-167).

Part 1: Overview

Simulation Development: Overview

Many rehabilitation education programs now include simulation as an instructional approach; however, simulation education itself is a well-established discipline with recognized standards of best practice. These standards of best practice in simulation education were developed by experts to ensure the provision of sound educational principles that take advantage of the capabilities of simulation modalities. The simulation practice standards can be applied to multiple professions and include programming that has successfully replaced clinical experiences with simulation-based experiences (INACSL Standards Committee, 2021; Watts et al., 2021). In addition to educational components, best practice recommendations include unifying and supportive components that address the infrastructure and terminology used in a simulation program (Motola et al., 2013; INACSL Standards Committee, 2016; Figure 13-1). There are several key best practice components of a simulation program. They are described, outlined, and reviewed in the following text.

Curriculum design is the first step to designing a simulation program. Figure 13-1 represents how a simulation program can be designed using best practice, beginning with curriculum design and extending through the debriefing. While many educators believe that simulation begins with the creation of a scenario, best practice in simulation education starts with the curriculum design to ensure that there is a thoughtful integration of simulation that meets the learning needs of the students and the program. An additional initial consideration is how training for faculty and others involved in the simulation will be provided on an ongoing basis.

The simulation does require an investment of resources—it can be time and program intensive. Remember to include simulation in your strategic plan. Think about simulation as a program that contributes to student learning experiences, rather than a single scenario or series of scenarios. It is important to connect simulation with the learning requirements or educational standards of the program. Connecting simulation to a course or curricular objective rather than a one-time simulation event or research study promotes learning. Learning through simulation can fill curricular gaps, augment or replace clinical learning, and provide varied learning opportunities for all students (INACSL Standards Committee, 2016, 2021).

Resources, including faculty time, should be built-in to the strategic plan for growth. As part of your curricular integration, plan scheduled times for simulation program review to enhance accountability. As the simulation program evolves, established times for review with faculty, staff, administration, and other key stakeholders will be necessary to ensure that the program is unfolding as planned and to control for challenges and take advantage of opportunities. As the role of simulation becomes established, it needs to be supported by securing resources, such as simulation equipment or supplies (see Chapter 12: Simulation on a Budget). Sustained simulation programs create an environment where simulation is considered as a teaching strategy—not a "one and done" approach to learning.

Educational objectives are the next consideration when creating a simulation program. Simulations should be designed to support course and clinical objectives with opportunities for individualized learning. The simulation program must have clear outcomes and benchmarks, i.e., what the learner can expect to gain by participating in the program.

Simulation design should be purposeful. The simulation should begin with clearly defined learning outcomes derived from course objectives that are a valid representation of clinical practice. A simulation learning objective should be measurable, specific, observable, relevant, and able to be completed within the time allotted. Typically, simulations should have between one to four learning objectives and allow for repetitive or deliberate practice (McGaghie et al., 2011). Deliberate practice allows the learner to focus on clinical skills and key elements embedded in the simulation (McGaghie et al., 2011). See the sidebar for information about deliberate practice in simulation. Table 13-1 is a list of simulation design aspects to include and avoid.

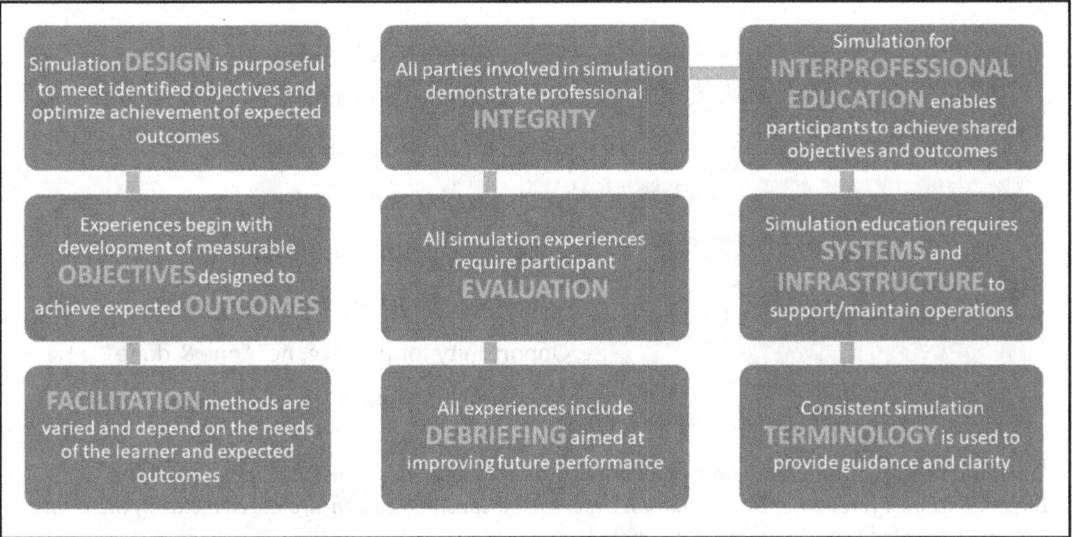

Figure 13-1. Overview of best practice standards. (Adapted from INACSL Standards Committee, 2016, 2021.)

Table 13-1. Critical Features for Effective Use of Simulation in a Health Professional Curriculum

To Include and Achieve	To Avoid
Opportunities for repetitive practice	Inconsistent scenarios, practice environments
Clinical variation	Erratic variations in levels of difficulty
Integration into the curriculum	Content that is not included in course objectives
Controlled environment	
Clearly defined learning outcomes	Vague, subjective expected outcomes
Valid representation of clinical practice	Unrealistic representations of clinical practice
Adapted from Issenberg et al., 2005.	

Assessment measures are the next step in implementation of a simulation program. These measures must comprise individual student learning experiences of each simulation, including performance on specific learning outcomes. The assessments must also examine how the simulation program is performing within the curriculum as a whole. This should include an assessment by the learners and faculty. There should also be an assessment to determine the validity of the simulations themselves—do the simulations assess what they are meant to assess? How well does the simulation reflect reality? See Chapter 7 for more information about assessments used to assess a variety of behaviors and skills used in simulation encounters.

Debriefing is the last step of integration, as this is where learning becomes concrete. Debriefing should occur after each experience, and may occur during the simulation, too. In addition to the reflection that occurs during debriefing, the feedback provided during and after simulation also contributes to learning. See Chapter 15 for information about debriefing.

These five categories of best practice in simulation program development occur simultaneously and individually during implementation, as reflected by the arrows in Figure 13-2. The following section provides detailed information about simulation scenario development.

Motivated Learners	Link to course assignments
Well-defined Learning Objectives	Objective outcome
Appropriate Levels of Challenge	Founded on curricular objectives
Repetitive Practice	Post-Classroom/lecture activity
Feedback from instructors	Feedback and debriefing provided
Learner Self-correction	Include video/chance for auto-examination
Desire to master a Task...And then	Opportunity for practice, nor "one & done"
Move onto a more challenging task	Embed other challenges

Simulation incorporating deliberate practice relies on the elements in the left column; therefore, as the simulationist (creator of the simulation experience), consider and ensure the elements in the right column. (Adapted from Issenberg et al., 2005.)

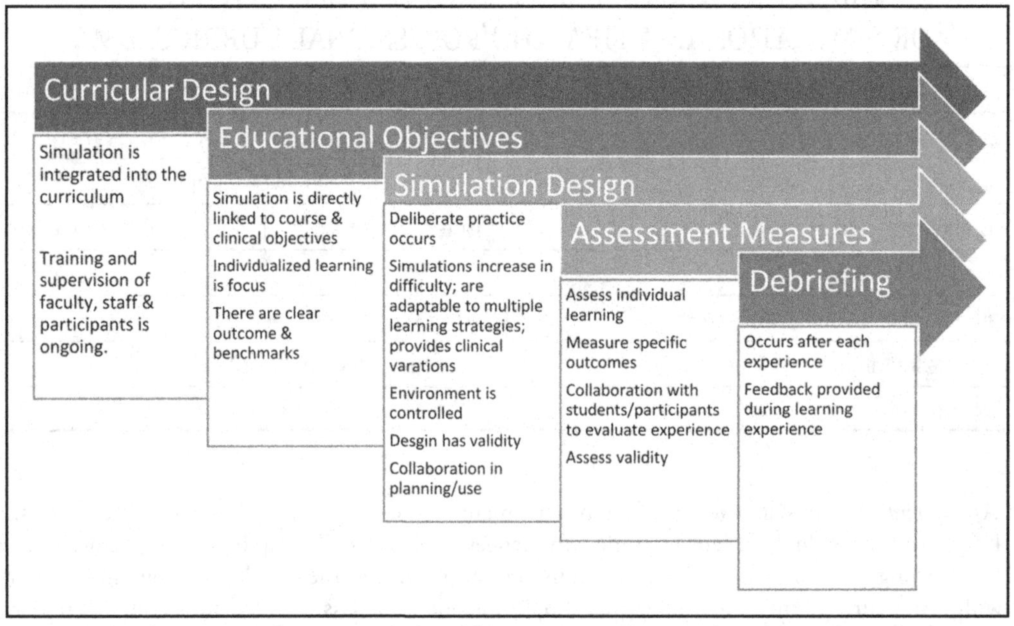

Figure 13-2. Simulation program best practice. (Adapted from Bremner et al., 2006 and Issenberg et al., 2005.)

Part 2: Scenario Development and Implementation

Learning Objectives

1. Describe key components of clinical simulation used to facilitate learning.
2. Identify and describe the roles of key personnel needed for clinical simulation.
3. Identify space, materials, equipment, and supplies needed for simulated activities and rationale.
4. Formulate strategies to address challenges associated with clinical simulation used in health professional curriculum.
5. Discuss how to integrate formative and summative assessment measures of clinical simulation processes for quality improvement.

Simulation Development: Creating the Experience

Begin with the learning objectives first. Many novice educators begin simulation design by considering a clinical scenario rather than starting with learning objectives. Rigorous simulation design always begins with problem identification at the curriculum level. For example, using Kern's Model for development, the first step is to determine the unmet needs of the program that can best be met through simulation (Kern et al., 1998). The next step is a targeted assessment of what the needs of the learner are. What does the learner know and what does the learner need to know? This can provide the focus for specific simulation education topics. Following this, the outcomes and learning objectives of the simulation should be established. Outcomes are the measurable results of the learners' progress. Refer to Chapter 6 for more details about this process. It is only once these steps are complete that a clinical scenario is considered.

Developing the Scenario

Scenario development includes staging the simulation, so think of the "big picture." This is an iterative process that requires the simulationist (expert simulation team/faculty creator) to revisit, review, and revise the foundational elements needed for creating the simulation encounters. Developing the scenario is more than just the identifying the learning objectives and assessments and creating the case and necessary documents. Strategic and thoughtful planning is needed to ensure all the resources are available on the day(s) of your simulation encounter.

The first step of scenario development is to identify the desired outcomes and learning objectives of the simulation, the assessments that will be used. Table 13-2 lists guiding questions to consider during this phase of development. These questions will provide the foundation for the simulation and should be answered concretely, before moving the simulation story or scenario.

Create the Learning Environment

Once you have answered the previous questions and have concrete learning objectives, decided upon formative or summative assessment measures for learners, and how to assess the simulation effectiveness itself, the next step is to consider the learning environment and how to best prepare the learner.

To create the best learning environment, consider the fidelity needed to meet the learning objectives (see Chapter 6) and which simulation modality would be best suited for your outcomes. Table 13-3 contains guiding questions in this area.

Table 13-2. Does Simulation Make Sense?

- What are your one to four observable, quantifiable, measurable learning objectives?
- What specific attitudes and skills-based knowledge are needed to meet these objectives?
- Provide a rationale that supports the simulation modality required to meet the learning objectives.
- Is simulation the best educational strategy? The learning objectives must match the observed actions, attitudes, and skills explicitly.
- How will you assess the learner? Consider a formative assessment as part of the educational components of a prelicensure program or a summative assessment as part of prelicensure competency or credentialing.
- How will you assess the simulation? Consider evaluating the simulation experience as a teaching strategy after the formal event, remember to include learners' perceptions of simulation as part of the simulation evaluation. Standardized assessments are available.

Table 13-3. Creating the Learning Environment

- Consider the simulation modality (e.g., standardized patient [SP], manikin, task trainer, virtual): Which simulation modality will provide the best learning experience by directly supporting the learning behaviors expected from the objectives?
- Consider the simulation environment: Describe all aspects of the available spaces (a classroom, laboratory, simulated apartment, home or clinic, mock hospital room, the hallway, virtually created areas). Which environment will provide the best learning experience by directly supporting the learning behaviors expected from the objectives?
- Consider the fidelity: Describe the types of fidelity that would be most important. How much realism is too much? Not enough? The environment should balance immersion with recognition of the elements of safety. What type and degree of fidelity will provide the best learning experience by directly supporting the learning behaviors expected from the objectives?

Prebriefing: Preparing the Learner

Setting up the simulation encounter for the learner is critical to their success and involves more than just creating the scenario and environment. The learner should understand that simulated clinical experiences are complex and require application of accumulated knowledge and skills from many aspects of their curriculum. Learners need to be aware of all the professional content that is associated with the objectives, including the curricular location (i.e., courses) associated with the content. For example, learners should be directed to the specific classroom lectures, readings, videos, and additional resources approved by the instructor that address simulation content and learning objectives. Table 13-4 provides guidance for connecting learners with curricular resources to that they are prepared for the simulation.

Prebriefing: Create Support Materials

For the simulation to resemble the clinical setting and to provide learners with an overall consistent experience, support materials are necessary. These are the documents (written and virtual) that the learner and the simulation team will refer to before, during, and after the simulation. These deliverables are needed for clear communication among all personnel involved in the simulation and are realistic in the clinical setting.

Table 13-4. Preparing Learners Through Curricular Resources

To reinforce procedural and psychomotor skills, remind the learner of:

- Classroom laboratory demonstrations by instructor/faculty
- Classroom laboratory peer practice
- Faculty feedback sessions
- Instructor-approved videos available for study/practice

To reinforce the professional behaviors and affective skills remind the learner of:

- The use of clinical reasoning to support actions, including quick thinking and problem solving
- The importance of remaining calm during unexpected events and spontaneous conversations
- The constructs of communicating clearly and confidently with others, which will include the SP, manikin, simulated patient, etc.

Table 13-5. Examples of Support Documents

Document	Purpose	Used By
Case scenario	This is the simulation story; it explains the expected scene and events of the simulation	Simulation team
Scripts	Details verbal or nonverbal communication and cues expected from SP, manikin voice over, others involved in the simulation	Simulation team
Sample radiological reports and images	Used to support clinical case	Learners and simulation team
Medical record documents, such as evaluations, interventions, reports of past medical history, etc.	Used to support clinical case	Learners and simulation team
Feedback and assessment forms	Used to support learner performance, SP performance, the perception of the simulation itself	Facilitator, SP, learner

When developing the scenario and materials for the learners, consider using templates from the clinic. For example, creating a client profile, a formal assessment report, documentation notes from team members, etc. Simulation activities allows for the intentional exposure of these materials and enhances the fidelity of the experience. See Table 13-5 for examples of supporting documents and their purpose.

Preparing to Implement

After developing the scenario, implementation is the next step. However, implementation does not mean immediate use with the learner. Implementation is composed of many tasks, all designed to assure success when the simulation scenario is used as part of the course. These tasks include resource identification, readiness, and preparation, as well as piloting the planned simulation. Table 13-6 provides key areas for consideration in each of these domains.

Table 13-6. Simulation Preparation

Key Area I: Readiness and Preparation

While innovating, think about what the simulation will need to be successful and how those needs will be met. Here are some key areas that will help identify the resources needed.

- Who will your learners be, exactly? This will lead to decisions about:
  - Space needed (e.g., number and type of rooms)
  - Length (time) of each simulation
  - When the simulation will occur (one day or several days, overall duration of simulation day[s]), during class time, during laboratory time, during specially scheduled time)
  - Type and amount of materials, equipment, and supplies
  - Location of materials, equipment, and supplies and if these items will need to be moved into different rooms during the simulation
  - Number of faculty to train and in what respective role/s (e.g., observers, SPs, debriefers, assistance with set-up/clean-up)
- What will the simulation schedule look like? Scheduling can be a challenge. Consider the following factors when making decisions:
  - Availability of everyone involved, including faculty, SPs, manikin training team, learners, simulationists
  - The academic schedules of the learners
  - The simulation design (group or individual encounter/scenario)
  - Faculty/simulationist time needed during the simulation, before the simulation, and after the simulation
  - Additional time, if required, for postsimulation debriefing, remembering that a good rule of thumb is that the debriefing sessions should be at least as long as the actual scenario
  - Time for set-up and clean-up, as well as resetting the simulation space between learners, if needed
  - Training time for faculty, staff, and others who will assist: Remember to include SPs (see Chapter 14)
  - Simulation center availability, including specific areas (e.g., medical theater rooms, classrooms) and the flow between areas that will be needed for learners to move through the simulation
    - → When possible, having overhead announcements play during the simulation can enhance the likelihood of everyone staying on the schedule
    - → Typical announcements include:
      - › *2 minutes before the encounter* (learners are outside the room; SPs are setting up and getting into initial position)
      - › *You may enter the room* (learners knock on the door, enter the room, and begin encounter)
      - › *You have 5 minutes remaining* (a cue to assist with pacing of the session)
      - › *Encounter over; please exit the room* (learner completes final task and closes the session with the SP)
  - Simulation center staff and equipment availability
  - SP availability and cost; some programs have additional fees for nonbusiness hours, such as evenings and weekends

(continued)

Table 13-6 (continued). Simulation Preparation

- Other space availability (waiting room area, clinical apartment, or in situ clinical area, i.e., an acute care treatment area or rehabilitation gym/clinic)

- How will the connection between the simulation encounter and other learning experiences in the course and/or curriculum be illustrated? Consider how you will do the following to assure a strong connection between the simulation, the course, and the learning objectives:
  - Align the feedback/assessment forms with the learning objectives by using similar language
  - Access to electronic or paper feedback and assessment forms for the learner and the faculty
  - Collect completed assessment and feedback forms from learners, SPs, and faculty
  - Follow up with learners who did not perform well or who received significant amounts of feedback from their evaluator/grader/SP
    - → *Note:* Simulations, especially if the learner is alone, are personal. Feedback is very powerful so it should be framed as a learning moment.
- Record the simulation encounter. If the simulation is recorded, consider the following elements:
  - Identify the personnel responsible for recording
  - Create a secure method of storage and policy for storage, security, and review of video and when video is permanently removed from storage platform
  - Plan for a recording malfunction, and if this happens, how will the learner be informed
  - Develop a plan for the learner to view their recording; address if a faculty facilitator will be present or if the student will do an independent review
- Determine how this plan, including how the recording information (e.g., the playback medium, location, time available, people involved) will be communicated to the learners
- Consider having the learner sign a waiver that includes the rationale for being recorded

Key Area II: Identifying Resources

- Decide which materials, equipment, and supplies will be needed. Doing this now will save countless time, worry, and money later. Consider exactly what the simulation needs to run successfully:
  - Materials, equipment, and supplies
    - → Examples: hospital beds, x-ray machines, ultrasound machines, reachers, IV bags, IV poles, pulse oximeter, sphygmometer, wheelchairs, walkers
    - → Space (for storage of equipment and for the simulation encounter)
- Consider training and the training time needed to use the equipment, software associated with any technology, and for working with personnel
  - Training is needed to operate equipment safely and properly (i.e., for high-fidelity manikins)
  - Training is required for standardized or simulated patients
  - Training is needed for the specialized personnel regarding program specific content and activities (simulation tech or operations tech)
- Consider funding/financial support for the simulation program
  - Charges may include room fees, equipment fees, charges to purchase materials/supplies, payment for SPs
  - Determine who will provide additional resources
    - → Simulation center
    - → Personnel/human resource department

(continued)

Table 13-6 (continued). Simulation Preparation

→ Another department within the organization

→ An outside organization

Key Area III: Identifying and Training the Team

Simulation is a team sport. While it can be done well with single faculty involvement, typically simulation involves multiple faculty members, instructors, and often individuals outside of academic departments. In these situations, every team member must receive education and training to work together to operationalize the simulation so each learner can achieve the learning objectives identified. See the following table for a list of personnel and responsibilities.

List of Personnel and Responsibilities

Team Member	*Role*	*Responsible*
Simulation center staff (simulation technologists, simulation coordinators, simulation educators, simulation coordinators)	Individuals who work solely with simulation education	Responsibilities vary and may include set-up for each encounter before, during, and help with clean-up after the encounter. Other responsibilities may include managing the technology related to the simulation including video equipment, setting up and running the manikins, or hiring SPs.
Faculty	Individual from an academic discipline, scientific field, or profession who may/may not have simulation expertise	Responsible for ensuring that the simulation is supported by curriculum design and course materials; typically responsible for assisting or creating simulation experience and ensuring fidelity.
Simulationist	Individual who designs, implements, and/or delivers the simulation	With documented expertise in simulation, responsibilities and background may vary; maybe an educator or someone with expertise in simulation or simulation technology.
Standardized patient	Individuals who have been coached and trained to accurately and realistically portray clients and clinical conditions	Responsible for assisting with teaching and assessing learners, may include providing feedback and assessment with training.

Adapted from INACSL Standards Committee, 2021; Lopreiato et al., 2016; and Oxford Dictionary, 2010.

Training Faculty, Academic, or Clinical Staff

While faculty, academic, and clinical staff have expertise in clinical areas, most do not have expertise in simulation. Thus, preparation will focus on simulation management. During this meeting, it is also important that those involved understand how the learners were prepared for the simulation. This includes didactic materials used, the learner's level of progression through the curriculum, and the exact expectations for participation. It is important for each team member to understand their role for there to be consistency.

- Clarify faculty and staff roles:
    - Assign specific tasks for everyone, for example:
        - → Preparation of materials and the simulation environment

(continued)

TABLE 13-6 (CONTINUED). SIMULATION PREPARATION

- → Assist with the briefing/prebriefing
- → Assist with clean-up and set-up between the simulations to ensure standardization of the scenario
- → Specific scripted communications, tasks, or actions during the scenario and strategies to avoid interfering with learner actions
- → Supportive roles to act as impromptu actors when needed to interrupt a clinical scenario if safety becomes a concern or the clinical scenario is going significantly awry (a simulation lifesaver)
- → Observation of the simulation in person or remotely through a live video feed for assessing learner performance or gathering information to use during the debriefing session

- Provide training to ensure a rigorous, quality experience for the learner
    - → Trained facilitators can assist with leading debriefing sessions
        - Training to support the debriefing in a healthy way is imperative. Elements of a well-facilitated debriefing session include support for a learners' mental health, diffusion of initial affective responses postsimulation, and discussion of the learner's challenges and strengths related to clinical skills (Fanning & Gaba, 2007; INACSL Standards Committee, 2016, 2021)
    - → Training should address how to use simulation technology, including high-fidelity manikins if appropriate, to support the simulation experience

- Training should also include preparation for the following:
    - Simulation can be physically and emotionally exhausting
    - Simulation demands full attention and investment
        - → This is not a dual attention task, team members must fully attend
        - → This can be a challenge to diplomacy and instructional skills
- Training should include provision and review of all support materials, electronically and/or on paper. This may include:
    - Guidelines for the simulation
    - Equipment management procedures
    - The debriefing model, structure, and questions that will be used
    - Schedules for the learners, the team members, and the SPs
- Include opportunities for hands-on practice of tasks, such as:
    - Equipment management
    - Resetting the room
    - Managing the clock
- Provide extensive and clear scoring guidelines for assessment materials, predicated with a reminder that the goal of the simulation is to demonstrate achievement of the learning objectives, which is often to complete a clinical task at a specified level of competency. The focus is on:
    - Evaluation of learners' behavioral (observable) actions
    - Achievement of strong inter-rater reliability, which is critical to maintain academic rigor (and because learners are sensitive to their performance and will compare experiences)
- Build a cohesive team through training:
    - Train everyone together when possible

(continued)

Table 13-6 (continued). Simulation Preparation

- → Discuss the information shared during training sessions with other team members, such as SPs or simulation center staff members
- Prior to the simulation:
  - → Gather everyone, and introduce each team member
  - → Explain every member's role to provide a level of understanding of how responsibilities might articulate.
  - → This should be done well before the simulation, and again on the day of the simulation before the simulations begin and learners arrive
- After the simulation:
  - → Meet again as a team to allow time for formal sharing of experiences and feedback (see Chapter 16)

Training Simulation Specialists

Simulation centers have on-site staff to assist with the training and development of the simulation. They often assist with usage of equipment such as task trainers, manikins, video capture systems, and associated environmental systems. This may also include SPs. Simulation center staff are experts in simulation, equipment use, and simulation technology; however, they have minimal knowledge of specific educational program, clinical, course or curricular, or professional expertise. A partnership is needed to ensure that the simulation learning objectives are supported. During the training session, collaborate with the simulationists (faculty and simulation staff) to create and implement the simulation. This training should focus on the learning objectives and how/why the simulation is being used.

Training Learners

Learners also have to be prepared to engage in the simulation. Of all the individuals involved, it could be argued that learner training is the most important as their success is paramount. It is a true test of their ability to engage in their health professional role—even when there is no grade attached to the performance.

- Focus on clinical behaviors and skills: Simulation allows the learner to take actions that are being observed and directly assessed (behavior observed), while indirectly assessing the knowledge and reasoning that prompts the action (clinical and professional reasoning)
- Include key competency areas that exist during a clinical scenario
  - Communication skills
    - → Interpersonal interactions
    - → Therapeutic rapport
    - → Professional behaviors as defined for the scenario (i.e., the learning objective or within the curriculum)
  - Management of environment
    - → Managing objects such as materials, equipment, and technology within a given space (e.g., a patient room)
    - → Interacting with the SP in a given amount of space
  - Skill development in clinical assessment and clinical intervention
    - → Demonstrating clinical reasoning
    - → Demonstrating good judgement and problem solving
    - → Completing standardized assessments (including scoring)

(continued)

TABLE 13-6 (CONTINUED). SIMULATION PREPARATION

- → Performing specific manual clinical skills:
  - › Managing transfers and functional mobility activities with durable medical equipment (DME)
  - › Providing activities of daily living (ADLs) and instrumental activities of daily living (IADLs) assessments and interventions
  - › Assessing vital signs, including blood pressure
  - › Positioning SP properly for testing or procedure (e.g., ultrasound, x-ray, blood draw)
- → Responding to emergency situations, such as a client who "feels dizzy" upon standing (i.e., learner provides place for the SP to sit, takes blood pressure immediately, and calls for help)

Key Area IV: Planning

Planning is key to a successful learning experience and must include the learner and those involved to support the simulation. The following areas deserve significant consideration when planning.

- Identify team members and responsibilities; using a team approach can ease the workload
  - Include members from other disciplines, institutions, or community agencies to enhance collaboration/interprofessional simulation to allow the inclusion of different perspectives
  - Multiple members may aid in securing resources if many programs can utilize the same resources
- Address the availability of the team and simulation personnel during the simulation encounter
  - During debriefing sessions with the learners and an overall debriefing session with the simulation team for program evaluation
  - Consider requesting a simulation technologist or operations person to join your team if medical equipment or high-fidelity manikins, task trainers, or other technology equipment is being used.
  - Identify who will be responsible for managing technology, if needed. Is there additional training needed specific to the technology (e.g., high-fidelity manikin that can cry, speak, and demonstrate unstable vitals; simulated x-ray machine; simulated arm task trainer for drawing blood practice)?
  - Identify who will set up and reset the simulations. To ensure a uniform realistic learning experience, setting up the physical space, including the equipment and/or position of the SP, is critical. To create a standard learning environment for the simulation, find strategies to set up/reset the room quickly between learners to maintain a reliable and efficient schedule and learner experience.
  - Determine the length of time for each training session (e.g., prebriefing, SP training, simulation equipment training)
  - Consider specific training for the simulation operations, role play during the encounter, or debriefing afterward and define the elements needed for each
- Be aware simulation is "real life" to the learner. Skills and responses are completed in *real time*; therefore, preparation must:
  - Address timing
    - → Ensure that the learner has enough time to complete the activities. Consider adding buffer time for learners who might benefit and others who would use it to further develop the therapeutic relationship.
    - → Include training with faculty, lab instructors, and SPs about how to ensure the learner's success by providing support rather than impeding behaviors; progression through the simulation should not be slowed because of actions other than the learner's

(continued)

Table 13-6 (continued). Simulation Preparation

- → Consider how time is allotted: the number of tasks the learner needs to complete, the location of the materials (i.e., onsite or outside of the simulation room), if/when breaks are scheduled
- → Consider if time will be limited and what the rationale for this would be

- Weigh factors that contribute to fidelity
  - Choose the location of the simulation that most closely replicates what the learner will experience in practice (e.g., classroom, laboratory, simulation center)
  - Define the elements of realism in the environment that are most important to the scenario and the expected behaviors and actions to take place
  - Decide what behaviors, skills, and tasks learners are expected to plan for in the encounter (e.g., starting an IV, teaching the patient a skill, conducting an assessment, administering a vaccine)
  - Consider the unexpected events that could be predicted by learner actions
    - → These unexpected events can be managed by simulation "lifesavers"—teaching faculty/simulation staff how to provide specific help if a predicted unexpected event occurs.
    - → For example, if a learner engages the SP in an unsafe task, the faculty member playing the role of a nurse can bring a note to the SP with instructions on how to give feedback to the learner that would be realistic in the clinical situation (i.e., SP is unsteady; SP states, "I'm scared"). The note is described to the student as a "phone message from a friend" that called in from the front desk.
    - → For example, if a learner forgets a piece of equipment, allow "aides" (the learners who are observing) to leave the room and procure the item.
- Consider the affective components of learning (see Chapter 12): Students may experience anxiety and uncertainty that influence their performance with:
  - Verbal communication skills
  - Clinical reasoning and "thinking on their feet"
  - Psychomotor skills (i.e., equipment management in a given space)

Key Area V: Piloting the Simulation

The last step before deployment with learners is to pilot the entire simulation. Piloting the simulation involves having the simulation team assembled and running through the entire simulation as planned without skipping any steps. The purpose of piloting the simulation is to work through any potential or obvious problems. The following section provides guiding questions about five key areas to consider during the pilot: space; materials, equipment, and supplies; personnel and training; scheduling and time; and the minimum essential elements.

- Space: During the pilot, pay special attention to the environment and use these guiding questions.
  - Does the type of space/environment used work well for the scenario(s), whether it is in a simulation center, a classroom, apartment, or a classroom laboratory?
  - Is there enough space for learners and personnel to access materials and complete tasks?
  - Has the simulation been scheduled far enough in advance that room reservations have been confirmed and the learner(s) are available and trained for the scenario?
- Materials, equipment, and supplies: Be sure to consider not just where the simulation will take place, but also what will be needed. The following questions should be answered before and after the pilot.
  - Will the equipment fit into the room?

(continued)

Table 13-6 (continued). Simulation Preparation

- What about storage before, during, and after the experience?
- Does the equipment work?
- If multiple pieces of equipment are used, will they be tested ahead of time in case more are needed?
- Who is responsible for making sure that the equipment is set up, in working order, ready, and then storing it?
- What is the process to order the appropriate amount and correct/appropriate types of materials, equipment, and supplies?
  - For example, if the scenarios require a specialized type of need for a blood draw, do you have enough? If SPs need to wear slipper socks, is there enough and extra in case of an emergency?
- How will materials and supplies be provided to and collected from learners? These can include schedules, pre- and postsimulation self-assessment forms, and postsimulation evaluation forms

- Personnel and training: This should have been a focus area prior to the pilot and should remain a focus area. Remember that the learner is part of your simulation team, too.
  - Has everyone received the needed training to do their role?
  - Does anyone need prebriefing with additional training or extra time just before the simulation?
  - Is there enough support (personnel) to run the simulation efficiently and effectively?
  - Do learners, faculty, staff, and other team members understand what is expected, how to meet those expectations, and the schedule they are to follow?
    - Consider creating customized schedules and responsibility documents for each role:
      - Faculty, simulation team, lab facilitators
      - Learner
      - Simulation operating personnel
      - SPs
- Scheduling and time: Scheduling and the time needed for preparation, planning, and training cannot be underestimated. Carefully consider the responses to the following questions and the suggestions provided.
  - Does the simulation schedule work as planned?
    - How much time is needed for set-up?
      - Set up space(s) the day or night before the event—simulations that require the use of multiple rooms and spaces especially benefit from this
    - How much time is needed to reset the simulation room between learners?
      - Identify who is responsible for the reset
      - For more efficient reset, leave visual cues to where items should be located (i.e. signs on the cabinet doors, or arrows, or "Xs")
      - If learners are transitioning between rooms, hallways, or different floors of a building, team members may need to help guide learners quickly so they are not late for the next activity.
      - If learners need clarification about what to do and where to go during the event, have faculty/staff stationed at key points in the space (hallways, stairwells) to assist with learners' transitions between activities

(continued)

Table 13-6 (continued). Simulation Preparation

- Does the simulation team need clarification about what to do and where to go?
  - → Develop a personalized schedule for each team member
  - → Create a one-page handout with key points for the day/role
- Is the time for the learner to complete the simulation tasks in the estimated time allotted realistic?
  - → Is the time allotted realistic for a seasoned clinician or novice learner?
    - › Allow extra time for a novice who may refer to notes during the experience or may be nervous
- Consider adding "buffer" time in the middle of the simulation experience lasting over 1 hour; this time can be used for learners to:
  - → Refresh and relax
  - → Share general thoughts about the experience
  - → Be updated about cases—changes in patient status or available personnel
- Is there time (and space and opportunity) between the end of the simulation activities and the debriefing session to segue into a group debriefing?
  - → Recognition of the accomplishment of the experience
  - → Refreshing and diffusing emotional tensions
  - → Collecting self-assessment or postsimulation evaluation surveys
  - → Sharing general thoughts about the experience

- The minimum essential elements: This section provides an extensive review of the overall simulation experience so that no critical components are omitted. Guiding questions and suggestions are provided here. It is suggested that this section is carefully reviewed prior to the pilot simulation and again after the pilot.
  - Describe how the simulation addresses the learning objectives
  - Identify the learning activities and how the prebriefing/briefing is designed to ensure that the learner knows what is expected and how to prepare
    - → This is the time—prior to the simulation—to orient the learner to the experience. The prebriefing includes defining expectations, explaining the simulation structure and logistics, assessment measures, and providing debriefing information.
  - Confirm that the simulation is designed to lead the learner to a predictable pathway for success with no unintended, negative secondary outcomes
  - Match the assessment and assessment tools with the simulation learning objective(s) and provide a rationale
  - Confirm personnel responsible for assessing are trained and understand expectations that meet the level of the learner
    - → Be sure they are properly trained to use the assessment tool
    - → Ensure consistency in expectations of learner performance by reviewing how the learner was prepared/trained
  - Identify how the assessment tool with be used within the encounter
    - → Decide if the assessment tool is electronic, online-web-dependent (internet-based), or paper-based
    - → Clarify process for submitting completed tool (e.g., submitted electronically, stored on a remote drive, reviewed with the student, given directly to the faculty course instructor)

(continued)

Table 13-6 (continued). Simulation Preparation

- → Describe the plan for technology glitches; if online/electronic submission, what is the plan if the computer shuts down
- → Describe the system for inter-rater reliability among graders or those providing feedback
- ◦ Identify the debriefing time, location, format, and personnel
  - → Clarify how debriefing will occur as close to immediately after the event as possible
  - → Consider the environment/location of the debriefing experience (i.e., is travel time needed to another building or is it in the same space as the event)
  - → Describe the debriefing format and training process for facilitators

Over time, scenarios should be modified to ensure fidelity to the examination or learner experience. If any information is vital to learner performance, consider that learners may share specific details related to simulation experiences across cohorts, so modification to simulation experiences can allow more novel experiences to occur.

Avoiding Pitfalls—Contingency Planning

Even after piloting a simulation, expect the unexpected. There are some important additional areas that warrant advanced planning.

- Expect last minute changes in participation. Learners can miss a simulation due to illness, oversleeping, or arriving late. Faculty, instructors, or SPs also may not be available due to an unexpected event.
- Be prepared if a learner, faculty member, or SP gets hurt or becomes ill and needs medical attention while on site.
- Identify the medical emergency guidelines for your center and secure basic first aid supplies.
- Identify any legal processes to ensure all departments are aware of the health emergency (e.g., human resources, simulation center director, director of employee health).
  - ◦ Know the resources needed to address equipment failure or problems with materials, supplies, or technology. Be prepared if a manikin or other equipment, technology, or software malfunctions during a simulation event.
  - ◦ Have extras of anything possible: materials, equipment, supplies … and even build in extra time in the schedule when feasible. This includes extra copies of assessments or simulation operation documents, equipment back-ups, personal protective equipment, and cleaning supplies.
    - → Additional time built into the schedule can be used to procure items, problem solve with the simulation, calm a student, catch up a simulation that is running behind, or provide extra time for someone who is late.
- Consider additional time if the learner or another member of the team needs clarification about the expectations. When will time for questions occur? If this is the case:
  - ◦ Consider using discussion boards or virtual meetings as additions to scheduled meetings and opportunities for communication outside the classroom.
- Grant time for additional requests or concerns.
  - ◦ A learner may want to practice skills prior to the simulation in a space that is specifically set up for the simulation. If so, consider informing the learner of the importance of independent practice with specific resources (i.e., instructor-approved videos and handouts) or designate specific practice times that do not interfere with simulation set-up.

Table 13-7. Strategies to Address Student Performance Concerns
These strategies can be suggested to students on the day of their simulation. They will help the learner remain "in character" during the simulation, while allowing needed time for clinical reasoning.

Remind the learner to:
• Take a breath and smile
• Use their notes and/or "aides" in the room (if available)
• Communicate with the patient, "Let me organize your room so we can access the equipment we need." During this time the learner can also refer to notes and/or collect their thoughts about the plan.
• Verbalize their plans/actions, "Now I am going to take your blood pressure while you are in bed, then I am going to sit you up and take it again ..." Thinking aloud provides another avenue for processing and will help finalize a decision.
• What if the learner begins to cry, becomes frustrated, or panics in the middle of the simulation? This situation should be addressed during team training. Strategies include:
  ∘ Having the facilitator or SP support the learner by calling a "time out" or otherwise slowing the scenario to a safe stopping point.
  ∘ For example, if a learner has not properly supported the SP during the transfer, the SP states, "I don't feel safe; I'm going to fall." If the learner does not respond appropriately by returning the SP to the initial position, the SP can tell the learner, "Just place me back on the bed [the initial start point].

- Learners may also approach the simulation coordinator or faculty member with concerns about their performance prior to the simulation and expresses their anxiety. In this situation, communication is critical.
  - → Begin with a review of the assessment tools and feedback forms.
  - → Consider providing the assessment/grading rubric so the learner can practice.
  - → Highlight the breaks between simulation activities in the schedule so the learner knows when they can relax.
  - → Additional strategies for students to use during the simulation are provided in Table 13-7.

Putting It All Together: Exemplars

This section of the chapter will provide an exemplar of how to provide skills training that prepares learners for a simulation program embedded into a course or curriculum. It can be used as a template for other simulation designs or to spur further thinking about simulation development.

To participate in the simulation, a learner must have already learned all the clinical skills needed in order to be successful in the clinical scenario (i.e., communication, interviewing, technical skills, managing IV's, managing adaptive equipment needed for the encounter, body movements, performing clinical skills, taking blood pressure, or operating equipment such as ultrasound machine or x-rays). This content is traditionally taught in lecture and laboratory learning venues. After being provided with this knowledge base, the learner must be encouraged to deliberately practice these skills to demonstrate some level of competency prior to their clinical intern placement (Miller, 1990). Using a clinical scenario with SPs or another high-fidelity modality allows learners to practice needed skills at a level approximating clinical placement before going to clinical placements or internships. Figure 13-3 provides an exemplar of how simulation can be embedded in a prelicensure curriculum to prepare students for clinical placement.

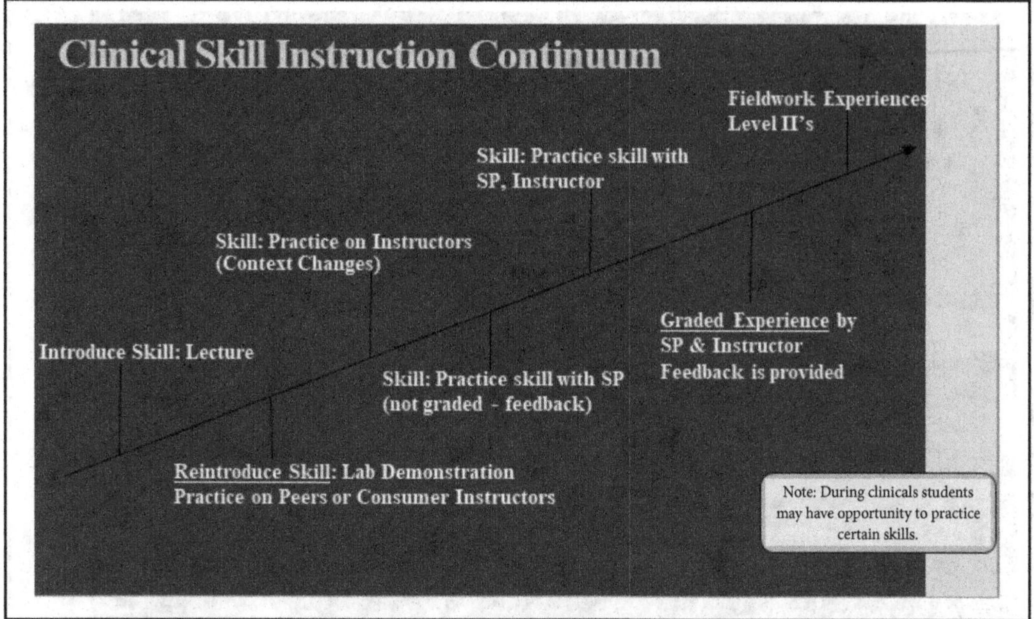

Figure 13-3. Embedding simulation activities into a health profession curriculum. (Adapted from Lorch and Zapletal, 2010 and Zapletal et al., 2016.)

The learner should take responsibility to prepare for the simulation. In addition to ensuring that the learners have learned the content, the learners have access to the clinical scenarios, learning objectives, and the tasks they will be expected to complete during the scenario. Learners are encouraged to practice other skills related to the scenario, such as designing treatment plans, writing goals, documentation, or suggesting a transition plan so that they fully understand the simulation and clinical case. Figures 13-4 and 13-5 show how specific learning activities precede and are paired with simulation experiences.

Learners should be provided with and understand the schedule; this includes how each activity relates to each other, where to report (i.e. which room), and at what time. Prior to the day of the simulation, the simulation is frequently discussed with the learners. Discussions include if the learner will be working with the SP individually or in a group so the learner can understand how the day will flow. Learners are provided with instructor-selected clinical skill videos to prepare for the simulation. Videos are to be selected by the instructor rather than allowing the learner to select from non-vetted internet-based videos, which may not support the specific skill protocol being taught. This consistency in teaching and training also helps the SP, who expects the learner to demonstrate specific skills based on a certain protocol.

Each simulation learning activity is accompanied by an opportunity for instructor, peer, and SP feedback, if appropriate, and assessment (either formative or summative). Debriefing occurs immediately after each simulation with trained facilitators. Students are progressed through the continuum across a series of courses or within a course in the curriculum, as planned to meet the program objectives and learning objectives. Students are also given opportunities to provide feedback about individual simulations, and the simulation program. This information is used to improve the program.

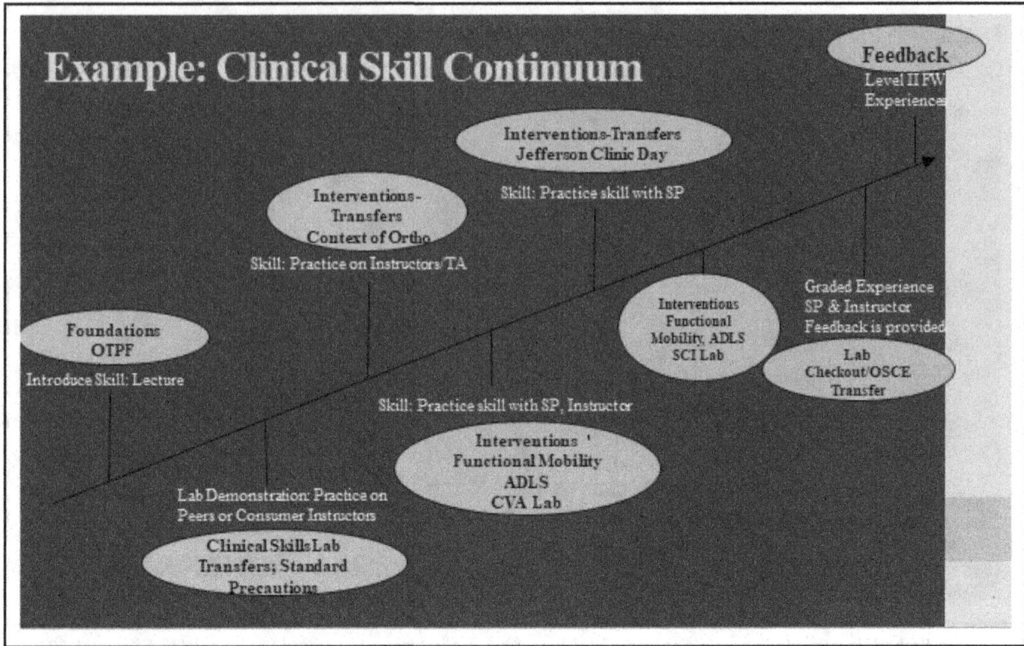

Figure 13-4. The white text indicates the learning anchors and activities associated with that part of the continuum; the black text reflects the skill addressed by the learning activities. Students are expected to master each skill in the continuum, from left to right, culminating in their lab checkout/OSCE. (Adapted from Lorch and Zapletal, 2010 and Zapletal et al., 2016.)

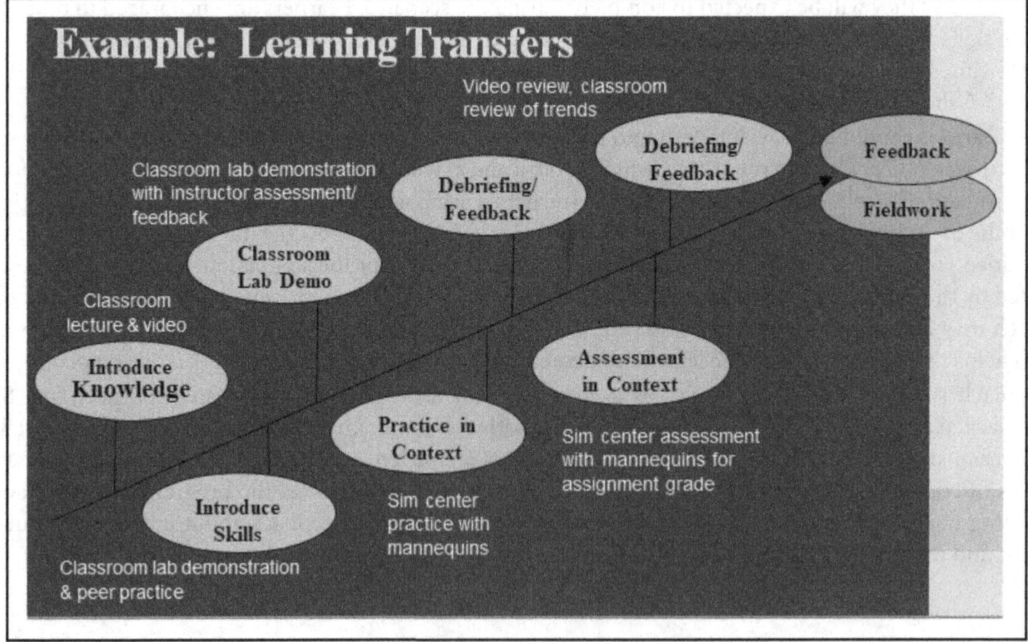

Figure 13-5. The white text indicates the learning anchors associated with that part of the continuum; the black text reflects the learning activities used to address each skill to help the student master the task of learning how to transfer clients. Students are exposed to each learning anchor in the continuum, from left to right, culminating in their laboratory performance assessment prior to attending their clinical assignments. (Adapted from Lorch and Zapletal, 2010 and Zapletal et al., 2016.)

References

Bremner, M. N., Aduddell, K., Bennett, D. N., & VanGeest, J. B. (2006). The use of human patient simulators: Best practices with novice nursing students. *Nurse Educator, 31,* 170-174. https://doi.org/10.1097/00006223-200607000-00011

Fanning, R. M., & Gaba, D. M. (2007). The role of debriefing in simulation-based learning. *Simulation in Healthcare, 2,* 115-125. https://doi.org/10.1097/SIH.0b013e3180315539

INACSL Standards Committee. (2016). INACSL standards of best practice: Simulation^{SM} Simulation design. *Clinical Simulation in Nursing, 12*(S), S5-S12. https://doi.org/10.1016/j.ecns.2016.09.005.

INACSL Standards Committee. (2021). Healthcare simulation standards of best practice. *Clinical Simulation in Nursing, 58,* 66. https://doi.org/10.1016/j.ecns.2021.08.018

Issenberg, S. B., McGaghie, W. C., Petrusa, E. R., Gordon, D. L., & Scalese, R. J. (2005). Features and uses of high-fidelity medical simulations that lead to effective learning: A BEME systematic review. *Medical Teacher, 27,* 10-28. https://doi.org/10.1080/01421590500046924

Kern, D. E, Thomas, P. A, Howard, D. M., & Bass, E. B. (1998). *Curriculum development for medical education: A six-step approach.* Johns Hopkins University Press.

Lopreiato, J. O. (Ed.), Downing, D., Gammon, W., Lioce, L., Sittner, B., Slot, V., Spain, A. E. (Associate Eds.), and the Terminology & Concepts Working Group. (2016). *Healthcare simulation dictionary.* Retrieved from http://www.ssih.org/dictionary.

Lorch, A. and Zapletal, A. L. (October, 2010) *The standardized patient encounter: An effective method for developing clinical competency in allied health students.* Presentation at the Association of Schools of Allied Health Professions Conference, Charlotte, North Carolina, October 21, 2010.

McGaghie, W. C., Issenberg, S. B., Cohen, E. R., Barsuk, J. H., & Wayne, D. B. (2011). Does simulation-based medical education with deliberate practice yield better results than traditional clinical education? A meta-analytic comparative review of the evidence. *Academic Medicine, 86,* 706-711. https://doi.org/10.1097/ACM.0b013e318217e119

Miller, G. E. (1990). The assessment of clinical skills/competence/performance. *Academic Medicine, 65*(9), 63-69. https://doi.org/10.1097/00001888-199009000-00045

Motola, I., Luke, D., Chung, H.S., Sullivan, J. & Issenberg, B. (2013). Simulation in healthcare education: A best evidence practical guide. AMEE Guide No. 82. *Medical Teacher, 35*(10), e1511-e1530, DOI: 10.3109/0142159X.2013.818632

Oxford Dictionary. (2010). Oxford University Press. Retrieved from http://oxforddictionaries.com/definition/ english/VAR

Watts, P., Rossler, K., Bowler, F., Miller, C., Charnetski, M., Decker, S., Molloy, M., Persico, L., McMahon, E., McDermott, D., & Hallmark, B. (2021). Preamble. *Clinical Simulation in Nursing, 58,* 1-4. https://doi.org/10.1016/j.ecns.2021.08.006

Zapletal, A., Herge, E. A., Van Oss, T., Prast, J., Baird, J., & Hoppe, M. *Innovative strategies for integration of clinical simulation into occupational therapy curriculum.* Institute Workshop presented at the American Occupational Therapy Association's Annual Conference, Chicago, IL. April 6, 2016.

PART 3: MANIKINS AND TASK TRAINERS

Learning Objectives

1. Define task trainers and manikins in the context of a simulation experience.
2. Compare and contrast the benefits and limitations of each modality.
3. Share evidence related to the use of these modalities in the context of simulation.

Task Trainers

Task trainers are physical or virtual models of body parts which may include non-anatomical experiences (virtual reality) that focus on the mechanics of biological concepts. Task trainers, sometimes referred to as partial task trainers, provide an opportunity to repeatedly practice a specific skill or set of skills to help the learner develop confidence and mastery. Depending on the learning objectives, they can break physical tasks down into specific steps to build on the desired skills necessary for competency. This form of simulation is a valuable adjunct to traditional education that allows educators to enhance cognitive and psychomotor skills in a safe environment and thereby improve practice (Lateef, 2010).

One of the benefits of a partial task trainer is that it can allow instructors to validate a skill prior to allowing a novice to perform that skill on a real person. This can protect the patient and allow trainees to have their first encounters with real patients when they are at higher levels of technical and clinical proficiency (Ziv et al., 2006).

Task trainers allow learners to practice one specific task, such as catheterization or monitoring vital signs, to establish or build competency in clinical skill(s). Health care staff can develop and refine their skills, repeatedly if necessary, using simulation technology without putting patients at risk (Lateef, 2010). While this form of simulation is useful when the goal is to practice a psychomotor skill in isolation, keep in mind that it can also be used with SPs or while role playing to allow learners to practice multiple professional and/or clinical skills. Some examples include using a task trainer that is an area of tissue with an invasive IV strapped to the arm of an SP or task trainer that is an area of tissue with staples/sutures strapped to the extremity of an SP. These combination modalities allow learners to combine technical psychomotor skills with clinical reasoning and communication skills during overlaying tasks, such as transfers, selfcare, or exercise. There are many other advantages to using a task trainer modality. Advantages and limitations of task trainers are outlined in Table 13-8.

Manikins

In contrast to task trainers, manikins represent an entire body. Full body manikins are sometimes also called "complex human patient simulators." They can actively simulate bowel sounds, as well as respiratory and cardiac functions. These functions are realistic and computer driven, allowing for programming of episodic critical events designed to enhance student learning. At the most complex level they interface with computerized systems allowing the learner to experience a virtual reality situation, such as a simulated surgery, wherein the manikin connects to a computer monitor with a programmed response. The learner performs an intervention/task and the computer responds to the interventions, thus if the simulated intervention is botched, the manikin responds with the appropriate medical or physical instability (McGaghie, et al., 2010).

There are many advantages, including the inability to induce any true harm to a human; thereby providing an environmentally appropriate situation without risk. The use of these inanimate simulators allows educators to create structured learning situations and outcome-based assessments (Isenberg et al., 2005; Lammers et al., 2008). Simulators used this way also allow educators to provide a consistent learning experience for each student (Issenberg et al., 2005; Rothgeb, 2008). They have strong fidelity due to

Table 13-8. Advantages and Limitations of Task Trainers

Advantages
Preparation for transition and application of skills on an actual client
Breaks task down into specific actions/steps to enhance competency for the whole process: • Allows the instructor to slow, stop, pause, and restart a physiological event • Allows focus on key elements—a specific task or technical skill • Provides physiological feedback to the learner • Helps learners develop confidence and prepare to transition to an actual client • Helps learners develop skill proficiency • Replicates clinical situations not otherwise possible, such as wounds or edema
Enhance the realism of the simulation encounter using moulage, a technique used to make skin look injured to enhance realism
Limitations
Does not represent clients from a global perspective
Works only for specific tasks
Provides limited opportunity for learner engagement
Has limited application to some health care professions as they were developed primarily for, and often used in, invasive tasks

their environmental components and unarguable, consistent responses. Manikins are often used to address manual and procedural psychomotor skills predicated on clinical reasoning and critical thinking. While they can be used to promote verbal communication skills, this may best be done with a verbal team interaction and simulation patients may be a better option for verbal patient communication.

Manikins (manikin patient simulators) may have a variety of features and may be either low or high technology. Low technology manikins do not replicate vital signs and are not programmable; they typically offer articulating joints and are anatomically correct. High technology manikins offer dynamic physiological features, ranging from vital signs to giving birth. They can be categorized as either tethered, which means that the manikin needs to be connected to a computer by cables, or tetherless, which means that the manikin will work for a time without cables connected. High technology manikins can be programmed using software that allows for physiological adjustments in response to the learner's actions. Table 13-9 provides a list of considerations when planning for manikins.

Just as in any simulation, when using a manikin as the simulation modality, the scenario must be driven by the learning objectives, with considerations for the environment. For new learning or novice learners, less learning objectives may be better; consider single-objective scenarios. Serial- or multiple-learning objective scenarios are best for intermediate/advanced learners. The environment should be realistic and should support and "stage" the experience so that the learner can realistically engage. Remember that simulations provide learning experiences for the developer too, so expect to revise scenarios over time.

Manikins have many advantages as simulation modalities. They also have many challenges. Manikins lack a "human" element. For example, manikins have tears but they do not cry. They can be programmed to unfold in a sequence of events (i.e., using prerecorded responses or a support person can provide a voiceover), but they do not talk, move their lips, or respond spontaneously. Manikins are not animated, they are fully dependent for physical tasks, and therefore the weight of the manikin needs to be known to design the encounter. Since manikins and task trainers are stationary, plans must be in place in a position for all learners to access desired body parts/areas for physical exam and clinical skills training. Manikins cannot assist with any physical interaction related to functional mobility or manipulation—which is also an advantage. Because manikins cannot provide verbal feedback, they do not address the affective and psychosocial aspects of learning outcomes as well as an SP might.

Table 13-9. Considerations for Use of Manikins

Consistency	Each manikin is anatomically the same, and the environmental set-up of the manikin can be standardized for each encounter—thus the same experience can be provided for all learners in the cohort.
Responsiveness	Manikins only respond to activity and manipulation (or gravity). They have no active listening, hearing, or emotions, and can be programmed for exact responses.
Safety	The manikin and materials cannot be harmed from the learners' interaction.
Cost Effectiveness	Manikins may be more cost-effective in the long run than scheduling SPs. For example, they do not need scheduled breaks and do not become fatigued.
Repeated Practice	Allow for development of motor skills through repeated practice (e.g., deliberate, distributed, mixed).
Availability	Depending on the situation, learners may be able to access the manikin for additional practice outside of the simulation or a clinical setting.
Objective Environmental Information	This includes dynamic tracking (i.e., vital sign data that can be recorded and/or synchronized to learner actions), vital sign data that is displayed on monitors and visual and auditory alarms synchronized to the manikin and monitor.
Programmable Situation/ Scenario	Prior to the simulation, parameters can be set so that each encounter will provide the same situation to each learner and the learner's response and interaction with the manikin determines the outcome. Manikin settings can be a mix of predictable (known changes) and unpredictable (unknown responses) for the scenario.
Environmental Versatility	Can be used in a lower technology setting, such as a classroom or apartment, or a higher technology setting, such as a simulated hospital room or clinic.

References

Issenberg, S. B., McGaghie, W. C., Petrusa, E. R., Gordon, D. L., & Scalese, R. J. (2005). Features and uses of high-fidelity medical simulations that lead to effective learning: A BEME systematic review. *Medical Teacher, 27,* 10-28. https://doi.org/10.1080/01421590500046924

Lammers, R. L, Davenport, M., Korley F., Griswold-Theodorson, S., Fitch, M. T., Narang, A. T., Evans, L. V., Gross, A., Rodriguez, E., Dodge, K. L., Hamann, C. J., & Robey, W. C. (2008). Teaching and assessing procedural skills using simulation: Metrics and methodology. *Academic Emergency Medicine, 15,* 1079-1087. https://doi.org/10.1111/j.1553-2712.2008.00233.x

Lateef, F. (2010). Simulation-based learning: Just like the real thing. *Journal of Emergencies, Trauma, and Shock, 3*(4), 348-352. https://www.onlinejets.org/text.asp?2010/3/4/348/70743

McGaghie, W. C., Issenberg, S. B., Petrusa, E. R., & Scalese, R. J. (2010). A critical review of simulation-based medical education research: 2003-2009. *Medical Education, 44,* 50-63. https://doi.org/10.1111/j.1365-2923.2009.03547.x

Rothgeb, M. K. (2008). Creating a nursing simulation laboratory: A literature review. *Journal of Nursing Education, 47,* 489-494.

Ziv, A., Wolpe, P.R., Small, S.D., & Glick, S. (2006). Simulation-based medical education: An ethical imperative. *Simulation in Healthcare, 1,* 252-256.

Part 4: Simulated Patients/Standardized Patients

Learning Objectives

1. Define SP in the context of a simulation experience.
2. Compare and contrast the benefits and limitations of use of SPs in curricula.
3. Share evidence related to the use of these modalities in the context of simulation.
4. Examine a simulation scenario incorporating an SP.
5. Describe components for SP training and rationale.
6. Discuss team-training strategies for large simulations with multiple cases and SPs.

Introduction and Background

SPs are individuals specially trained to portray a specific set of behaviors, physical movements, communication patterns, cognitive abilities, and/or attitudes (Herge et al., 2013; Lioce et al., 2020). SPs can be used for learning assessment or intervention skills (Lioce et al., 2020). SPs are a type of simulation modality that provide many advantages for health care professionals and are viewed by the learner to be the "gold standard" of simulation (Mavis et al., 2006). They allow for a physical interaction with the learner while adding an additional layer of complexity and realism, because the learner must respond to the genuine psychological and emotional responses. An SP simulation is a teaching/learning activity based on the realistic clinical scenario that incorporates the use of an SP (Lioce et al., 2020, p. 49).

Advantages and Disadvantages

Using SPs in simulations provides a dynamic environment in which the learner must constantly respond to the needs of another person. These needs include verbal and nonverbal communication that may also include an element of physicality; for example, the learner may need to touch the SP's hand if the SP demonstrates sadness as an emotion. Another advantage to using SPs is to provide access to populations that may be scarce in a particular region. SP simulations enhance training to be efficient and effective, and evidence indicates that using them actually improves clinical performance (Borghi et al., 2016; Giles et al., 2014; Haracz et al., 2015; Johnston, 2018). SP encounters offer invaluable opportunities for experiential learning and reflection, as well as feedback from multiple sources including faculty, lab instructors, peers, and SPs as compared to a traditional simulation lab or traditional teaching methods (Giles et al., 2014).

Using SPs increases the realism of the *situation,* whereby the simulation environment and the encounter mimic the real world. This situational realism makes SPs ideal to train health professional learners for medically complex patients when there is a shortage of clinical sites. SP simulations provide learners with the opportunity to practice essential clinical skills that impact patient safety, including communication, interpersonal skills, management of the environment, and technical skills of their health profession.

Just as with any simulation modality, SPs have limitations. There is evidence that learners feel that SP encounters and simulated events are stressful (Hardenberg & Tori, 2020; Neilsen & Harder, 2013); however, with exposure and becoming more confident in their health professional role, the stress level may decrease. Because simulation encounters with SPs can be challenging and complex, the debriefing session must be structured and facilitated by a well-trained debriefer who enables learners to express and diffuse any strong emotions to decrease the stress level of the learners (Abulebda et al., 2020; Fanning & Gaba, 2007; see Table 13-10).

While SP simulation can be a rigorous and efficient method to teach large numbers of learners and providing quality feedback, using this modality does require a high level of organization and significant planning. Table 13-11 outlines several key elements to consider when contemplating an SP simulation. Keep in mind that additional time will be required to develop the simulation experience because of these elements.

Table 13-10. Advantages and Limitations of Standardized Patients

Advantages
• Delivers real world, authentic interactions that learners must navigate • Provides unique opportunities to practice professional communication skills, clinical assessment, and intervention skills • Creates situational challenges to learner's clinical reasoning and problem solving • Allows for evaluative and unbiased feedback in desired standards of learner's performance and behaviors from trained SPs • Presents learners with the opportunity to navigate the environmental demands coupled with the human demands of the interaction (i.e., moving medical equipment or furniture in order to access the patient) • Awards opportunities to address unique cultural aspects to care in real time • Enhances the realism of the simulation encounter; SP may need to wear a costume/dress for the role and wear moulage for realistic wounds, abrasions, bruises, etc. • Costs less than academic staff/faculty; cost of SPs are variable based upon skill level and demand required in the performance of the simulation • Awards for high level of learner satisfaction after the encounter and impact on learning • Provides opportunity for practice and building confidence prior to transitioning to real patients • Reduces faculty's time in reviewing basic instruction, assessment, and intervention skills
Limitations
• Time required for recruitment, screening, and training • Available resources including cost of time for scheduling, recruiting, training, SPs, and coordinating all schedules (including the learner) and finances for SP encounter • Securing adequate space and materials for realistic environment • Be aware of liability/risk management for activities (i.e., dressing activities, inappropriate use of/discussion of topics during simulation, equipment failure, SP or student goes "off script")

Create the Clinical Scenario and Determine the Standardized Patients: Learner Design

Just as with any simulation modality, creating the clinical scenario begins with development of the learning objectives, determination of the outcome methods, and creation of the clinical scenario. Using SPs allows for multiple simulation designs that can be used to address the learning objectives and outcome methods, and to meet the needs of the learner. It is important to develop scripts for actors (SPs and protocol for learners). Also, remember that for all SP simulations the details of the environment (e.g., materials, equipment, supplies) should be described and clearly planned as part of the clinical scenario. Several SP simulation designs are listed in Table 13-12.

Training Standardized Patients

This section describes critical elements and strategies for an effective SP training session. Once the SPs have been selected and training day has been scheduled, many foundational items are needed for a successful training session (see Chapter 14 for more informations on training SPs).

TABLE 13-11. CONSIDERATIONS FOR STANDARDIZED PATIENT USE

Recruitment and Retention	Some SPs are also trained actors, so approaching community theaters and service organizations may be an option. Other options may be retired and current faculty or using advertisements. Regardless of background, SPs will require additional training.
Economic/ Financial	SPs are trained workers who must be compensated. Compensation varies among region and institutions within those regions. Financial compensation (hourly wage, honorarium, etc.) should be equitable to the skills needed for the desired work.
Quality Assurance/ Fidelity	SPs must be trained and perform accurately to ensure that the learner experience is of high quality and reflects workplace fidelity. Faculty training time, preparation, and set-up can be involved to ensure a safe, simulated-authentic experience.
Logistics	Once recruited and through general training, enough SPs for the actual encounter must be scheduled for the prebriefing, training, simulation, and debriefing. Another consideration is to assure that there is enough equipment and materials for the day(s) of training and the day(s) of the simulation.
Desired Outcome	Incorporating an SP encounter requires a thoughtful and intentional examination of the health professional curriculum and should be used to meet an unmet need. Crafting an encounter requires the simulationist to convey relevant information to all stakeholders involved. Communication skills are extremely important to ensure that learners are prepared appropriately, SPs are trained according to the learner's preparation and skill, and other team members (lab instructors, debriefers, etc.) have ample time to understand their role within the encounter.

TABLE 13-12. SIMULATION DESIGNS

Individual Learning Sessions	• One SP and one learner • 30-minute session to address specific clinical skills • *Example:* Patient and practitioner completing an interview regarding nutritional health needs
Learner Pairs/Group Sessions	• One SP and two learners • 15- to 25-minute session to address specific clinical skills • Example: Patient and practitioner complete transfer activities
Learner Pairs With Instructor Guidance	• One SP and two learners • Guided step-by-step by the instructor to learn specific clinical skills • 50-minute session to address specific clinical skills • *Example:* Patient and practitioners learning dressing skills/functional mobility/ bed mobility • *Example:* Learning how to conduct a clinical assessment
Objective Structured Clinical Examination	• One SP, one learner, one instructor • 30-minute session • Graded by the instructor and trained SP • Learner prepares for six different cases • Learner tested on one case that is multifaceted • Typically used for summative assessment/outcome • Design activities that will occur during the clinical scenario on a timeline • *Example:* Lab checkout

The SP session should have a set agenda and schedule. During the session, it is important to clearly set expectations for SPs (for example, they should have personality/emotions as written in scenario and should also be cooperative so that the simulation can move forward). If applicable, inform the team of any modifications from the prior year/simulation (especially if based on SP, learner, and/or faculty feedback), as communicating these modifications allows for the scenario and simulation day to run as intended and demonstrates the value of their experience and feedback. Similarly, time should be spent on a discussion of what is expected of the learner, what variations may manifest, and how these should be managed. For example, if the tasks include dressing, the order of the dressing activities could be shirt, pants, socks, shoes; or based on the position of the patient, the learner could decide to progress starting with socks, pants, shirt, then shoes. Neither is incorrect as long as the SP is safe and the learner articulates their clinical reasoning.

The training session should focus on SPs and should emphasize the "doing" part of the training. It is important that the SP have an opportunity to practice the entire scenario, ideally with another SP as the learner. Having SPs practice with faculty or clinicians can be misleading. Seasoned faculty/clinicians' skills are fluid and unintentionally set the expectations of the SP too high. As a result, learners may be unfairly graded.

A sample SP training agenda is provided in Table 13-13.

Training in Teams by Scenario

Training SPs with the assistance of colleagues and staff can help with efficiency. If this is an option, meet with the individuals (colleagues and staff) involved in the simulation (the simulation team) prior to the SP training. At this meeting, describe the purpose of the SP training and review the clinical scenarios and learning objectives, especially the expectations of the learner and SP. It is important that the simulation team helping with the training recognize the importance of providing feedback to the SP regarding their performance, as it ensures the consistency and quality of the simulation. Often training should focus on SP performance, as SPs can convincingly portray a client with less information about the clinical conditions, while they may need more information about the relevant behaviors to successfully play the part consistently.

Having access to multiple faculty members who can act as simulation trainers can greatly reduce the burden of training SPs. For example, if multiple clinical scenarios or SPs are planned, the practice portion of the session can be completed comfortably using a ratio of one faculty trainer to six SPs in about 60 to 90 minutes, depending on the complexity of the case. The introduction, overview, scenario description, and wrap-up portion of training can be done with the entire simulation team (faculty and SPs). This helps reduce the amount of training time required.

Table 13-13. Training Agenda

Introductions	• Introductions of team members, including role and experience in simulation • Team members include the cast, faculty, simulation staff, and anyone who is responsible for conducting the event
Overview	• Description of the health profession and overview of education for practice • Description of where the learners are in their health profession curriculum and the purpose of the course that the simulation experience is embedded in • Overview of the specific clinical simulation day and activities • Discussion of the structure of the day, including performance time, breaks, and any other details (i.e., use of backup/floats or replacement SPs throughout the day)
Scenario Description	• Describe and discuss the diagnoses involved, including a brief overview of the pathology, how the patient may have been diagnosed with the clinical condition, the signs and symptoms of the clinical condition and possible treatments, the tasks to be completed by the SP, and how much assistance the learner will or will not provide • Provide SPs time to discuss, review, and outline dress code (e.g., costumes) and explain the procedure and any materials, equipment, and supplies (e.g., props) that they will encounter or wear • Read through the case scenario, defining any clinical terminology and acronyms as needed; hearing the clinical terms helps SPs understand the language of the profession and clinical setting • Emphasize the observable behaviors needed from the SP, as well as any helpful hints to enact these behaviors
Practice	• Provide opportunities for the SP to practice their role using the props and equipment to ensure a smooth scenario and to help the SP better understand their role • Begin the training by providing a demonstration of the expected and important behaviors. Consider narrating the rationale and key points during this initial demonstration so that the SPs understand their role. Using videos of the scenario can emphasize specific issues and behaviors. • Next, the SPs should practice on each other, with one being the SP and the other being the learner so they can understand how and what is expected of both parties when a novice completes the tasks • It is helpful to use a clinical scenario with a sequential checklist of what is supposed to happen, as well as what activities are not desired for comparison • Provide feedback and additional practice to master the behaviors, movement patterns, emotions, communication, and pain levels • Review evaluation tools and feedback forms that will be used to assess the learner and use them during the practice session
Wrap-Up	• Allow time to address any questions, review the schedule, and ensure everyone understands what time to report on the day of the simulation • Share common issues evident in some learners, including professional behaviors or minimal preparedness • Consider having an SP-specific briefing on simulation day prior to the actual scenarios for any last-minute questions and to make sure everyone arrives on time

References

Abulebda K., Auerbach M., & Limaiem F. (updated 2020). *Debriefing techniques utilized in medical simulation*. StatPearls Publishing. Retrieved from https://www.ncbi.nlm.nih.gov/books/NBK546660/

Borghi, L., Johnson, I., Barlascini, L., Moja, E. A., & Vegni, E. (2016). Do occupational therapists' communication behaviours change with experience? *Scandinavian Journal of Occupational Therapy, 23*(1), 50-56. https://doi.org/10.3109/11038128.2015.1058856

Fanning, R. & Gaba, D. (2007). The role of debriefing in simulation-based learning. *Simulation in Healthcare, 2*(2), 115-125. https://doi.org/10.1097/SIH.0b013e3180315539

Giles, A. K., Carson, N. E., Breland, H. L., Coker-Bolt, P., & Bowman, P. (2014). Use of simulated patients and reflective video analysis to assess occupational therapy students' preparedness for fieldwork. *American Journal of Occupational Therapy, 68*, 57-66. https://doi.org/10.5014/ajot.2014.685S03

Haracz, K., Arrighi, G., & Joyce, B. (2015). Simulated patients in a mental health occupational therapy course: A pilot study. *British Journal of Occupational Therapy, 78*(12), 757-766. https://doi.org/10.1177%2F0308022614562792

Hardenberg, J., Rana, I., & Tori, K. (2020). Evaluating impact of repeated exposure to high fidelity simulation: Skills acquisition and stress levels in postgraduate critical care nursing students. *Clinical Simulation in Nursing*, 1-7. https://doi.org/10.1016/j.ecns.2020.06.002

Herge, E. A., Lorch, A., DeAngelis, T., Vause-Earland, T., Mollo, K. & Zapletal, A. (2013). The standardized patient encounter: A dynamic approach to prepare professional healthcare students for the workplace. *Journal of Allied Health, 42*(4), 229-235. Retrieved from https://www.ncbi.nlm.nih.gov/pubmed/24326920

Johnston, T. E. (2018). Assessment of medical screening and clinical reasoning skills by physical therapy students in a simulated patient encounter. *Internet Journal of Allied Health Sciences and Practice, 16*(2), 10. Retrieved from https://nsuworks.nova.edu/cgi/viewcontent.cgi?article=1735&context=ijahsp

Lioce L., Lopreiato J., Downing D., Chang T. P., Robertson J. M., Anderson M., Diaz D. A., Spain A. E., & the Terminology and Concepts Working Group (2020). *Healthcare Simulation Dictionary–Second Edition*. Agency for Healthcare Research and Quality; AHRQ Publication No. 20-0019. https://doi.org/https://doi. org/10.23970/simulationv2.

Mavis, B., Turner, J., Lovell, K., & Wagner, D. (2006). Faculty, students, and actors as standardized patients: Expanding opportunities for performance assessment. *Teaching and Learning in Medicine, 18*(2), 130–136. https://doi.org/10.1207/s15328015tlm1802_7

Neilsen, B. & Harder, N. (2013). Causes of student anxiety during simulation: What the literature says. *Clinical Simulation in Nursing, 9*(11), e507-e512. https://doi.org/10.1016/j.ecns.2013.03.003

Suggested Readings

Palaganas, J., Maxworthy, J. C., Epps, C. & Mancini, M. E. (2015). *Defining excellence in simulation programs*. Wolters Kluwer.

Smithson, J., Bellingan, M., Glass, B., Mills, J. (2015). Standardized patients in pharmacy education: An integrative literature review. *Currents in Pharmacy Teaching and Learning, 7*, 851-863. https://doi.org/10.1016/j.cptl.2015.08.002

Ulrich, B. & Mancini, M. E. (2014). *Mastering simulation: A handbook for success*. Sigma Tau International.

Wallace, P. (2007). *Coaching standardized patients for use in the assessment of clinical competence*. Springer Publishing.

Part 5: Sample Scenario Using Standardized Patients

Audrey L. Zapletal, OTD, OTR/L, CLA

Learning Objective

1. Illustrate the sequence of activities for a clinical simulation using SPs.

Case Example

The following section provides an example of an embedded simulation.

Student Clinic Day

Student Clinic Day is a half-day medical setting-based simulation for occupational therapy learners in their second year of study. Occupational therapy learners utilize knowledge and clinical skills from prior coursework to simulate being an occupational therapist for an SP. SPs are trained to depict a specific orthopedic or chronic neurological condition. All SPs have at least one piece of simulated-medical equipment attached to their body (peg tube, IV line with bag of saline, nasal cannula with tubing attached to an oxygen tank, etc.).

Learning Objectives and Competencies

- Demonstrate the use of clinical reasoning and problem solving in use of relevant occupations, purposeful activities, and preparatory methods and educational processes that support intervention goals, are client-centered, and appropriate to the activity demands and context.
- Demonstrate the ability to grade and adapt selected activities and occupations for therapeutic intervention utilizing clinical reasoning.
- Demonstrate the ability to integrate precautions into therapeutic intervention.
- Utilize clinical reasoning to apply principles of therapeutic adaptation to assist consumers in accomplishing purposeful activities including environmental adaptations, selecting orthotics, use of adaptive equipment, proper position, and other technologies.
- Plan and set up the therapeutic environment and maintain and organize treatment areas, equipment, and supply inventory utilizing clinical reasoning.
- Utilize appropriate professional behavior and verbal and written communication skills with the client, team members, and others (fieldwork educators, supervisors) and employ therapeutic use of self during the intervention process.
- Demonstrate knowledge of the teaching-learning process and the ability to select effective instructional strategies for clients, family, and others.

Prebriefing Phase

Learner Support Activities and Simulation Information

Prior to clinic day, learners are provided with the case descriptions, chart information, any assessment tools and results, and documentation from other professionals in order to prepare for the encounter. Learners should be instructed to:

- Review
  - Relevant pathological conditions
  - Bathroom safety, fatigue management, adaptive equipment for ADL interventions
  - Relevant readings
- View instructor-approved clinical skills videos: hand washing, universal precautions, clinical skills.
- Practice clinical skills from specific clinical skills lab and review specific knowledge from coursework.
- Using the case information and documents provided, learners need to:
  - Discern pertinent information from chart review
  - Understand evaluation results related to each case and how to perform expected interventions stated to perform
  - Create a one to two page patient education handout related to one case using evidence-based health literacy guidelines; this handout will be used during the simulation encounter
  - Practice the tasks associated with each case; i.e., by the end of the session, client will:
    - → Participate in a discussion about adaptive equipment to promote independent dressing
    - → Dress themself using adaptive equipment, with assistance as necessary
    - → Verbalize at least two reasons for the adaptive equipment and total hip precautions
    - → Transfer to the wheelchair with assistance
    - → After the simulation, the learner will document the session using assigned documentation format

Simulationist, Simulation Team Including Standardized Patients, and Faculty/Lab Instructors Support Activities and Simulation Materials

Prior to *clinic day*, SP and faculty/lab facilitators training session(s):

- Conduct 3 hours of training time for each SP character.
- Training agenda includes:
  - Introductions of all team members and roles
    - → Suggest an opportunity to share previous experiences with simulation activities
  - Discuss the role of occupational therapy as a health profession and within the setting of the simulation (e.g., hospital, school, team meeting)
  - Share the background of learners: description of the curriculum, course, level of the learner, and expectations during the performance
  - Describe and provide handouts showcasing the structure for the day (e.g., start and end time, bathroom/lunch breaks)
  - Review of the cases (e.g., understanding diagnoses and associated behaviors)
  - Practice specific skills included in the simulation scenario:
    - → Transfers, hand placement
    - → Set-up and use of adaptive equipment and durable medical equipment
    - → Precautions included/expected and how the demonstration of poor safety awareness might be included to promote learner skill
    - → Specific behaviors associated with simulation scenario (e.g., impulsivity, breaking precautions, demonstration of increased pain)
    - → Common challenges and how to navigate them during the scene
  - Review feedback and assessment forms

Example Schedules of Simulation

	SP: Joe	SP: Carla	SP: Ted	SP: Martin
8:30-8:55	Students Meet in the Rehab Gym - surveys and announcements			
9:00-9:35	**Sarah**, John, Tamera, Erna	**Pete**, Tanisha, Caryn, Emily	**Lynne**, Melissa, Talia, Mark	**Kathryn**, Jessie, Todd, Erin
9:35-9:45	SP complete Student Feedback Forms and Prep; Student Therapists return to Rehab Gym			
9:45-10:20	Kathryn, **Jessie**, Todd, Erin	Sarah, **John**, Tamera, Erna	Pete, **Tanisha**, Caryn, Emily	Lynne, **Melissa**, Talia, Mark
10:20-10:30	SP complete Student Feedback Forms and Prep; Student Therapists return to Rehab Gym			
10:30-11:05	Lynne, Melissa, **Talia**, Mark	Kathryn, Jessie, **Todd**, Erin	Sarah, John, **Tamera**, Erna	Pete, Tanisha, **Caryn**, Emily
11:05-11:15	SP complete Student Feedback Forms and Prep; Student Therapists return to Rehab Gym			
11:15-11:50	Pete, Tanisha, Caryn, **Emily**	Lynne, Melissa, Talia, **Mark**	Kathryn, Jessie, Todd, **Erin**	Sarah, John, Tamera, **Erna**
11:50-12:00	SP complete Student Feedback Forms and Prep; Return Equipment to Rehab Gym			
12:00-12:15	Complete Surveys & Post-Simulation Announcements			
12:15-1:00	Debriefing with Faculty			

Figure 13-6. Example schedule of simulation (clinic day).

Scenario Organization and Support Materials

Figure 13-6 is an example of a simulation schedule involving four scenarios. Learners rotate among four SPs, each of whom has a different condition/scenario, during a half day experience. The bolded name among the group of four names represents the "student therapist" and the others are observers or "life-lines" who can assist upon request. The schedule also informs the SP when to complete the feedback form and instructs the learners when to return to the "rehab gym" for more information, to complete the program surveys, and to debrief.

Briefing Phase: Clinic Day (Simulation Day) Information

Expectations upon arrival to the simulation center and start room:

- Learners dress in appropriate attire with their name present and any materials they would like to bring to the scenario, such as case notes. Learners may bring their own notes into the clinical scenario; however, it is made clear that they are expected to interact with the SPs and complete the activities. Therefore, they are not to rely on their notes to conduct the simulation.
- When learners arrive at the simulation center, they report to a specific room that represents a rehabilitation gym.
- Once the learners arrive, the faculty simulationist can role play a nurse/rehab manager to orient the learners to the gym and the necessary components of the day such as the rehabilitation gym, location of the patient rooms, and the schedule for the day. Learners should know where equipment is located in the treatment area/room or in the rehabilitation gym, including personal protective equipment (disposable gowns, face masks, etc.).
- After this information is provided, the hard copy schedules and any other materials are provided for the learners.
- Simulation activities begin!

During the Simulation

All personnel are performing their roles:

- Lab instructors/faculty are observing the simulations in the video-viewing room
- Simulation operations technicians are managing the cameras in all rooms
- SP coordinator is supporting SPs during breaks by answering questions or refreshing equipment
- Simulationist/faculty responding to learner questions, issues, and helping students navigate through the experience
- Learners are interacting with their case-specific SPs

Just After the Learner's Simulation Performance

Learners report back to the main room for a brief congratulations! This is important so learners can recognize their achievement and begin to process the encounter. This includes:

- Sharing of general feedback about the experience and learners can share their perspectives about their experience. This is not a debriefing session; however, it does allow for some learners to diffuse their emotions, which is important (see Chapter 15 for more details).
- Completing program-specific or self-assessments are conducted and collected at this time.
- Returning of the equipment, collecting their belongings, and transitioning to the debriefing room (usually conducted in small groups using multiple rooms in the building).

Debriefing Session

This session is done with learners and lab instructors who viewed the performance.

- See Chapter 15 for instructions about debriefing.

Debriefing and Program Evaluation

This session is done with the simulation team, faculty/lab instructors involved, and SPs.

- See Chapter 16 for more information related to program evaluation.

Part 6: Designing and Implementing Simulation

Worksheet 13-1
Developing Your Simulation Activities

Date: ______________________________

Title of the simulation: ______________________________

Brief description of the simulation encounter (one to two sentences): ______________________________

____

____

Setting: ______________________________

____

Simulation modality/ies (SP, task trainers, manikin, other): ______________________________

____

Using the space following, begin to outline how your simulation could unfold. Use the following guiding questions/topics and your learning objectives and assessment ideas to help you structure the development process.

1. Name of the simulation: ______________________________
2. Course/class: ______________________________
3. Number of students: ______________________________
4. Number of instructors/faculty: ______________________________

Staging the Simulation

5. Location needed for simulation:

6. Type of simulation: task trainers, manikin, student role play, SPs (actors):

7. Do you have a simulation team that is knowledgeable about how to use simulated products, including recruiting/training actors? If No, will this impact your simulation activity?
   - ☐ Yes
   - ☐ No

8. Brief description of the simulation activity (one to two sentences).

9. What are the primary clinical skills being addressed?

(continued)

Worksheet 13-1 (continued)

Developing Your Simulation Activities

10. Draft schedule of simulation encounter:

Activity	*Student Time*	*Faculty Time*	*Standardized Patients*
Prior to Simulation			
Set up simulation activities (simulation space, training of SP or simulation staff with equipment, other activities)			
Simulation Day			
Premeeting (optional, may include preassessments)			
Simulation activity			
After simulation meeting			
Debriefing			
Simulation team/faculty post-meeting			
After Simulation			
Edits to simulation activity		Variable	
Data collection and analysis		Variable	
Thank you notes		Variable	

11. Describe the student preparation that will ensure they can meet the most expectations. Which class(es) will prepare them for this experience?

12. Describe the room that is needed for the simulation. Include materials and equipment you will need to make this activity realistic to practice (e.g., gloves, bed with clean sheets/pillows, catheters, chair for client, stool for student).

(continued)

Worksheet 13-1 (continued)
Developing Your Simulation Activities

13. Describe how many high-fidelity simulation materials will you need:
- Task trainers (body part):
- Medical equipment:
- Manikins (and if need special function):
- SPs (may consider having one extra due to sickness, SP fatigue, etc.):
- Other:

14. Describe the student's attire (dress code) and professional expectations for the simulation activity.

Creating the Scenario and Materials

(See samples in the Appendices.)

15. Describe your simulation encounter. If you have multiple activities (e.g., clients with different conditions), describe each one separately.

Case #1: Patient Name and Condition

Student Preparation

16. What materials will your students need prior to the encounter (evaluation, brief history, purpose of the encounter, orders from the physician, etc.)?

17. What learning assignments should students complete prior to the simulation encounter (patient education handout that could be incorporated into the simulation, review health conditions, etc.)?

18. What clinical skills should they practice prior to the simulation encounter (be specific)?

Simulation Preparation

19. Who do you contact to have access to the equipment? Or does the department need to buy and store the equipment?

(continued)

Worksheet 13-1 (continued)

Developing Your Simulation Activities

20. Do you know how to operate the simulation equipment or set up the medical equipment?

21. If you are using trained actors, who will recruit the actors:
    - What characteristics would be preferred: age, body composition, gender, ethnicity/racial backgrounds?
    - Describe the acting skill needed to perform simulation. Will they be passive (e.g., coma patient) or be very emotional, demonstrate physical behaviors of impairment, etc.?

Need to schedule simulation training and create materials. (See the Appendices for more information.)

Other Faculty

22. What is their availability for assisting with simulation training and implementation?

Simulation Day

23. What forms/information will the students need for the event (e.g., personal/group schedule, learning activities, last-minute changes)?

24. What forms/information will the SPs need for the event (e.g., schedules, assessments)?

25. What forms/information will the faculty/simulation team need for the event (e.g., schedules, video schedule, assessments)?

26. Will students be observing each other? Form for peer assessment (example):
    - ☐ Strength: ______________________________
    - ☐ Constructive comment: ______________________________

27. Debriefing—see Chapter 15.

Worksheet 13-2
Reflecting on Your Simulation Design in Order to Minimize Learner's Stress

Date: ____

Title of the simulation: ______________________________________

Brief description of the simulation encounter (one to two sentences): ____________________

____

____

Setting: ____

____

Simulation modality/ies (SP, task trainers, manikin, other): ____________________

____

Preparing for Your Simulation Encounter

1. In the space provided here, draw a sketch of the space in which you are planning to use for your simulation. Space includes the floor plan with the designated room(s), bathrooms, and waiting areas labeled.

2. List all of your materials, equipment, and supplies needed for each room. Include any signage that should be created and location for posting in the hallways and doors. Consider copying this list onto another document and printing it for each simulation room. Having the supply list on each door during set-up can decrease set-up time and increase communication among team members.

3. In the space here, draw a sketch of how each room(s) should be set up. Having this layout for other team members can decrease your set-up time.

4. List the strategies for mitigating student stress that will be incorporated into this simulation.

14

Recruit, Screen, and Train Standardized Patients

Audrey L. Zapletal, OTD, OTR/L, CLA
Chalia Bellis, MS, OTR/L
Madeleine Clements, MS, OTR/L

Learning Objectives

1. Discuss the strategies for recruiting, screening, and training standardized patients (SPs) in health care education.
2. Create SP training session using best practice guidelines.

Kern's Model of Program Development

The content in this chapter articulates Step 5 of Kern's Model: Implementation. Information in this chapter explains the specific simulation modality of SPs. This articulates with how to identify and obtain the resources needed for the simulation program.

Zapletal, A. L., Baird, J. M., Van Oss, T., Hoppe, M. M., Prast, J. E., & Herge, E. A. *Clinical Simulation for Health Care Professionals* (pp. 169-174).

One of the most common challenges in establishing a simulation program is financing, recruiting and training the SPs (Calhoun et al., 2008). However, investing time and money into the hiring of SPs is necessary for quality assurance (Adamo, 2003; Pascucci et al., 2014). Evidence suggests that experienced actors may be more likely to offer thoughtful feedback to students following encounters and may be more likely to participate in future simulations (Pascucci et al., 2014); however, trained nonhealth professionals and laypeople are just as valuable and sometimes have more consistent availability. The Association of Standardized Patient Educators developed best practice guidelines to facilitate the professional and safe use of SPs in simulation encounters (2017). In addition, this organization provides professional development for those interested in learning more.

Recruitment

Recruitment is fundamental to ensuring a quality SP program. For large scale programming, the goal is to secure a blend of professionally-trained actors and nonprofessionally-trained actors who exhibit a variety of ages, gender identities, ethnicities, religious beliefs, lifestyles, and professional/personal backgrounds. Recruitment venues can include a range of sources such as professional agencies, alumni, and retired health professionals, and may impact the financial compensation required (Bosek et al., 2007; Pascucci et al., 2014). Investing resources, including time and money, into the recruitment process ensures a high quality simulation (Adamo, 2003; Pascucci et al., 2014).

As part of the recruitment process, it is critical to fully explain the experience of being an SP upfront in order to ensure commitment to the experience (Ker et al., 2005). For example, potential SPs need to understand the purpose of the role and the importance of being punctual to the experience; this can prevent unnecessary administrative challenges such as the cost to find a replacement SP or the time to rearrange schedules (Ker et al., 2005; Pascucci et al., 2014). In addition, SPs should be aware of specific wardrobe requirements and/or if they will be asked to remove clothing during the encounter and how their dignity will be preserved. Overall, certain populations (e.g., individuals 20 to 50 years of age) may be more challenging to recruit and this should be taken into account when preparing scenarios (Cleland et al., 2009). See the following section for further details about the specific venues for recruitment that are commonly employed.

Venues for Recruitment

- *General Public:* Advertise in local newspapers or online to recruit from the general public (Ker et al., 2005). Brochures can also be left at public places such as libraries and coffee shops (Cleland et al., 2009).
- *Professionally Trained Actors:* Actors can serve as an excellent source of SPs (Pascucci et al., 2014). Amateur dramatic groups from the community playhouse or elsewhere provide reliable SPs (Cleland et al., 2009). Furthermore, the use of actors can increase the fidelity of the experience because of their advanced training (Mavis et al., 2006).
- *Theater Students:* Some academic institutions offer credit courses specifically designed to train undergraduate or graduate theater students as SPs. Course topics may include developing empathy, believability, verbal communication, and nonverbal communication. These programs offer theater students job opportunities/skills while simultaneously producing a pool of reliable SPs (Swift & Stosberg, 2015).
- *Actual or Former Patients:* Real patients can be recruited as SPs through outpatient appointments and through general practice (Ker et al., 2005). When recruiting individuals with any condition, mental energy and physicality must be considered to ensure capacity to sustain the role for longer durations and for all required learners.
- *Word of Mouth:* Current SPs can also recruit future SPs through word of mouth (Cleland et al., 2009).
- *Standardized Patient Bank:* Once an SP program has been established, the best practice for recruiting new SPs is to recruit from an already established bank (Cleland et al., 2009; Ker et al., 2005). This promotes efficiency as past encounters can be tracked through the bank and future encounters can be based off of past experiences (Ker et al., 2005). In addition, schools with multiple departments

utilizing SPs can centralize the program through the bank to allow for a variety of experiences (Adamo, 2003). Retention is critical to the efficacy of the bank. In order to promote consistent participation, Cleland et al. (2009) recommend finding ways to recognize the efforts of the SPs such as with receptions, thank you cards, and certificates of recognition.

Tips for Recruitment

- Consider recruiting 1.5 to 2 months in advance.
- Hold auditions or screening for the specific role(s) at least 1 week ahead of the simulation.
- Hire at least one additional SP to help ensure smooth operations on the day of the encounter in the event that an SP has an unforeseen conflict or illness (Wallace, 2006).

Screening

After recruiting potential SPs, it is important to screen candidates for certain qualities or attributes. This process should be aimed at maximizing students' educational gains while protecting their safety (Ker et al., 2005.) The screening process may include an interview, an online questionnaire, a background check, or a drug screen depending on your institution (Cleland et al., 2009; Hansel, 2013; Ker et al., 2005). Members of the screening team may include a program director and a trainer/coordinator, as well as experienced SPs and faculty directly involved in the simulation encounter (Hansel, 2013).

Screening Process

The screening process may include several steps from submitting an intake form with medical history to completing an online quiz (Cleland et al., 2009; Husson & Zulkosky, 2014). In-person and telephone interviews are other methods to ensure the applicant demonstrates the appropriate characteristics for the position (Hansel, 2013; Ker et al., 2005). During the interview process, the applicant should share their interest in being an SP, as well as the nature of their previous health care experiences (Cleland et al., 2009; Husson & Zulkosky, 2014). This information can help determine if their interest is genuine (see section Desired Characteristics for more information). This is also an opportunity for the staff to help clarify the role. Additionally, applicants should be given the opportunity to view a training session so they understand what to expect should they be hired as an SP (Cleland et al., 2009).

A group interview (no more than 10 people per group) is an efficient method for screening multiple candidates and providing an opportunity to experience a training session. The training session includes a clinical case as well as an evaluation of the candidate's skill in giving reflective, individualized feedback (Hansel, 2013). During the "training session," the hiring team (e.g., the SP coordinator and involved faculty) observes verbal and nonverbal interactions as well as acting skills, this shows retention of clinical scenarios.

Before hiring candidates the team provides detailed information about the position, including a description of the activity and an anticipated time commitment (Cleland et al., 2009; Husson & Zulkosky, 2014). It may be important to have a trial period to allow both the recruiters and SPs the option to dissolve the agreement more easily should problems arise (Cleland et al., 2009). Table 14-1 outlines important considerations for the interview and screening process.

Desired Characteristics

In order to standardize hiring decisions, the interviewer may choose to use a checklist when evaluating the presence of positive or negative characteristics (Hansel, 2013). The checklist can include positive characteristics, such as reliability, conscientiousness, trustworthiness, and punctuality, in addition to role-related characteristics such as believability, accurate recollection, and adaptability (Cleland et al., 2009; Liao et al., 2015; Pascucci et al., 2014; Wallace, 2006). Additionally, the ideal candidate should be interested in their character, inquisitive, passionate about taking part in the educational process, highly

Table 14-1. The Interview and Screening Process

Example Interview and Screening Session	
Part 1	Logistics → Benefits of position, financial compensation, purpose of SP
Part 2	Warm-up activity → Retention and recall games, personality, participants' flexibility
Part 3	Sample clinical scenario → With guiding checklist of behaviors
Part 4	Closing → Reminders of the time/day of performance, dress code, etc.

Adapted from Wallace, 2007 and Wilson and Rockstraw, 2012.

communicative, reflective, and detail-oriented when providing feedback (Liao et al., 2015; Pascucci et al., 2014; Wallace, 2006). If the case has already been developed, recruiters should attempt to match the characteristics (e.g., ethnicity, age, gender) of the actor to the case as much as possible (Wallace, 2006). It may be necessary to modify characteristics of the case to better match the SP (e.g., such as gender identity, or changing a name from Ernie to Ernestine). If any element of the SP is changed throughout the process, be sure to inform the learners prior to the encounter.

In addition to screening for desired characteristics, the interviewer should note characteristics or attitudes that could provide students with negative experiences. For instance, a potential SP should be excluded if they hold negative views of health care professionals based on past experiences (Pololi, 1995). Students early in their education may be especially vulnerable as they have not yet built their confidence as clinicians (Ker et al., 2005). Additionally, potential SPs should be excluded if they appear susceptible to "character shading," in which the actor/SP begins to embellish the clinical scenario to the point of de-standardization (Hargraves, 2011). This usually happens when the actor/SP is bored or fatigued.

Training

Importance

Training is an integral component of the SP experience, contributing greatly to the educational value and fidelity of the encounter (Cleland et al., 2009; Lewis et al., 2017; Liao et al., 2015). With consistent and thorough training, SPs can provide reliable and valid assessment of student learning (MacLean et al., 2018). Proper training will ultimately ensure each student is presented with the same or comparable experiences (Boursicot & Roberts, 2005; Lewis et al., 2017).

Best Practices

Developing and maintaining an SP database provides the simulationist with detailed information about the SP's performance abilities both efficiently and effectively (Ker et al., 2005). Acting skills can be divided into three categories, which can be helpful for casting across simulation programs (Hargraves, 2011):

1. SP is able to perform verse body movements and gestures.
2. SP is able to communicate and respond to simple learner interactions and demonstrate appropriate physical and gross motor types of movements.
3. SP is able to memorize complicated scripts, demonstrate complex body movements over long periods of time accurately and consistently, incorporate emotions into the clinical scenario, and respond to learners appropriately.

Training SPs can be a costly endeavor, therefore retaining reliable, trained, and committed SPs can lessen the costs of future encounters (Keiser & Turkelson, 2017; Zhang et al., 2018). The timeline for training varies based on the nature of the encounter, but a recommended protocol for basic training is four 2-hour sessions (Ker et al., 2005). The first block should include observing an experienced SP and discussing observations (Ker et al., 2005). It may also be prudent to include information on policies and procedures during this time in addition to expectations regarding reliability and punctuality (Keiser & Turkelson, 2017). Future blocks should give the SP the opportunity to practice (Keiser & Turkelson, 2017; Ker et al., 2005). For example, the second block can provide them with an opportunity to try out a script with a clinician and the third block can provide a video analysis of the SP's encounter. The final block should simulate a true encounter and can include the SP attempting a script with a few students and receiving feedback (Ker et al., 2005). Piloting the case with the SPs involved is worthwhile time spent, answering their questions, crafting feedback scripts, and developing their confidence as well.

Training for specific encounters will vary greatly depending on the nature of the encounter (Boursicot & Roberts, 2005). However, generally, the SP should be sent the scenarios in advance to allow for ample practice time (Boursicot & Roberts, 2005). They may also benefit from time spent practicing together in the presence of a clinician/faculty simulationist in order to collaborate and, ultimately, effectively portray their role (Boursicot & Roberts, 2005). Time spent in structured training includes ensuring accuracy in role portrayal, communicating feedback and developing inter-rater reliability among SPs, and an opportunity to share programmatic feedback with the faculty/simulations (Lewis et al., 2017; Zhang et al., 2018).

Other Considerations

Adolescent Standardized Patients

Over the last decade, institutions have started recruiting SPs as young as 7 years old (Cleland et al., 2009) with the goal of improving clinical competence and confidence working with adolescent patients (Blake et al., 2000; Macdonald et al., 2014). Indeed, Blake et al. (2000) found that medical students' psychosocial interviewing skills improved significantly following feedback from an adolescent SP and their parent, a phenomenon they suggest may not have occurred had the parent alone provided feedback. While an adult could portray an adolescent SP, the portrayal is not immersive or believable, detracting from the experience and educational gains associated with the experience (Blake et al., 2000; Macdonald et al., 2014). To increase believability during the encounter, the SP's age should closely match the case they are portraying (within 2 to 3 years; Cleland et al., 2009).

However, as children are a vulnerable population, their safety and well-being is a priority and the child's parents/school should be fully involved during the recruitment and screening process. Blake et al. (2006) suggested conducting an information session with candidates and their parents to answer questions about the process and obtain consent and assent. During this time, young SPs should also be informed that they can leave at any time should they become uncomfortable (Blake et al., 2006).

Additionally, it is important to consider whether a role could be psychologically stressful to the young SP, causing lower mood and/or higher anxiety (Blake et al., 2006). Brown et al. (2005) determined that children as young as 9 years old were capable of stepping into psychiatric roles, and Blake at al. (2006) reported no adverse events from adolescent females ages 13 to 15 portraying risk-taking roles (e.g., reported drug use and sexual activity).

Blake at al. (2006) reported that the adolescent SPs were most concerned about forgetting their character during the encounter. Therefore, when training young SPs to play a role and provide feedback, consider using visual aids such as mind-maps to enhance memory (Blake et al., 2006).

Cultural Diversity

Cultural competency is an important part of health care education. Simulation may be used to increase students' cultural competency. However, such programs are few and far between, and culturally diverse SPs are largely underrepresented (Livesay et al., 2017). Therefore, recruiting and retaining SPs must be intentional and inclusive of a wide array of ethnicities, disabilities, languages, sexual identities, gender identities, and religions (Livesay et al., 2017). Livesay et al. (2017) suggests adopting an intersectionality framework to represent the full spectrum of diversity and to move beyond stereotyping.

Training SPs should include aspects of cultural humilty and competemility in addition to general information about simulation and the role of the SP (Campinha-Bacote, 2018; Livesay et al., 2017). SPs should also receive opportunities to practice providing feedback aimed at enhancing cultural humility, either through role play or after watching "trigger videos" that portray culturally insensitive interactions (Livesay et al., 2017).

References

Adamo, G. (2003). Simulated and standardized patients in OSCEs: Achievements and challenges 1992-2003. *Medical Teacher, 25*(3), 262-270. https://doi.org/10.1080/0142159031000100300

Blake, K. D., Gusella, J., Greaven, S., & Wakefield, S. (2006). The risks and benefits of being a young female adolescent standardised patient. *Medical Education, 40*(1), 26-35. https://doi.org/10.1111/j.1365-2929.2005.02343.x

Blake, K. D., Mann, K., Kaufman, D., & Kappelman, M. (2000). Learning adolescent psychosocial interviewing using simulated patients. *Academic Medicine, 75*(10), 556-558. https://doi.org/10.1097/00001888-200010001-00018

Bosek, M. S., Li, S., & Hicks, F. D. (2007). Working with standardized patients: A primer. *International Journal of Nursing Education Scholarship, 4,* Article 16. https://doi.org/10.2202/1548-923X.1437

Boursicot, K., & Roberts, T. (2005). How to set up an OSCE. *The Clinical Teacher, 2*(1), 16-20. https://doi.org/10.1111/j.1743-498X.2005.00053.x

Brown, R., Doonan, S., & Shellenberger, S. (2005). Using children as simulated patients in communication training for residents and medical students: A pilot program. *Academic Medicine, 80*(12), 1114-1120. https://doi.org/10.1097/00001888-200512000-00010

Calhoun, B. C., Vrbin, C. M., & Grzybicki, D. M. (2008). The use of standardized patients in the training and evaluation of physician assistant students. *The Journal of Physician Assistant Education, 19*(1), 18-23. Retrieved from https://journals.lww.com/jpae/pages/default.aspx

Campinha-Bacote, J. (2018). Cultural competemility: A paradigm shift in the cultural competence versus cultural humility debate—Part I. *The Online Journal of Nursing, 24*(1). https://doi.org/10.3912/OJIN.Vol24No01PPT20

Cleland, J. A., Abe, K., & Rethans, J. J. (2009). The use of simulated patients in medical education: AMEE Guide No 42. *Medical Teacher, 31*(6), 477-486. https://doi.org/10.1080/01421590903002821

Hansel, A. (2013). Program innovations abstract professionalizing the simulated participant recruitment and hiring process (Submission #1029). *Simulation in Healthcare, 8*(6), 443. https://doi.org/10.1097/01.SIH.0000441434.42025.a5

Hargraves, R. (2011). Standardized patient training. In L. Wilson & L. Rockstraw (Eds.), *Human simulation for nursing and health professions* (pp. 37-44). Springer Publishing Company, LLC.

Husson, N., & Zulkosky, K. D. (2014). Recruiting and training volunteer standardized patients in the NCSBN national simulation study. *Clinical Simulation in Nursing, 10*(9), 487-489. https://doi.org/10.1016/j.ecns.2014.05.001

Keiser, M. M., & Turkelson, C. (2017). Using students as standardized patients: Development, implementation, and evaluation of a standardized patient training program. *Clinical Simulation in Nursing, 13*(7), 321-330. https://doi.org/10.1016/j.ecns.2017.05.008

Ker, J. S., Dowie, A., Dowell, J., Dewar, G., Dent, J. A., Ramsay, J., Benvie, S., Bracher, L., & Jackson, C. (2005). Twelve tips for developing and maintaining a simulated patient bank. *Medical Teacher, 27*(1), 4-9. https://doi.org/10.1080/01421590400004882

Lewis, K., Bohnert, C., Gammon, W., Holzer, H., Lyman, L., Smith, C., Thompson, T., Wallace, A., & Gilva McConvey, G. (2017). The Association of Standardized Patient Educators (ASPE) Standards of Best Practice (SOBP). *Advances in Simulation, 2*(10). http://dx.doi.org/10.1186/s41077-017-0043-4

Liao, C.-S., Kao, S.-P., Liang, S.-Y., & Hsieh, M.-C. (2015). Training actors as standardized patients. *Tzu Chi Medical Journal, 27*(2), 96-97. https://doi.org/10.1080/0142159040000488210.1016/j.tcmj.2015.04.001

Livesay, K., Lau, P., McNair, R., & Chiminello, C. (2017). The culturally and linguistically diverse SPs' evaluation of simulation experience. *Clinical Simulation in Nursing, 13*(5), 228-237. https://doi.org/10.1016/j.ecns.2017.01.004

Macdonald, M., MacCuspie, J., Mann, K., & Blake, K. (2014). Improving medical student's confidence regarding adolescent interviewing. *Pediatrics & Therapeutics,* 4(4). https://doi.org/10.4172/2161-0665.1000218

MacLean, S., Geddes, F., Kelly, M., & Della, P. (2018). Simulated patient training: Using inter-rater reliability to evaluate simulated patient consistency in nursing education. *Nurse Education Today, 62,* 85-90. https://doi.org/10.1016/j.nedt.2017.12.024

Mavis, B., Turner, J., Lovell, K., & Wagner, D. (2006). Faculty, students, and actors as standardized patients: Expanding opportunities for performance assessment. *Teaching and Learning in Medicine, 18*(2), 130-136. https://doi.org/10.1207/s15328015tlm1802_7

Pascucci, R. C., Weinstock, P. H., O'Connor, B. E., Fancy, K. M., & Meyer, E. C. (2014). Integrating actors into a simulation program: A primer. *Simulation in Healthcare: Journal of the Society for Simulation in Healthcare,* 9(2), 120-126. https://doi.org/10.1097/SIH.0b013e3182a3ded7

Pololi, L. H. (1995). Standardised patients: As we evaluate, so shall we reap. *The Lancet, 345*(8955), 966-968. https://doi.org/10.1016/S0140-6736(95)90706-8

Swift, M. C., & Stosberg, T. (2015). Interprofessional simulation and education: Physical therapy, nursing, and theatre faculty work together to develop a standardized patient program. *Nursing Education Perspectives, 36*(6), 412-413. https://doi.org/10.5480/15-1652

Wallace, P. (2006). *Coaching standardized patients: For use in the assessment of clinical competence.* Springer Publishing Company.

Wilson, L. & Rockstraw, L. (2012). *Human simulation for nursing and health professions.* Springer Publishing Company.

Zhang, S., Soreide, K., Kelling, S., & Bostwick, J. (2018). Quality assurance processes for standardized patient programs. *Currents in Pharmacy Teaching, and Learning,10*(4),523-528. https://doi.org/10.1016/j.cptl.2017.12.014

Section VI

Kern's Model Step 6
Evaluation and Feedback

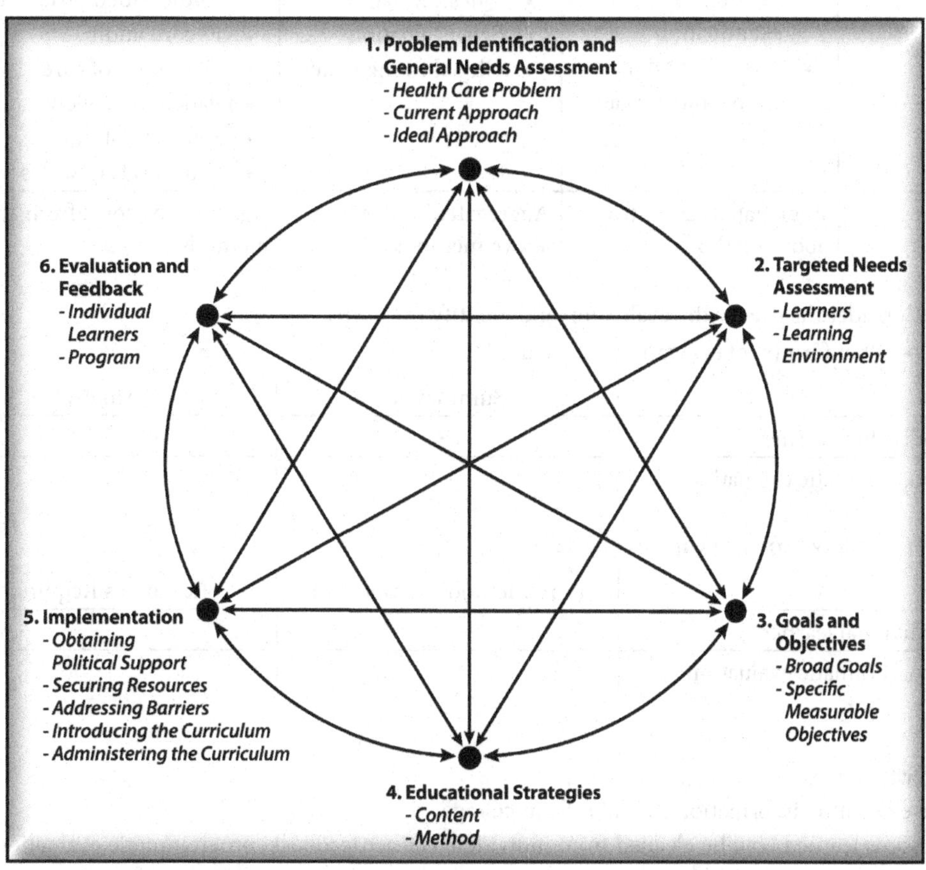

- The purpose of this step is to determine if goals and objectives were met.
- Evaluation includes individual assessment and overall program evaluation.
- This step will provide information to improve the curriculum/program and assess individual learner achievement.
- Determine the type and method of collecting data, as well as the resources required.
- Evaluation questions and measurement methods must match the learner objectives and be feasible.
- Obtaining outcome measures can satisfy accreditation requirements and garner support for upcoming changes.

- Consider whether the learner evaluations will be formative (i.e., during or within instruction) or summative (i.e., following, to sum up results).
- Ideally, assessors use multiple measurement methods to evaluate learner and program outcomes.

- Evaluation methods:
  - Assess the achievement of objectives and continuous improvement.

	Measurement Methods for Assessing ***Cognitive Objectives/Knowledge***	Measurement Methods for Assessing ***Affective Objectives/Attitude***	Measurement Methods for Assessing ***Psychomotor Objectives/Skills and Behaviors***
Learner	• Oral examination • Written examination • Case discussion • Global rating scale	• Learner interview • Questionnaire • Self-evaluation • Global rating scales	• Direct observation • Audio/video observation • Record audit • Outcomes of care • Patient interview • Self-evaluation • Global rating scales
Program	Aggregated scores from above methods	Aggregated scores from above methods	Aggregated scores from above methods

  - Consider the use for the evaluation and identify the users.

    → What form(s) of evaluation will be used?

	Summative	Formative
Individual learner		
Programmatic evaluation		

    → What type of data will be collected?

	Type/Method of Evaluation	Resources Required
Individual learner		
Programmatic evaluation		

After this step:

- The evaluation information should inform change.
- "Lessons learned" can be gleaned from individual learner feedback, programmatic evaluations, and informal observation.
- Management of change, resource management, and sustaining progress should be considered.

Suggested Readings

Farnan, J., & Schindler, N. (2013). *Curriculum development and evaluation guide resident as teacher: A mutually beneficial arrangement APPD/COMSEP pre course 2013.* Retrieved from: https://www.appd.org/meetings/2013SpringPresentations/PCWS1Handout.pdf

Kern, D. E. (2014). *Curriculum development: An essential educational skill, a public trust, a form of scholarship, an opportunity for organizational change.* Weill Cornell College of Medicine, Qatar. Retrieved from: https://dnnyqetna.blob.core.windows.net/portals/15/Six-Step%20Approach%20to%20Curriculum%20Development.pdf?sr=b&si=DNNFileManagerPolicy&sig=9sAOUX/lzfZQsN6QKLOpWJ46YLRuXmQwOghR7ptxnFw=

Khamis, N. N., Satava, R. M., Alnassar, S. A., & Kern, D. E. (2016). A stepwise model for simulation-based curriculum development for clinical skills, a modification of the six-step approach. *Surgical Endoscopy,* 279-287. https://doi.org/10.1007/s00464-015-4206x

15

Debriefing

Developing the Debriefing Session

Joanne M. Baird, PhD, OTR/L, CHSE, FAOTA
Tracy Van Oss, DHSc, MPH, OTR/L, FAOTA, CHSE

Learning Objectives

1. Define debriefing and describe its importance to simulation education.
2. Examine characteristics of effective debriefing.
3. Recognize commonly used debriefing methods.
4. Describe various methods for self-reflection that promote optimal learning outcomes.

Kern's Model of Program Development

The content in this chapter articulates Step 6 of Kern's Model: Evaluation and Feedback. Information in this chapter describes methods to help learners determine if they met individual simulation goals and objectives. This information supports individual assessment and learner evaluation.

Zapletal, A. L., Baird, J. M., Van Oss, T., Hoppe, M. M., Prast, J. E., & Herge, E. A. *Clinical Simulation for Health Care Professionals* (pp. 177-196).

Debriefing Versus Feedback: Is There a Difference?

Debriefing is a semi-structured conversation based on guided reflection (Lopreiato et al., 2016). The goal of debriefing is to have the learner identify areas in need of reinforcement and areas in need of improvement. Often in simulation, much of the learning occurs during the debriefing. Debriefing itself is a teaching strategy and serves many purposes, including helping learners master skills learned and organizing information for future application (Cantrell, 2008; Johnson-Russel & Bailey, 2010). Debriefing is considered a teaching strategy and an essential part of simulation directly related to learning objectives (Fanning & Gaba, 2007; see Chapter 6 for more information about learning objectives). Debriefing is a critical component of simulation education, requiring the active participation of learners.

Debriefing is not the same as feedback. While debriefing is interactive and based on the bidirectional flow of conversation using guided reflection, feedback is information given to the learner regarding their performance (Cheng et al., 2017; Voyer & Hatala, 2015). Often this information is designed to address how the learner's performance can be improved to achieve benchmark standards (Archer, 2010). Feedback should occur throughout the simulation experience as the learner experiences the consequences of his actions. Remember that feedback does not have to be overt, verbal, or through a facilitator. Feedback should provide information for future improvement and may include praise about what should be continued or repeated. Praise based on ego-involvement and feedback about performance that does not move learning forward should be avoided.

Chang et al. (2014) pointed out that debriefing should reflect the simulation activities and include discussion or assessment of:

- Events that occurred
- Decisions that were made
- Actions that were taken
- Consequences for choices
- Possible alternatives
- Suggestions to modify behavior/improve performance
- Cognitive, affective, and psychomotor skills demonstrated

Debriefing is used to enhance learning, heighten self-confidence, increase understanding, promote transfer of knowledge to the clinical setting, and identify best practice. By doing so, debriefing promotes safe quality patient care and lifelong learning (INACSL Standards Committee, 2021). Therefore an effective debriefing session:

- Requires expert facilitation
- Recognizes and process all aspects of the simulation experience: emotional, cognitive, and psychomotor
- Aims to close the gap between learner knowledge and skills
- Explains, analyzes, and synthesizes information

Debriefing Logistics: How It Is Done

Debriefing can be done either within the simulation by the facilitator or after the simulation by the facilitator or even by the learners themselves (Fanning & Gaba, 2007). The debriefing facilitator has a critical role, one that even experienced simulation educators find challenging (Voyer & Hatala, 2015). The role of the facilitator is to guide the conversation to ensure that learning objectives are discussed, and that discussion remains on track and progresses. A facilitator may also serve as a subject matter expert if experienced in the simulated area, or if they have expertise or training.

Self-guided debriefing occurs when participants facilitate the debriefing themselves. This type of debriefing happens after, not during, the simulation. The facilitator can be an external "co-learner" who can facilitate the debriefing for those directly involved in the simulation. When self-guided debriefing is done, some type of cognitive support, such as teamwork evaluation forms or cue cards, is used for structure and to ensure that the simulation learning objectives are addressed. Evidence suggests that self-guided peer debriefing is as effective as facilitator-led debriefing for behavioral skills training (Voyer & Hatala, 2015).

If debriefing occurs during the simulation, "micro-" or "stop-action" debriefing techniques can be used. In this method, the facilitator stops participants as errors are noted. Facilitation of reflective learning is the aim of the discussion, and then the simulation is paused and/or rewound just prior to the error so that the learner has an opportunity to try again. Evidence suggests that this pause/rewind/try again format is effective for deliberate practice of specific skills, but may not be effective with retention of these manual skills (Eppich et al., 2015; Xeroulis et al., 2007). In general, debriefing that occurs after the simulation appears more effective than debriefing done during simulation (Dufrene & Young, 2014; Levett-Jones & Lapkin, 2012).

Video-assisted debriefing is another method used in simulation. In this method, simulations are recorded and video playback is incorporated during debriefing by the facilitator. Video-assisted debriefing can be effective to reinforce hands-on clinical skills (Chronister & Brown, 2012). Many studies indicate that it is not as effective as once thought, with recent research suggesting that facilitator-only debriefing is as effective for long-term learning as facilitator and video-assisted debriefing in achieving learning outcomes (Levett-Jones & Lapkin, 2012, 2014; Lorello et al., 2014; Reed et al., 2013).

Best Practice: Essential Debriefing Elements

There are several steps to include in a simulation to assure the success of a debriefing session. For example, before debriefing it is necessary to ensure the psychological safety of the learner. To promote reflective learning, the debriefing environment must not threaten the learner or make them feel defensive or exposed (Decker et al., 2013; Dreifuerst, 2012; Rudolph et al., 2014). There are several methods to promote psychological safety, including: clarity related to simulation goals, boundaries, and the expectations of and from the learner; use of a fiction contract (see Chapters 3 and 8); and respect for the learner (Rudolph et al., 2014). For example, expectations typically include verbal confidentiality agreements and some institutions or simulation centers require a signed confidentiality agreement. See Figure 15-1 and Table 15-1 for specific examples of these methods.

Additional methods to promote positive learning environments include defining a debriefing stance and basic assumptions prior to engaging in the debriefing (i.e., that all participants offer relevant, objective feedback related to improving performance on the simulation learning objectives). This also includes establishing rules for debriefing so that learners know what to expect (Sawyer et al., 2016).

Debriefing should be done as close to the time of the simulation as feasible with sufficient time allotted; recommendations for debriefing times vary but can be up to equal to the time of simulation or more. Immediate debriefing positively influences learner knowledge and confidence (Hall & Tori, 2017; Dufrene & Young, 2014; Levett-Jones & Lapkin, 2012). During the debriefing, all participants should be involved; this may include observers, note-takers, standardized patients, students, professionals, and faculty (Sawyer et al., 2016). The debriefer should have directly observed the simulation and should have formal debriefing training (Decker et al., 2013; Dufrene & Young, 2014; Edgecombe et al., 2013). Even the debriefing environment should be considered. Generally, unless additional demonstration using equipment is needed, debriefing after the simulation is best done in a different room to allow learners to refocus.

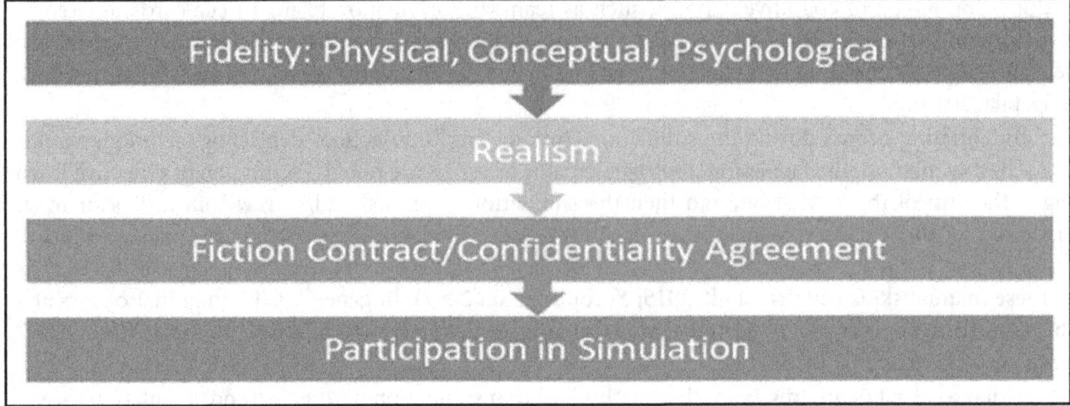

Figure 15-1. Building blocks for success: considerations for psychological safety and reflective learning. (Adapted from Rudolph et al., 2014.)

Table 15-1. Methods to Promote Learning Through Psychological Safety

Learners are explicitly made aware of the following elements (through written materials, discussion, electronic resources, demonstration, and explanation):

Course Objectives	If there will be observers	Expected professional behaviors	Length of simulation
Expected Learning Outcomes	Pre- and postsimulation activities	How to manage confidentiality	If/when breaks are scheduled
Goals of Simulation	Assessment method and instrument	The value of their perspective	The use of social media and electronic devices
Properties of Equipment	How simulation performance will influence progress in program/course	The role of the instructor to create an engaging environment	The instructors' interest in promoting learning

Adapted from Rudolph et al., 2014.

Debriefing Models: Which Is Best?

There are many models of debriefing and limited rigorous comparative research has not indicated that a single method is superior to another method (Decker et al., 2013; Dreifuerst, 2012; Hall & Tori, 2017). While there are many debriefing formats to choose from, during the debriefing the following elements should be present (Sawyer et al., 2016):

- Use a structured framework to recapitulation of key events of the simulation that establish a shared mental model (Decker et al., 2013; Edgecombe et al., 2013)
- Focus on key learning objectives (Decker et al., 2013; Rudolph et al., 2008)
- Aim to move the learner through the phases of debriefing: reaction, analysis, and summarization/planning (Hall & Tori, 2017)

A sample of some specific debriefing formats are provided later in this chapter.

Useful Tips

- *Debriefer must be trained not to provide feedback or over talk*
- *Debrief immediately after the simulation*
- *Smaller groups may enhance participation*
- *Use guided questions or scripts to facilitate the process for group; can make the focus specific for individual learners*
- *Be comfortable facilitating a discussion*
- *Focus on reflection of learning objectives*
- *Redirect as needed, remain on task*
- *Encourage responses when there are none or they are limited*
- *Use open-ended questions and silence to promote reflection*

Best Practice: Effective Debriefing and Feedback

To ensure effectiveness, debriefing should include an assessment component. The assessment should include the effectiveness of the debrief facilitator as well as the debriefing experience itself. The facilitator's effectiveness should be assessed using multiple methods, including learner input, practice, and formal assessment instruments (Cheng et al., 2017; Decker et al., 2013; Hall & Tori, 2017). A few formal assessment instruments are listed here (see Chapter 7 for additional information on assessments):

- Debriefing Experience Scale (Reed, 2012)
- Debriefing Assessment of Simulation in Healthcare (DASH; Brett-Fleegler et al., 2012)
- The Objective Structured Assessment of Debriefing (OSAD; Arora et al., 2012)
- TeamGAINS (Kolbe et al., 2013)

These criteria-based assessments offer debriefing facilitators clear descriptions of competency areas and highlight the differences between perceived and actual performance, providing a valuable tool for professional development (Cheng et al., 2017).

Reflection

Debriefing is a major component of simulation and should occur with each and every encounter. Unfortunately, sometimes logistically a full debriefing does not occur. If this is the case, reflection can be used as an alternative to foster learning. Writing reflections and providing feedback from the reviewer can lead to significant gains in personal growth (Sanders et al., 2015). The purpose of the reflection exercise is to allow the learner to gain insight about personal strengths and areas for improvement.

Reflection may occur as part of a group, in pairs or alone. There are a plethora of methods for learners to participate in reflection exercises. Katznelson (2014) described reflective functioning when a person reflects on experiences, then will draw an inference on own behavior from these reflections. Those inferences are then used to construct and develop a representation of their own self. Self-reflective reasoning can affect self-concept development and identity (Dishon et al., 2017).

Some self-reflection methods may include:

- Video review
- Peer debriefing
- Guided self-reflection
- Worksheets

In addition to considering what type of reflection method to use, it is also important to consider where the reflection will take place. Reflection may be done anywhere, pending the learner's preference and the structure of the simulation. Individual reflection may occur while the learner is alone in a quiet nondistracting environment or with background noise. Reflection may be done with others in a common area or part of a social gathering over a meal.

It is imperative to deliberately include reflection when planning the simulation, especially if debriefing may not be a part of the experience. The timing of the reflection can have a strong impact on the learner. Reflection can occur before the simulation activity to help the learner imagine what to expect and provide mental practice, or the reflection can be part of the actual simulation experience to help the learner ponder the process or the outcome. Keeping track of the time spent on reflection can be a good strategy for faculty to assess if the desired outcomes were achieved, or if other strategies need to be implemented for future assignments.

Reflection can be done either in writing or orally. Whether written or oral, a reflection can be completed by individual students privately or done in a group setting, and can be led by a preceptor as a guided reflection. With any written reflection it is important for instructors to provide written feedback. It is beneficial for students to go beyond the surface in responses and respond "why" for more in-depth responses. Responses can begin orally and be completed as a written assignment to allow students some time to respond thoughtfully and with introspection.

Self-reflection can be a powerful tool to allow an individual the ability to portray personal perception of performance rather than an external perspective. It can be used for insightful thinking and learning. Using reflection as part of a clinical simulation experience can enhance the student outcome by allowing time to ponder some specific written or oral questions. Start by coming up with general questions and include questions specific to roles played or how it felt to be a client. After participating in a simulation encounter have each student write a SOAP or narrative note pertaining to the session and a one-page reflection of the session.

Conclusion

It is vital to plan and prepare for debriefing for optimal learning to occur following a simulation experience. Debriefing can solidify the established learning objectives and outcomes created for students. Deliberate debriefing can allow students to share insight on one or many of the skills acquired. The use of reflection can also foster personal growth.

Worksheet 15-1
Debriefing

Guided reflection time: ______ minutes
Write a list of questions you would ask the learner based on the simulation encounter linked to the learning objectives.

General Debriefing Example

The following questions are general debriefing questions not specific to a format that could be used during facilitation:

- How did perceptions of roles change from beginning to end of activity?
- How did you feel throughout the simulation?
- What do you feel went well?
- What do you feel did not go well?
- Describe the objectives you were able to achieve.
- What do you feel you got out of the experience?
- What are the take-home points of the simulation?
- What do you plan to incorporate into your practice?

Specific Debriefing Example

The following questions are specific to a simulation role and can be used to facilitate discussion during a debriefing.
Questions directed to those portraying a patient/client:

- What was your initial reaction to the professionals coming into your room?
- Discuss what it was like being a patient in this environment?
- What did you learn?

Questions directed to those portraying a significant other/family member:

- Describe what you were thinking during the visit.
- Describe your perception of the visit from your initial reaction to the end.
- What did you learn?

Questions directed to those portraying a health care professional:

- What were your initial thoughts and reactions when entering the room?
- What did you observe about the environment?
- What was your thought process for the assessment and interventions you provided?
- If you were able to do this again, what would you do differently?
- What did you do that went well?
- What did you learn?

The following are examples of debriefing models.

(continued)

Worksheet 15-1 (continued)
Debriefing

Model 15-1.

Component Areas	Excellent (92% to 100%)	Above Average (85% to 91%)	Average (83% to 84%)	Needs Improvement (82% or below)	Total
Reflective Analysis of Performance (20 points)	Self-analysis of clinical simulation includes completed rubric with comprehensive detailed qualitative comments and numeric score for each performance area. Student identifies three key learnings from experience and opportunities for change with future client interactions.	Self-analysis of clinical simulation includes completed rubric with several qualitative comments with details and numeric score for most performance areas. Student identifies two key learnings from experience and at least one opportunity for change with future client interactions based on clinical simulation experience.	Self-analysis of clinical simulation includes completed rubric with some qualitative comments with limited details and numeric scores for each performance area. Student identifies two key learnings from experience. Insight into opportunity for change with future client interactions based on clinical simulation experience not adequately described.	Self-analysis of clinical simulation is missing multiple components of assignment.	

(continued)

Worksheet 15-1 (continued)
Debriefing

Model 15-2.

Component Areas	Excellent (92% to 100%)	Above Average (85% to 91%)	Average (83% to 84%)	Needs Improvement (82% or below)	Total
Application of Learning to Level II Fieldwork (20 points)	Self-analysis of clinical simulation experience demonstrates insight into areas for further review preparatory to Level II fieldwork and application to future fieldwork success, as well as noting most valuable aspects of the clinical simulation process to student learning.	Self-analysis of clinical simulation experience demonstrates insight into areas for further review preparatory to Level II fieldwork based on clinical simulation experience with some connections made relevant to future fieldwork success.	Self-analysis of clinical simulation experience identifies areas for further review preparatory to Level II fieldwork with limited connection to clinical simulation learning experience or application to future fieldwork success included.	Self-analysis of clinical simulation experience does not include relevant insight into areas for further review preparation for Level II fieldwork and/or application to future fieldwork success.	
Mechanics and Style (10 points)	Self-analysis is typed and in APA format with no more than two grammatical or APA errors.	Self-analysis is typed and in APA format with no more than four grammatical or APA errors.	Self-analysis has more than five grammatical or APA errors.	Self-analysis contains excessive grammatical/APA errors. Student needs to make an appointment with course instructor to discuss.	
Comments:				Total Points:	

(continued)

Worksheet 15-1 (continued)
Debriefing

Model 15-3. 3D Model of Debriefing

This model of debriefing allows the learner to explore their reactions and responses and then synthesize their learning by connecting new knowledge and skills to application.

Step 1: Defuse

Let the learner vent/process the emotions associated with the simulation:
How did that feel? NOT How do you feel that went?
Then can ask for an SBAR (Situation, Background, Assessment, Recommendation) to put everyone involved on the same page.

Step 2: Discover

Analyze the learner's performance by using reflection to discover the mental model the learner used to make decisions.
Use the "5 Whys" model. Ask "Why?" neutrally and nonthreateningly five times in response to the learner to get to the true underlying thinking associated with the decisions made and actions taken.
Q: Why did you ____________?
A: The client demonstrated ____________ and ____________.
Q: Given that information, help me understand why you chose X instead of Y.
A: I thought ____________.
Q: Why did that lead you to Z?
A: I learned in class that if you see ____________ then you should ____________.
Q: Why did you decide to use this approach, given ____________?
A: I thought this would be the best because of ____________.
Q: Why did the client have ____________?
A: Oh, so if the client has ____________, I should have used ____________ instead.

Step 3: Deepen

Make connections to practice through application of the lessons learned through the simulation. Discuss how the simulation relates to "real world" performance.
How would you do this differently next time?
What is one thing you can take away from this experience that you can use in practice tomorrow?
How would you use this in real life?

Remember to focus not just on actions and behaviors that would be changed, but also on actions/behaviors that would be reinforced.

Adapted from Zigmont, J. J., Kappus, L. J., & Sudikoff, S. N. (2011). The 3D model of debriefing: Defusing, discovering, and deepening. *Seminars in Perinatology, 35*, 52-58. https://doi.org/10.1053/j.semperi.2011.01.003

(continued)

Worksheet 15-1 (continued)
Debriefing

Model 15-4. Structured and Supported Debriefing

Step 1: Gather

Invite the learner to decompress by sharing their thoughts and feelings. You are using this time (i.e., approximately 25% of the total debriefing time) to identify the gaps between the learner's perception of the performance compared with those of their actual performance as viewed by the facilitator.

What are your thoughts?

How did that make you feel?

Step 2: Analyze

Begin with a one- to two-sentence summary of the intended course of action for the scenario, delivered in a nonjudgmental manner. Use this to segue to the learning objectives, which are the focus of discussion for this step. The facilitator's role is to have the learner reflect upon and provide an analysis of their actions. Use open-ended questions to close the gap between perceived performance and actual performance. This section should be approximately 50% of the total debriefing time.

I noticed ... Tell me more about ... What were you thinking when ... I understand, however, tell me about _____________ aspect of the scenario.

Let's refocus: What's important is not who is right but what is right for the client.

Step 3: Summarize

The facilitator's goal is to promote identification and review of the lessons learned. Learners identify positive actions and aspects of behaviors as well as behaviors that require change. A summary comment or statement is obtained (~25% of the total debriefing time).

List two actions or events that you felt were effective or well done.

Describe two areas that you think you/team need to work on.

Adapted from O'Donnell, J., Rodgers, D., Lee, W., et al. (2008). *Structured and supported debriefing using the GAS method.* Presented at the Second Annual WISER Symposium for Nursing Simulation, Pittsburgh, PA, December 4, 2008.

(continued)

Worksheet 15-1 (continued)
Debriefing

Model 15-5. Advocacy Inquiry or Debriefing with Good Judgment

Step 1: Reaction

This phase is composed of feelings and facts. The facilitator provides an opportunity to clear the air and relax, validate emotional responses, and clarify critical facts of the scenario.
How did that feel?
Give the "punchline" of the situation up front.
Let's present the facts of the case. This scenario involved a patient who recognizes that things might not be the same for them at home since he has had a stroke.

Step 2: Analysis

This phase lets the facilitator and learner work together to identify gaps between desired and actual performance and investigate the basis for this, as well as discuss how to close the gaps. The facilitator must be curious and use this curiosity to drive an understanding about the learner's frame of reference so that the reasons why decisions were made are brought to light.

First, specific questions are used to advocate for the cognitive dissonance noted.
I observed ____________ (concrete example of what you observed that was pertinent to a learning objective and how this may illustrate a performance gap).
I'm concerned about ____________ (concrete example of what you observed that was pertinent to a learning objective and how this may illustrate a performance gap).
I was pleased about ____________ (concrete example of what you observed that was pertinent to a learning objective and how this may illustrate a performance gap).

Then open-ended questions are used for inquiry; to understand the learner's reasoning.
What was on your mind at that time?
How did you view that?
What were your concerns then?

The process in its entirety looks like this: *I noticed that you* ____________ *when* ____________ *was happening. I think that this may have caused* ____________.
How do you see it?

Step 3: Summary

This phase lets the facilitator allow the learner to share insights and complete the analysis of past and future performance. The goal is for the learner to summarize and implement a plan for using this knowledge when it is needed in practice.
As our debriefing session comes to a close, I'd like to invite you to share your thoughts about what went well, as well as what you might hope to change or improve in the future.

Adapted from Rudolph, J. W., Simon, R., Dufresne, R. L., & Raemer, D. B. (2006). There's no such thing as "nonjudgmental" debriefing: A theory and method for debriefing with good judgment. *Simulation in Healthcare: Journal of the Society for Simulation in Healthcare, 1,* 49-55.

(continued)

Worksheet 15-1 (continued)
Debriefing

Model 15-6. PEARLS Using the +/Δ Method

This is a combination of frameworks, with the +/Δ used as the analysis tool. You may choose to just use +/Δ. It is easy to use, nonthreatening and particularly useful for focusing on specific behaviors or with resistant learners. The +/Δ method can be beneficial when there is limited time for debriefing (Levine et al., 2013). It can, however, be more superficial and not always facilitate the most reflective learning.

Step 1: Reaction

Allow the learner to respond/react to the simulation.
How did that feel?

Step 2: Description

Allow the learner to describe the simulation in their own words. This allows the facilitator to gain insight into the learner's point of view.
Can someone summarize what the case was about from a clinical point of view?
What were the main issues?

Step 3: Analysis

This is where +/Δ comes in. This is the learner's self-assessment. You can do this in writing or verbally.
What aspects of the case do you think you managed well?
What aspects of the case would want to change?

What went well during this event? (+)	What areas are noted for improvement? (Δ)

Step 4: Summary

This step should ultimately be learner-driven, with the goal of identifying application to clinical practice.
Before we close, are there any outstanding issues we haven't discussed?
I'd like to close the debriefing by having everyone state one or two take-away points that will help you in the future.

Adapted from Eppich, W., & Cheng, A. (2015). Promoting excellence and reflective learning in simulation (PEARLS): Development and rationale for a blended approach to health care simulation debriefing. *Simulation in Healthcare: The Journal of the Society for Simulation in Healthcare, 10,* 106-115. https://doi.org/10.1097/SIH.0000000000000072

(continued)

Worksheet 15-1 (continued)
Debriefing

Model 15-7. TeamGAINS

Used specifically to debrief teams/groups of learners; combines other established approaches. This method incorporates the use of Advocacy-Inquiry, which lends itself to team learning (Hall & Tori, 2017).

Step 1: Reaction

To allow learners to release tension associated with the simulation and to obtain information about what mattered to the learner about the simulation.
How did you feel?
If the response includes comments that refer to specific clinical skills or behaviors: *These are important aspects of the simulation and we are going to address them in the next part of our discussion.*

Step 2: Discussion of Clinical Component

To establish a clear understanding of the clinical situation, procedure, problem, and expected outcome. Different approaches can be used.
Narrative: *What happened?*
Advocacy-inquiry: *I'd like to discuss ____________. I noted that you ____________ and this resulted in the need for ____________. I think that if you had done ____________, the client could have ____________ independently. So, I am wondering what was on your mind when you chose ____________.*
Guided team self-correction: *What other approach could you have used?*
Systemic-constructivist (circular question): *If your fieldwork educator/instructor/professor had been present at that moment, what would they have recommended to the student?*

Step 3: Transfer From Simulation to Reality

The goal here is to link what happened in the simulation to real clinical work.
What aspects of this scenario are familiar to you? What aspects can you apply to the clinical setting?

Step 4: Discussion of Behavioral Skills

The purpose of this step is to establish a thorough understanding of how behaviors, clinical skills, performance outcomes, and team interactions are linked. This is where the facilitator again reintroduces the learning outcomes and systematically discusses the behavioral skills and their relationship to clinical practice, using any of the following approaches.
Guided team self-correction: To elicit reflection about positive behavior: *Let's talk about the ____________ learning objective. Give me an example of how you addressed ____________. What did you do?*
Systemic question: To elicit the meaning of behavior: *Having anticipated that the client would ____________, how did this help you later?*
Advocacy-inquiry: *Let's talk about ____________. During that time, I saw you ____________ and I was concerned whether each of you knew about each other's plan for the next step. What was on your mind? What did you know about the other team member's plan in that situation?*

(continued)

Worksheet 15-1 (continued)
Debriefing

Circular question: To another learner: *How would it have been useful for them to know what you were about to do and what you needed?*
Guided team self-correction: To elicit reflection about positive behavior: *As heard earlier, ____________ can be used with good results when ____________. Describe an instance when one of you used this (technique/assessment/intervention) ____________.*
Advocacy-inquiry: *In that situation my impression was ____________. I was concerned about ____________. What was on your mind?*
Observer-perspective, circular questions using a reflecting team (to students/learners who observed the scenario): *What do you think they might have needed from you to speak up in that situation?*

Step 5: Summary

This step allows the learner to develop clarity about what the learning that occurred during the simulation.
What was the most important take-away point?
Overall, if someone else had observed you, what could they have learned?

Step 6: Supervised Practice of Clinical Skill (If Needed)

The purpose of this step is to practice skills that were not optimally performed during the simulation.

Adapted from Kolbe, M., Weiss, M., Grote, G., Knauth, A., Dambach, M., Spahn, D. R., & Grande, B. (2013). TeamGAINS: A tool for structured debriefings for simulation-based team trainings. *BMJ Quality and Safety, 22,* 541-553. https://doi.org/10.1136/bmjqs-2012-000917

(continued)

Worksheet 15-1 (continued)
Debriefing

Model 15-8. Health Care Simulation After-Action Review (DEBRIEF)

This is an adaptation of the U. S. Army's debriefing format. *Identifying what actually happened and Examining why* should take 50% of the debriefing time, 25% of the debriefing time is spent focusing on *Formalizing the learning*, and the remaining 25% is split among the other steps.

- *D*efine rules: How are we going to do this debriefing? Emphasize that this is a discussion, not a lecture. Focus on full participation from everyone and the benefits of peer learning.
- *E*xplain learning objectives: What was this simulation designed to teach? Learners will want to know what they need to know to be successful; make learning objective explicit.
- *B*enchmarks for performance: What performance standards were evaluated? Identify what had to happen for optimal performance and success; what were the benchmarks?
- *R*eview what was supposed to happen: What did the facilitator intend to happen? Outline the scenario, expected actions of the learner, and what their expected results were supposed to have been.
- *I*dentify what happened: What actually happened?
- *E*xamine why: Why did things happen the way they did? These steps are done simultaneously, with an aim at recreating what happened to identify any performance gaps.
- *F*ormalize learning: What went well, what did not go well, and what would you do differently next time? The learner draws conclusions to apply what happened/what was learned to real life.

Adapted from Sawyer, T. L., & Deering, S. (2013). Adaptation of the US Army's after-action review for simulation debriefing in healthcare. *Simulation in Healthcare: The Journal of the Society for Simulation in Healthcare, 8*, 388-397. https://doi.org/10.1097/SIH.0b013e31829ac85c

(continued)

Worksheet 15-1 (continued)
Debriefing

Model 15-9. Debriefing for Meaningful Learning

This debriefing method uses Socratic questioning (using the tenets of inquiry—who, what, where, when, how, why) to reveal the thought processes associated with learner's actions, which are sometimes based on assumptions, ill-conceived conclusions, or on a single prior experience that was erroneously thought to apply to all future associated situations. Debriefing is done using individual worksheets, verbal discussion, and group notes on a chalkboard/whiteboard, if appropriate. While each step is identified discreetly, during the debriefing many steps occur simultaneously. Debriefing for meaningful learning has been found to have a positive effect on the development of clinical reasoning skills (Dreifuerst, 2012).

Step 1: Engage
Learners transition from the simulation and focus on the clinical situation. Using a worksheet, learners: 1) name the client, 2) note the first thing that comes to mind about the clinical encounter, 3) note what went right and why, 4) note what did not go well or could have been done differently and why, and 5) outline what happened—the client's story.

Step 2: Explore
Learners discuss their version of the client's story and focus on issues for the instructor/facilitator to consider. Together, they review the simulation (or clinical experience) from their perspectives. Using the Socratic method and noting responses on a worksheet, the desired clinical/learning outcome is identified. The clinical actions that were taken and behaviors/skills used are noted, as are the associated client responses. The purpose of this step is to uncover the learner's ability to generalize, synthesize, and apply knowledge in a contextually appropriate manner to determine what the learner really does/does not understand. This identifies and corrects errors, thus providing critical prevention from harm.

Step 3: Explain
The learner and facilitator interact and articulate their thought processes that underpin the learning objectives/client care principles. This can include assessment, assumption, interpretation, decisions, actions, and outcomes. The processes of deduction, analysis, and inference are a focus. This step is solely verbal. Use What-if ____________? and Tell-me-more-about ____________ questions.

Step 4: Elaborate
Emphasize knowledge, skills, and attitudes that were evident and explain what was missing. Share one thing that went well and why. Tell me your thoughts about ____________. Use a chalkboard and code comments.

Step 5: Evaluate
The learner and facilitator interact and articulate what did not go well. This often occurs simultaneously with prior stages. The focus is on the decisions, reasoning, and mental models used that led to the actions taken. Ask learners to consider parallel situations/cases and identify if their actions would be the same or different by asking *What if ____________?*

(continued)

Worksheet 15-1 (continued)
Debriefing

Step 6: Extend

The debriefing concludes by challenging the learner to extend what was learned from this simulation to actual practice.

Adapted from Dreifuerst, K. T. (2015). Getting started with debriefing for meaningful learning. *Clinical Simulation in Nursing, 11*(5), 268-275. https://doi.org/10.1016/j.ecns.2015.01.005

References

Archer, J. C. (2010). State of the science in health professional education: Effective feedback. *Medical Education, 44*(1), 101-108. https://doi.org/10.1111/j.1365-2923.2009.03546.x

Arora, S., Ahmed, M., Paige, J., Nestel, D., Runnacles, J., Hull, L., Darzi, A., & Sevdalis, N. (2012). Objective structured assessment of debriefing: Bringing science to the art of debriefing in surgery. *Annals of Surgery, 256,* 982-988. https://doi.org/10.1097/SLA.0b013e3182610c91

Brett-Fleegler, M., Rudolph, J., Eppich, W., Monuteaux, M., Fleegler, E., Cheng, A., & Simon, R. (2012). Debriefing assessment for simulation in healthcare: Development and psychometric properties. *Simulation in Healthcare, 7,* 288-294. https://doi.org/10.1097/SIH.0b013e3182620228

Cantrell, M. A. (2008). The importance of debriefing in clinical simulations. *Clinical Simulation in Nursing, 4*(2), e19-e23. https://doi.org/10.1016/j.ecns.2008.06.006

Cheng, A., Eppich, W., Grant, V., Sherbino, J., Zendejas, B., & Cook, D. A. (2014). Debriefing for technology-enhanced simulation: A systematic review and meta-analysis. *Medical Education, 48*(7). 657-666. https://doi.org/10.1111/medu.12432

Cheng, A., Grant, V., Huffman, J., Burgess, G., Szyld, D., Robinson, T., & Eppich, W. (2017). Coaching the debriefer: Peer coaching to improve debriefing quality in simulation programs. *Simulation in Healthcare, 12,* 319-325. https://doi.org/10.1097/SIH.0000000000000232

Chronister, C., & Brown, D. (2012). Comparison of simulation debriefing methods. *Clinical Simulation in Nursing, 8*(7), e281-e288. https://doi.org/10.1016/j.ecns.2010.12.005

Decker, S., Fey, M., Sideras, S., Caballero, S., Rockstraw, L., Boese, T., & Borum, J. C. (2013). Standards of best practice: Simulation standard VI: The debriefing process. *Clinical Simulation in Nursing, 9*(6), S26-S29. https://doi.org/10.1016/j.ecns.2013.04.008

Dishon, N., Oldmeadow, J. A., Critchley, C., & Kaufman, J. (2017). The effect of trait self-awareness, self-reflection, and perceptions of choice meaningfulness on indicators of social identity within a decision-making context. *Frontiers in Psychology, 8,* 2034. https://doi.org/10.3389/fpsyg.2017.02034

Dreifuerst, K. (2012). Using debriefing for meaningful learning to foster development of clinical reasoning in simulation. *Journal of Nursing Education, 51,* 326-333. https://doi.org/10.3928/01484834-20120409-02

Dreifuerst, K. T. (2015). Getting started with debriefing for meaningful learning. *Clinical Simulation in Nursing, 11*(5), 268-275. https://doi.org/10.1016/j.ecns.2015.01.005

Dufrene, C., & Young, A. (2014). Successful debriefing—Best methods to achieve positive learning outcomes: A literature review. *Nurse Education Today, 34*(3), 372-376. https://doi.org/10.1016/j.nedt.2013.06.026.

Edgecombe, K., Seaton, P., Monahan, K., Meyer, S., LaPage, S., & Erlam, G. (2013). *Clinical simulation in nursing: A literature review and guidelines for practice.* Aotearoa: AKO National Centre for Tertiary Teaching Excellence. Retrieved from https://www.researchgate.net/publication/276060426_Clinical_simulation_in_nursing_a_literature_review_and_guidelines_for_practice

Eppich, W., & Cheng, A. (2015). Promoting excellence and reflective learning in simulation (PEARLS): Development and rationale for a blended approach to health care simulation debriefing. *Simulation in Healthcare: The Journal of the Society for Simulation in Healthcare, 10,* 106-115. https://doi.org/10.1097/SIH.0000000000000072

Eppich, W. J., Hunt, E. A., Duval-Arnould, J. M., Siddall, V. J., & Cheng, A. (2015). Structuring feedback and debriefing to achieve mastery learning goals. *Academic Medicine, 90,* 1501-1508. https://doi.org/10.1097/ACM.0000000000000934

Fanning, R. M., & Gaba, D. M. (2007). The role of debriefing in simulation-based learning. *Simulation in Healthcare, 2,* 115-125. https://doi.org/10.1097/SIH.0b013e3180315539

Hall, K., & Tori, K. (2017). Best practice recommendations for debriefing in simulation based education for Australian undergraduate nursing students: An integrative review. *Clinical Simulation in Nursing, 13,* 39-50. https://doi.org/10.1016/j.ecns.2016.10.006

INACSL Standards Committee. (2021). Healthcare simulation standards of best practice. *Clinical Simulation in Nursing, 58,* 66. https://doi.org/10.1016/j.ecns.2021.08.018

Johnson-Russell, J., & Bailey, C. (2010). Facilitated debriefing. In W. Nehring & F. Lashley (Eds.), *High-fidelity patient simulation in nursing education* (pp. 369–384). Jones and Bartlett.

Katznelson, H. (2014). Reflective functioning: A review. *Clinical Psychology Review, 34,* 107-117. https://doi.org/10.1016/j.cpr.2013.12.003

Kolbe, M., Weiss, M., Grote, G., Knauth, A., Dambach, M., Spahn, D. R., & Grande, B. (2013). TeamGAINS: A tool for structured debriefings for simulation-based team trainings. *BMJ Quality and Safety, 22,* 541-553. https://doi.org/10.1136/bmjqs-2012-000917

Levett-Jones, T., & Lapkin, S. (2012). The effectiveness of debriefing in simulation-based learning for health professionals: A systematic review. *JBI Database of Systematic Reviews and Implementation Reports, 9*(64), 1-16. https://doi.org/10.11124/jbisrir-2011-317

Levett-Jones, T., & Lapkin, S. (2014). A systematic review of the effectiveness of simulation debriefing in health professional education. *Nurse Education Today, 34*(6), e58-63. https://doi.org/10.1016/j.nedt.2013.09.020

Levine, A. I., DeMaria, S., Schwartz, A.D., & Sim, A.J. (2013). *The comprehensive textbook of healthcare simulation.* Springer.

Lopreiato, J. O. (Ed.), Downing, D., Gammon, W., Lioce, L., Sittner, B., Slot, V., Spain, A. E. (Associate Eds.), and the Terminology & Concepts Working Group. (2016). *Healthcare simulation dictionary.* Retrieved from http://www.ssih.org/dictionary.

Lorello, G. R., Cook, D. A., Johnson, R. L., & Brydges, R. (2014). Simulation-based training in anaesthesiology: A systematic review and meta-analysis. *British Journal of Anaesthesia, 112*(2), 231-245. https://doi.org/10.1093/bja/aet414

O'Donnell, J., Rodgers, D., Lee, W., et al. (2008). *Structured and supported debriefing using the GAS method.* Presented at the Second Annual WISER Symposium for Nursing Simulation, Pittsburgh, PA, December 4, 2008.

Reed, S. J. (2012). Debriefing experience scale: Development of a tool to evaluate the student learning experience in debriefing. *Clinical Simulation in Nursing, 8,* e211-e217. https://doi.org/10.1016/j.ecns.2011.11.002

Reed, S. J., Andrews, C. M., & Ravert, P. (2013). Debriefing simulations: Comparison of debriefing with video and debriefing alone. *Clinical Simulation in Nursing, 9*(12), e585-e591. https://doi.org/10.1016/j.ecns.2013.05.007

Rudolph, J. W., Raemer, D. B., & Simon, R. (2014). Establishing a safe container for learning in simulation: The role of the pre-simulation briefing. *Simulation in Healthcare, 9,* 339-349. https://doi.org/10.1097/SIH.0000000000000047

Rudolph, J. W., Simon, R., Dufresne, R. L., & Raemer, D. B. (2006). There's no such thing as "nonjudgmental" debriefing: A theory and method for debriefing with good judgment. *Simulation in Healthcare: Journal of the Society for Simulation in Healthcare, 1,* 49-55.

Rudolph, J. W., Simon, R., Raemer, D. B., & Eppich, W. J. (2008). Debriefing as formative assessment: Closing performance gaps in medical education. *Academic Emergency Medicine, 15*(11), 1010-1016. https://doi.org/10.1111/j.1553-2712.2008.00248.x

Sanders, M., Van Oss, T., & McGeary, S. (2015). Analyzing reflections in service learning to promote personal growth and community self efficacy. *Journal of Experiential Education 39*(1), 73-88. https://doi.org/10.1177/1053825915608872

Sawyer, T. L., & Deering, S. (2013). Adaptation of the US Army's after-action review for simulation debriefing in healthcare. *Simulation in Healthcare: The Journal of the Society for Simulation in Healthcare, 8,* 388-397. https://doi.org/10.1097/SIH.0b013e31829ac85c

Sawyer, T., Eppich, W., Brett-Fleegler, M., Grant, V., & Cheng, A. (2016). More than one way to debrief: A critical review of healthcare simulation debriefing methods. *Simulation in Healthcare, 11,* 209-217. https://doi.org/10.1097/SIH.0000000000000148

Voyer, S., & Hatala, R. (2015). Debriefing and feedback: Two sides of the same coin? *Simulation in Healthcare, 10,* 67-68. https://doi.org/10.1097/SIH.0000000000000075

Xeroulis, G. J., Park, J., Moulton, C.A., Reznick, R. K., Leblanc, V., & Dubrowski, A. (2007). Teaching suturing and knot-tying skills to medical students: A randomized controlled study comparing computer-based video instruction and (concurrent and summary) expert feedback. *Surgery, 141,* 442-449. https://doi.org/10.1016/j.surg.2006.09.012

Zigmont, J. J., Kappus, L. J., & Sudikoff, S. N. (2011). The 3D model of debriefing: Defusing, discovering, and deepening. *Seminars in Perinatology, 35,* 52-58. https://doi.org/10.1053/j.semperi.2011.01.003

16

Simulation Program Evaluation

Audrey L. Zapletal, OTD, OTR/L, CLA

Learning Objectives

1. Discuss the value of conducting a simulation program evaluation.
2. Describe methods of seeking feedback from various stakeholders.

Kern's Model of Program Development

The content in this chapter articulates Step 6 of Kern's Model: Evaluation and Feedback. Information in this chapter contributes to creation of formal simulation program assessment. This articulates with gathering simulation feedback and assessment data to evaluate learner and program effectiveness.

Zapletal, A. L., Baird, J. M., Van Oss, T., Hoppe, M. M., Prast, J. E., & Herge, E. A. *Clinical Simulation for Health Care Professionals* (pp. 197-201).

At the end of every simulation encounter, it is important for the faculty/simulation team to gather information from multiple stakeholders regarding the experience to ensure the fidelity and integrity of the simulation experience (INACSL Standards Committee, 2021). Stakeholders include:

- Learners
- Standardized patients (SPs)
- Lab instructors (teaching team members)
- Clinical educators
- Other faculty
- Simulation staff (e.g., SP trainer, SP coordinator, simulation operations specialist)

The following text describes methods of how to collect these stakeholder's feedback.

Learners

At the end of the simulation encounter:

- Hold a 10 to 15 minute debriefing session, acknowledging their accomplishments and sharing some of the challenges posed by the simulation experience. Challenges can include minimal knowledge or comfort with skills related to the health professional's role, or challenges created by the simulation process (e.g., not enough time between encounters, lack of equipment, inadequate prebriefing about the process, poor debriefing process). This session is not the formal debriefing or feedback given to the learner—this method allows for a quick assessment of the production.
- Learners complete a written evaluation of the experience.
  - Questions can include procedural items (i.e., have you been exposed to the content related to the goals of this session prior to this experience) and/or their perception (i.e., tell us some of the challenges of the experience).
- Self-evaluation forms.
  - Learners can complete a self-evaluation of their performance. This provides you with their perception of their areas of strength and growth. If time permits in the curriculum, acknowledging the areas of growth and modifying the curriculum to include opportunities for practice would enhance performance in the clinical setting.

Standardized Patients

- Learner feedback form
  - Each SP completes a learner evaluation form that contains procedural and qualitative questions related to the experience. This information helps you know if learners were prepared or did not have enough time to complete the activities.
- After the encounter debriefing session
  - After the simulation encounter, spending time with the SPs provides valuable insight into how they perceived the experience
  - Consider asking questions about the procedure
    - → Scheduling adequate time between learners to change clothes, set up the room, and complete the feedback form
    - → Feeling comfortable in their role during the performance (pertains to training effectiveness)

Lab Instructors/Clinical Educators

- Provide debriefing opportunities for them to share their perceptions while observing the encounters or after learners complete a clinical rotation in the field
- Consider their ideas to enhance the teaching/simulation sequence, including adding more current clinical techniques used in practice

Other Faculty

- Provide an opportunity to enhance simulation design or process
- Provide an opportunity to enhance the curriculum
- Provide the opportunity to showcase the relationship of the simulation encounter to a variety of courses
- Including faculty as observers or participants provides an opportunity to understand the dynamic process

Simulation Staff/Standardized Patient Trainer/ Simulation Operations Specialist

- Provide opportunities to discuss the simulation process and how it can be improved upon
- Debriefing formally with the simulation team is not always done; however, it is worthwhile when building a relationship and to learn new skills outside of the health professional skill set

There are many methods used to gather feedback from these stakeholders. The debriefing models shared in Chapter 15 can be modified and used for these purposes.

A simple form of debriefing with stakeholders is the +/Δ model. This model consists of two parts:

- +: An opportunity to share positive aspects of the simulation
- Δ: An opportunity to share suggestions or recommendations

It is an effective method to create a meaningful conversation for those who have invested in the student experience and simulation instructional method without focusing on the specific challenges that could be student-specific or variables that cannot be changed (Kim & Kim, 2017; Motola et al., 2013). For example, a simulation program is scheduled for Thursdays because the resources are available to the department, but a stakeholder would prefer to work on Tuesdays and shares the hardships of rearranging their personal schedule.

Simulation encounters are dynamic and complex yet very rewarding; they require high levels of planning and communication for all learners and team members to be on the same page. Using the +/Δ model ensures that stakeholders have a clear opportunity to provide meaningful constructive feedback. At the end of the meeting, the facilitator can summarize the discussion and list the considered suggestions for the future.

As a faculty/simulationist member, it's important to build relationships with all stakeholders. Their input enhances a variety of aspects of your program. As the simulationist, you have a unique lens of the process, the learners, learning objectives, and the desired outcomes. Therefore, not all feedback should be acted upon. Keep in mind the learners' development through the curriculum, understanding that becoming a health professional takes deliberate practice and feedback through multiple encounters in a variety of learning settings.

Ultimately, your simulation program should be embedded into the educational philosophy and design of your program. Meeting your program outcomes should indicate if simulation methods are enhancing your learners' success in the field.

Worksheet 16-1

Reflecting on Your Simulation Design in Order to Minimize Learner's Stress

Date: ____

Title of the simulation: ____

Brief description of the simulation encounter (one to two sentences): ____________________

____

____

Setting: ____

____

Simulation modality/ies (SP, task trainers, manikin, other): ____________________

____

Simulation Program Evaluation Form

Attendance:

Topic	Comment/Suggestion	Rationale/Background Information
+ (Strengths)		
Δ (Suggestions)		

References

INACSL Standards Committee, Bowler, F., Klein, M., & Wilford, A. (2021). Healthcare Simulation Standards of Best Practice™: Professional integrity. *Clinical Simulation in Nursing, 58,* 45-48. https://doi.org/10.1016/j.ecns.2021.08.014.

Kim, M., & Kim, S. (2017). Debriefing practices in simulation-based nursing education in South Korea. *Clinical Simulation in Nursing, 13*(5), 201-209. https://doi.org/10.1016/j.ecns.2017.01.008

Motola, I., Luke, D., Chung, H. S., Sullivan, J., & Issenberg, B. (2013). Simulation in healthcare education: A best evidence practical guide. AMEE Guide No. 82. *Medical Teacher, 35*(10), e1511-e1530. https://doi.org/10.3109/0142159X.2013.818632

17

Simulation and Research

Tracy Van Oss, DHSc, MPH, OTR/L, FAOTA, CHSE

Learning Objectives

1. Describe the benefits of using reliable and valid assessment tools in simulation research.
2. Illustrate the steps to plan and prepare a research project using simulation.

Kern's Model of Program Development

The content in this chapter articulates Step 6 of Kern's Model: Evaluation and Feedback. Information in this chapter illustrates how assessment tools and research can promote program evaluation. These methods contribute to the evaluation of learners and the simulation program.

Zapletal, A. L., Baird, J. M., Van Oss, T., Hoppe, M. M., Prast, J. E., & Herge, E. A. *Clinical Simulation for Health Care Professionals* (pp. 203-205).

Planning a new research project can be an exhilarating or daunting task to get started. Including simulation as part of a research project offers several possibilities to gain insightful information that can be used to foster student learning. There is a plethora of literature linking learning that occurs in simulation has led to *positive student learning outcomes* in a variety of disciplines. Researchers should be aware of and follow the institutional process for approval from the Institutional Review Board prior to the start of any research project to protect all participants.

When choosing an assessment tool for use in your research project, the process is the same as selecting a tool for your simulation encounter. Understand the psychometrics of the tool including its intended use, reliability, and validity. A tool that has inter-rater reliability or inter-observer reliability has two or more raters coming to the same conclusion. A valid tool will simply measure what it is intended to measure. Be mindful to use a tool that has inter-rater reliability and validity (Bannigan & Watson, 2009) and collaborate with others to consider an interprofessional research project.

Planning will take some considerable time, along with scheduling the multiple components of the research project, so it is important to get started early. Building a solid proposal can be beneficial if considering seeking external funding requests for support to fund a research project in simulation. There are a multitude of task trainers, simulation accessories, or payment for standardized patients to consider. Also, decide on selecting just a few students for a pilot or an entire class/cohort from one or more disciplines to be in the study. You may also include students in the research project itself to develop scripts and scenarios for future use in curriculum. There are a multitude of resources on research design that are recommended prior to the start of any formal research project. The following is a brief outline on steps related to simulation.

Steps to Begin

- Institutional Review Board approval
- Approval to use the assessment (if necessary) obtained
- Standardized patients are trained (inter-reliability if >1)
- Students have learned the skills needed to be assessed
- Student verbal/written agreements completed
- Prebriefing with focus on learning objectives
- Simulation encounter
- Video capture of the simulation encounter for future review, feedback, and learning.
- Debrief should occur after the learner completes the simulation learning experience and any post-assessment methods should also conclude at this time
- Work on analysis of data (e.g., qualitative, quantitative, mixed)

As with any educational pedagogy there are instances when clinical simulations go really well, and other times they do not go as planned. This can be for a variety of reasons, but here are some related specifically to the topic of using assessment tools in simulation.

Steps to Avoid

- Did not get permission to use the assessment tool for a planned research project
- Students did not complete the assessment in its entirety
- Did not use a valid or reliable assessment tool
- Did not plan/schedule ahead of time for optimal outcome

Simulation encounters can provide valuable information regarding the current status of a student in the learning continuum. Clinical scenarios can be created and assessed to learn about a student's non-technical skills of communication, professionalism, or student confidence. This type of learning can also be beneficial to assess particular performance skills. In any case, simulation ultimately helps students prepare for future clinical work. Learning how simulation learning experiences were helpful to prepare for fieldwork experiences is another possible research project ... so get going, there is a lot of work to do!

Reference

Bannigan, K., & Watson, R. (2009). Reliability and validity in a nutshell. *Journal of Clinical Nursing, 18*(23), 3237-3243. https://doi.org/10.1111/j.1365-2702.2009.02939.x

Initial Standardized Patient Encounter for Athletic Training Students

A

Quinnipiac University
Susan Norkus, PhD, ATC

How Are Students Prepared?

- Provided with the expectations in advance
- Provided access to watch a simulation experience of another student
  - Allows them to see the space
  - Allows them to see a good example (e.g., modeling professional behaviors)
- Given the rubric and Master Interview Rating Scale (MIRS) in advance

How Are Students Assessed?

This is a 50-point assignment (very low stakes).

- 30 points are the patient encounter itself, 20 points are from reflective exercises
- Patient encounter points (30% history taking, 30% physical exam, 30% MIRS/communication, 10% documentation/SOAP note rubric)
- Reflective assignments in Flipgrid (www.flipgrid.com)
  - *Initial reflection:* Post within 24 hours of the experience and reply to a minimum of two classmate's posts
    - → *Prompt:* Last semester, you read a paragraph about the importance of the medical interview. Research shows interviewing generates the information necessary for dx *more often* than the exam and lab studies combined. Overall, the clinician's ability to explain, listen, and empathize can have a profound effect on health outcomes as well as patient

Zapletal, A. L., Baird, J. M., Van Oss, T., Hoppe, M. M., Prast, J. E., & Herge, E. A. *Clinical Simulation for Health Care Professionals* (pp. 207-214).

satisfaction. Reflect on today's encounter and talk about how you feel you did communicating with your patient? What went really well? Share your positive thoughts!

- *After watching video; reflection:* Videos are released 24 hours after the experience. Students are to view their videos and then respond on Flipgrid to the prompt below. They are then to respond with thoughtful and complete responses to a minimum of 2 DIFFERENT classmates.
  - → *Prompt:* Video lets us see what happens. They are genuine. It shows our strengths and weaknesses. In the moment, it is difficult to see because we are so focused. Watching ourselves provides an opportunity to look again and reflect using a broad lens. It lets us see where we can improve, become better practitioners, and push our practice. After watching your simulation experience, reflect on what you learned about your communication skills. You can also discuss how your initial perceptions compared to what you watched.

Training

The faculty member meets with the director of the standardized patient (SP) center and lead SP to review the case. Faculty member performs and is filmed conducting the assessment on the lead SP. The lead SP uses this information to train the SPs.

Standardized Patient Encounter—Athletic Training Students

This will be 25 minutes total.

- 15 minutes for physical exam
- 5 minutes to document findings
- 5 minutes for feedback from SP

Case Title (Name + Clinical Issue)	Tory Mathers + ankle/leg injury
Author(s)	Susan Norkus
Brief Case Summary	You are a patient (intramurals) with right ankle and leg pain. You landed on someone's foot earlier today during a game (<1 hr).
Standardized Patient Demographics	• Gender: Any • Acceptable SP age range: College student through adult (coach, faculty, staff) • Incompatible features (scars?): None

Doorway Information

**Do not remove or write on.

Patient name: Tory Mathers
Age: 21 years old (college age students)/SP age (faculty, staff, coach)
Gender: (SP gender inserted here)
Reason for visit: R ankle and leg pain
Clinical setting: Athletic training clinic

Tasks for learner to accomplish:

1. Perform an evaluation and provide treatment recommendations for a musculoskeletal injury
2. Perform a thorough physical exam
3. Discuss a plan of care with the patient and answer their questions
4. Complete a SOAP note on the computer found outside the room

**Close placard when done reading.

General Patient Characteristics, Appearance, and Behavior

Name: Tory Mathers
Age: 21 years old (athletes)/SP age (faculty, staff, coach)
Gender: Your gender will be given on doorway instructions
Dress/attire: Athletic gear (shorts and t-shirt)

- They will need to be able to examine both feet/ankles and legs up to your knee.

Where patient should sit at start of encounter: Exam table
Physical behaviors at the start: Comfortable at rest
Affect: Concerned
Body language: See above
Eye contact: Normal
Voice (level, tone): Normal

History of Present Illness

You play intramural basketball with your friends/co-workers one afternoon each week. You injured your right ankle/leg during a game today (in the rec center; sport court flooring). You were going for a rebound after a free throw and came down on someone's foot, causing your ankle to roll.

You fell to the ground and had immediate pain. At the time, it hurt on the outside of your leg, from the ankle all the way up to just below your knee (on outside of leg only). Now it mostly hurts toward the ankle on the outside of your leg and a little at the outside of the ankle itself. You were able to get up, but couldn't continue playing. After the game was over, your teammates brought you here to get looked at.

The pain was initially 6/10 but has decreased with time, and it is currently 4/10 at rest. The pain is dull and achy and sometimes sharp. It is difficult to walk without limping, and you needed a little bit of help from your friends to get to the athletic training room.

The pain is now mostly on the outside of your leg (lower third), and a little on the outside of your ankle (just below the outside ankle bone).

No other areas of pain.

Scripted Responses to Begin Encounter

<table>
<tr><th>Scripted Response</th><th colspan="2">Chief Concern</th></tr>
<tr><td>Scripted response to possible opening student question/statement #1:
What brings you in today? How can I help you? What seems to be the problem? What symptoms are you experiencing? What would you like to talk about today?</td><td colspan="2">"I hurt my ankle/leg playing intramural basketball."</td></tr>
<tr><td>Scripted response to initial open-ended question:
Tell me more about your symptoms. Can you describe this in more detail? What else can you tell me about that?</td><td colspan="2">"I was jumping for a rebound, and when I came down I landed on someone's foot."</td></tr>
<tr><td rowspan="10">Standard qualifier questions of symptoms</td><td>Onset of symptoms: Time</td><td>"Less than an hour ago."</td></tr>
<tr><td>Duration</td><td>N/A</td></tr>
<tr><td>Location (of pain)</td><td>"The pain is mostly on the outside of my ankle and leg."</td></tr>
<tr><td>Course:
Changed? Constant or intermittent?</td><td>"The pain has been constant, but seems to be getting better."</td></tr>
<tr><td>Quality/description of pain or symptoms (sharp/dull)</td><td>"The pain is achy and dull but sometimes sharp."</td></tr>
<tr><td>Intensity of symptoms</td><td>"I would say the pain was initially 6/10 but now is 4/10 when I'm just sitting still."</td></tr>
<tr><td>What makes it better</td><td>"When I'm just sitting here or not walking on it, it feels better."</td></tr>
<tr><td>What makes it worse</td><td>"It's worse when I walk on it."</td></tr>
<tr><td>Associated symptoms</td><td>"Nothing else."</td></tr>
<tr><td>Radiation</td><td>"The pain sort of goes up my leg on the outside."</td></tr>
<tr><td>Patient perspective of illness:
What are your thoughts on this illness? What do you think the cause may be?
Impact of illness on patient:
How is this affecting your life?</td><td colspan="2">"I'm worried I may have broken my ankle."
"I need to be able to get around to class/work and really want to keep playing intramurals (or get to my work and function at my job, which involves lots of standing/walking)."</td></tr>
<tr><td>Information to hold back unless specifically asked about</td><td colspan="2">Previous injuries—sprained same ankle once in junior high</td></tr>
<tr><td>Review of symptoms</td><td>Positive symptoms (+)
• Right ankle pain (outside)
• Right leg pain (outside)
• Swelling (none)
• Painful to walk (antalgic gait) and pain with weight bearing on right foot</td><td>Negative symptoms (–)
• No fevers or chills
• No headache or injury
• No other musculoskeletal pain or injuries
• No numbness</td></tr>
</table>

Simulated Physical Examination Findings

- You have the most pain when the student palpates outside of your foot and lower leg, behind your ankle (5/10) when they directly press on it.
- You are also sore if they palpate higher up the leg, but not the top third.
- There is NO PAIN if the student palpates the outside ankle bone.
- After palpating but before having you move the ankle, the student should rule out a fracture—they may bump your heel, squeeze your leg, or both. You can express discomfort when these are done but NO PAIN.
- During the squeeze test, *if they squeeze over where you stated it was painful prior, then you should report pain where they are squeezing your leg.*
- If asked, the pain is where they hit (heel) or squeezed (upper leg). You have NO PAIN in your leg or ankle with these maneuvers.
- If they squeeze your foot across your foot bones (i.e., arch)—you have NO PAIN.

Range of Motion Assessment

- The student should assess your range of motion:
    - Actively (they will ask you to move it)—they should ask you "is that as far as you can go?" to ensure you have moved it through the full range
    - Passively (they will ask you to relax and move it for you)—they should ask you to relax so they can move it for you
    - Resisted (i.e., checking your strength)—they should explain they are going to resist you through the same motion
- The motions they should assess are:
    - Dorsiflexion (pull your foot up)
    - Plantar flexion (push your foot down)
    - Inversion (turn your foot inward)
    - Eversion (turn your foot outward)
- Active, passive, and resisted dorsiflexion (pulling your foot up) is full and pain free.
- Active and passive plantar flexion (stepping on the gas pedal) is full and pain free.
- Against resistance, pushing your foot down (plantar flexion) is sore on the outside.
    - NOTE: Make sure the student actually resists. If the resistance is minimal and you can't really feel it, then it's not painful.
- Active and resisted inversion (pulling your ankle in) is full and pain free.
- Pulling your ankle in while you are relaxed (passive inversion) is painful on the outside of your leg (where the pain was when they palpated)—4/10.
    - NOTE: Be sure the student moves your ankle all the way to the inside. Only report pain once the student gets to the end of the range and meets some resistance. It will only hurt once the student gets to that point in the motion. If they do not get to the end, then please report no pain.
- Active eversion (turning your foot out) is painful (4/10).
- Pulling your ankle outward while you relax (passive eversion) is not painful.
- Turning your ankle outward against resistance (resisted eversion) is the most painful (6/10).
- If the student asks, the pain is on the outside of your leg.

Manual Muscle Tests

- The student should recognize the injury is to a muscle and should do a few tests to figure out which muscle is injured.
- The student will ask that you put your foot into a specific position and will ask you to hold it there ("don't let me move you").
- The following position will elicit pain:
    - If they ask you to point your foot down and turn it outward at the same time
    - Once they offer you resistance in this motion—you should report significant pain (6/10) and say that's the pain you have been feeling
    - If they have you pull your foot up and turn your ankle outward at the same time → resistance to this motion will be "sore" but not painful
    - You can perform heel raises without pain (a little sore at the end range, all the way up on your toes)
    - If they ask you to turn your ankle in and resist → you have no pain

The student should end the evaluation at this point; however, they may decide to rule out ligamentous injury by performing a few special tests.

- They may perform an inversion stress test—this will cause pain on the outside of your leg, in the same area as previous. You have no pain on the outside of your ankle. The student must ask where the pain is.
- You will have NO PAIN if the student performs a talar tilt test; tilting your ankle inward or outward. Both are pain free.
- You should have NO pain if the student performs an anterior drawer test.
- You have a "painful" gait. You are unable to fully push off when walking because of pain. It is okay if you are just standing, but walking hurts. You cannot run.
- NOTE: Anytime the student places a hand or finger on the outside of your leg, you should report pain because of their pressure over those sore areas.

Information Sharing Phase of the Encounter

The athletic training students are expected to share a basic plan of care with you and answer your questions.

Potential question for the student:

- Do I need to see a doctor?

Standardized Patient Evaluation Checklist Items

Section weighting toward overall score:
History: 30% Physical exam: 30% Communication: 30% SOAP note: 10%

Nine History Items and Associated Item Point Value—Yes/No	
Asked about onset of pain/when injury occurred.	1
Asked about mechanism of injury (must inquire or obtain the direction of the ankle/foot motion)	1
Asked about quality of pain (i.e., describe pain)	1
Asked about location of pain (point with one finger)	1
Asked if experiencing anything other than pain (tingling, numbness, etc.)	1
Asked about intensity of pain (1 to 10 scale)	1
Asked what makes the pain better/worse	1
Asked if taking any medications	1
Asked about previous injury and treatment	1

Twelve Physical Exam Items and Associated Item Point Value—Correct/Incorrect/Not Done	
Washed hands (soap/water or hand sanitizer, one time)	1
Palpated leg, ankle, and foot (not just where the pain was)	1
Palpated purposefully (with enough pressure to identify painful areas, did not use multiple fingers simultaneously)	1
Ruled out fracture (did squeeze or bump test or both)	1
Tested active, passive, and resisted range of motion into *dorsiflexion* (moving ankle up)	1
Tested active, passive, and resisted range of motion into *plantar flexion* (pushing ankle down)	1
Tested active, passive, and resisted range of motion into *inversion* (turning ankle inward)	1
Tested active, passive, and resisted range of motion into *eversion* (turning ankle outward)	1
Performed manual muscle test (down and out)—hold/don't let me move	1
Performed manual muscle test (up and out)—hold/don't let me move	1
Performed exam (palpations, fracture, range of motion, and special tests) on both sides (uninjured side first)	1
Asked where pain was during a variety of the assessments	1

Nine Communication Items (MIRS) and Associated Item Point Value—Scale	
Introduction	1
Pacing	1
Types of questions	1
Nonverbal facilitation skills	1
Lack of jargon	1
Empathy (acknowledge and support)	1
Achieves a shared plan (mentions crutches and ice, compression, elevation)	1
Encouragement of questions	1
Closure	1

Feedback

Please focus the feedback on the student interaction, communication with you, and overall process/system (i.e., was it fluid/smooth). Do not share with them the actual diagnosis/injury. Your perspective as patient is preferred regarding bedside manner—feedback on the communication, instructions, plan of care, and overall student confidence.

Reference

Theresa A. Thomas Professional Skills Assessment & Teaching Center, Eastern Virginia Medical School. (2010). *Master Interview Rating Scale: The clinical conversation and interview. The training manual for standardized patients*. Author.

B

National League for Nursing Simulation Design Template

National League for Nursing

Zapletal, A. L., Baird, J. M., Van Oss, T., Hoppe, M. M., Prast, J. E., & Herge, E. A. *Clinical Simulation for Health Care Professionals* (pp. 215-229).

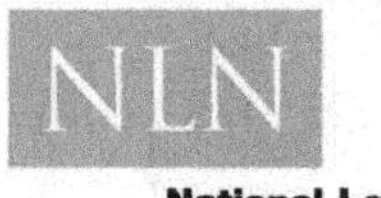

National League *for* **Nursing**

Simulation Design Template

Date: **Discipline:** Nursing **Expected Simulation Run Time:** Approx. 15 mins. **Location:** Community Clinic or Primary Healthcare Provider Office	**File Name:** Care to the Trans* and Gender Non-Conforming Identified Patient **Student Level:** Adapted to Cover All Levels **Guided Reflection Time:** Approx. 45 mins. **Location for Reflection:**

Admission Date: | **Today's Date:** XX/XX/XX

Brief Description of Client

Name: Joe Ramirez

Gender: FtMTG **Age**: 25 **Race**: n/a **Weight**: n/a **Height**: n/a

Religion: n/a

Major Support: Parents & Girlfriend **Support Phone:** 301-XXX-XXXX

Allergies: NKDA **Immunizations:**

Primary Care Provider/Team: No current primary provider. Has been under the care of an endocrinologist, Samuel Gordon, MD, for masculinizing hormone therapy treatments.

Past Medical History: Relatively healthy. Taking testosterone therapy for over 1 year.

History of Present Illness: Presents today to obtain a flu shot and annual physical.

Social History: In a committed heterosexual relationship for approximately 2 years. Feels supported in relationship with his girlfriend. Otherwise history unremarkable.

Primary Medical Diagnosis:

Surgeries/Procedures & Dates: Mastectomy and Chest Reconstruction

Nursing Diagnoses: Discuss with participants in debriefing.

Note: This simulation encounter is reprinted in its original form. The authors would make the following additions to the demographic section of the chart: (1) Pronouns would be included near the patient's name (Joe Ramirez), and (2) Assigned Sex At Birth (ASAB) would be included next to Gender as an additional descriptor.

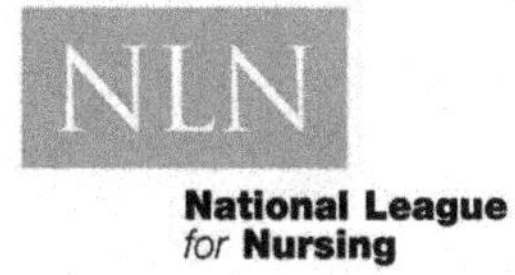

National League
for Nursing

Psychomotor Skills Required Prior to Simulation:

Review and practice effective interprofessional communication tools and strategies; namely, ISBARR
Review strategies for therapeutic communication in the patient care setting, and practice those strategies
Review and practice patient assessment skills

Cognitive Activities Required Prior to Simulation:

[i.e. independent reading (R), video review (V), computer simulations (CS), lecture (L)]

I. Pick at least one (1) of the following nursing articles to read prior to the simulation.

Caring for....Transgender Patients:
http://www.nursingcenter.com/cearticle?an=00152258-201411000-00006

Addressing Health Care Disparities in the Lesbian, Gay, Bisexual, and Transgender Populations: A Review of Best Practices
http://journals.lww.com/ajnonline/Fulltext/2014/06000/CE__Addressing_Health_Care_Disparities_in_the.21.aspx

Culturally Sensitive Care for the Transgender Patient:
http://www.nursingcenter.com/cearticle?an=01271211-201505000-00005&Journal_ID=682710&Issue_ID=3106455

Open the Doors for LGBTQ Patients:
http://www.nursingcenter.com/cearticle?an=00152193-201308000-00014&Journal_ID=54016&Issue_ID=1573627

Providing Care to GLBTQ Patients:
http://www.nursingcenter.com/cearticle?an=00152193-201212000-00009&Journal_ID=54016&Issue_ID=1467700

Treating Transgender Patients With Respect:
http://www.americannursetoday.com/viewpoint-treating-transgender-patients-respect/

Nursing Care of Transgender Patients:
http://nursing.advanceweb.com/Features/Articles/Nursing-Care-of-the-Transgender-Patient.aspx

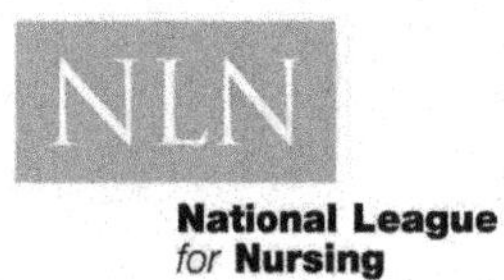

II. Review the information contained in *Injustice at Every Turn: A Report of the National Transgender Discrimination Survey* (2011). This is a most comprehensive investigation and published report on transgender and gender non-conforming matters related to health and the social determinants of health; namely, education, employment, family life, housing, public accommodation, identification and documentation, policing and incarceration. Please pay particular attention to the identified health section, although all factors addressed in this report have health implications:

Injustice at Every Turn: A Report of the National Transgender Discrimination Survey:
http://www.thetaskforce.org/static_html/downloads/reports/reports/ntds_full.pdf

Simulation Learning Objectives

General Objectives:

1. Describe barriers faced by transgender and gender non-conforming patients in the context of receiving care in a community health clinic;

2. Identify the various roles of a nurse in the context of providing care to a transgender patient in the context of a community health clinic;

3. Evaluate the effectiveness of the nurse in carrying out those roles in the context of patient care in this interaction;

4. Identify tools to incorporate into nursing care to develop a practice that is sensitive, informed, affirming, and empowering to the transgender and gender non-conforming patient.

Simulation Scenario Objectives:

1. Demonstrate therapeutic communication skills with the patient;
2. Recognize and demonstrate behaviors that create a safe, welcoming and professional working environment;
3. Demonstrate effective communication within the context of interprofessional collaboration (Identify, Situation, Background, Assessment, Recommendation, Read back);
4. Demonstrate proper assessment techniques in carrying out the tasks of providing care to the trans* identified and gender non-conforming patient;
5. Identify primary nursing diagnoses and/or collaborative issues in the context of the scenario.

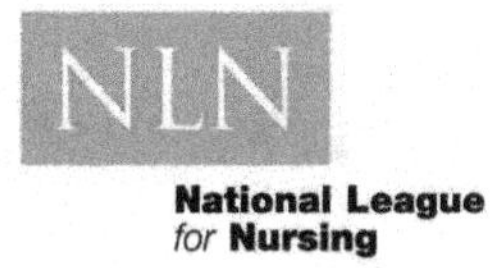

References, Evidence-Based Practice Guidelines, Protocols, or Algorithms Used for This Scenario:

Coleman, E., Botking, W., Botzer, M., Cohen-Ketteris, P., DeGuypere, G., & Feldman..., J. (2012). *Standards of Care for the Health of Transsexual. Transgender and Gender Non- Conforming People, 7th version.* Retrieved 2015, from http://www.wpath.org/site_page.cfm?pk_association_webpage_menu=1351&pk_association_webpage=3926

Hein, L., & Levitt, N. (2014). Caring for... Transgender patients. *Nursing Made Incredibly Easy!*, (12)6, 29-36. doi:10.1097/01.NME.0000454745.49841.76

Hill, M., & Mays, J. (2013). *The gender book* (1st ed.). Houston, Texas: Marshall House Press.

Makadon, H., Mayer, K., Potter, J., & Goldhammer, H. (2015). *The Fenway guide to lesbian, gay, bisexual, and transgender health* (2nd ed.). Philadelphia, Pennsylvania: American College of Physicians.

Teich, N. (2012). Transgender 101: A Simple Guide To A Complex Issue. New York: Columbia University Press.

Resiner, S., Bradford, J., Hopwood, R., Gonzalez, T., Makadon, H., Todisco, D., Cavanaugh, T., VanDerwarker, R., Grasso, C., Zaslow, S., Boswell, S., and K. Mayer (2015). Comprehensive Transgender Healthcare: The Gender Affirming Clinical and Public Health Model of Fenway Health, Journal of Urban Health (92) 3. doi:10.1007/s11524-015-9947-2

Schroth, L. (Ed.). (2014). *Trans bodies, trans selves: A resource for the transgender community (1st ed.).* New York, New York: Oxford University Press.

The Agency for Healthcare Research and Quality: Improving Cultural Competence to Reduce Health Disparities for Target Populations (2016) Retrieved 2016 http://www.ncbi.nlm.nih.gov/books/NBK361126/

The health of lesbian, gay, bisexual, and transgender people building a foundation for better understanding. (2011). Washington, DC: National Academies Press. Retrieved 2015, from http://www.nationalacademies.org/hmd/Reports/2011/The-Health-of-Lesbian-Gay-Bisexual-and-Transgender-People.aspx

The Joint Commission: Advancing Effective Communication, Cultural Competence, Patient- and Family- Centered Care: A Field Guide. (2014). Oak Brook, IL: The Joint Commission. Retrieved 2016 from https://www.jointcommission.org/lgbt/

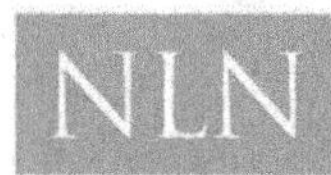

National League for Nursing

Fidelity (choose all that apply to this simulation)

Setting/Environment:

- ☐ ER
- ☐ Med-Surg
- ☐ Peds
- ☐ ICU
- ☐ OR / PACU
- ☐ Women's Center
- ☐ Behavioral Health
- ☐ Home Health
- ☐ Pre-Hospital
- ■ Other: Primary Care Setting—Health Clinic or Physician's Office

Simulator Manikin/s Needed:

Props:

Signage to create an environment that looks like a clinic setting;
Legal Identification Cards: Driver's License for a gender other than the person playing the role of the patient.

Equipment Attached to Manikin:

- ☐ IV tubing with primary line fluids running at ☐ mL/hr
- ☐ Secondary IV line running at mL/hr
- ☐ IV pump
- ☐ Foley catheter ☐mL output
- ☐ PCA pump running
- ☐ IVPB with running at ☐ mL/hr
- ☐ 02 ☐
- ☐ Monitor attached
- ☐ ID band
- ☐ Other:

Equipment Available in Room:

- ☐ Bedpan/Urinal
- ☐ Foley Kit
- ☐ Straight Catheter Kit
- ☐ Incentive Spirometer

Medications and Fluids: (see chart)

- ☐ IV Fluids
- ☐ Oral Meds
- ☐ IVPB
- ☐ IV Push
- ☐ IM or SC

Diagnostics Available: (see chart)

- ☐ Labs
- ☐ X-rays (Images)
- ☐ 12-Lead EKG
- ☐ Other:

Documentation Forms:

- ☐ Provider Orders
- ☐ Admit Orders
- ☐ Flow Sheet
- ☐ Medication Administration Record
- ☐ Graphic Record
- ☐ Shift Assessment
- ☐ Triage Forms
- ☐ Code Record
- ☐ Anesthesia / PACU Record
- ☐ Standing (Protocol) Orders
- ☐ Transfer Orders
- ■ Other: New Patient Intake Forms

Recommended Mode for Simulation:
(i.e. manual, programmed)

Student Information Needed Prior to Scenario:

- ☐ Has been oriented to simulator
- ☐ Understands guidelines /expectations for scenario
- ■ Has accomplished all pre-simulation requirements
- ☐ All participants understand their assigned roles
- ☐ Has been given time frame expectations
- ☐ Other:

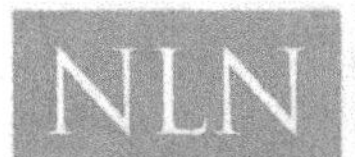

National League for Nursing

☐ Fluids ☐ IV start kit ☐ IV tubing ☐ IVPB Tubing ☐ IV Pump ☐ Feeding Pump ☐ Pressure Bag ☐ 02 delivery device (type) ☐ Crash cart with airway devices and emergency medications ☐ Defibrillator/Pacer ☐ Suction ☐ Other:

Roles/Guidelines for Roles:	**Important Information Related to Roles:**
■ Primary Nurse ☐ Secondary Nurse ☐ Clinical Instructor ☐ Family Member #1 ■ Administrative Clerk/Secretary- this role is played by a standardized patient ■ Observer/s: Patient's in the waiting room (Student roles) ☐ Recorder ■ Physician/Advanced Practice Nurse – played by faculty running sim ☐ Respiratory Therapy ☐ Anesthesia ☐ Pharmacy ☐ Lab ☐ Imaging ☐ Social Services ☐ Clergy ■ Nursing Student Assistant ☐ Code Team	

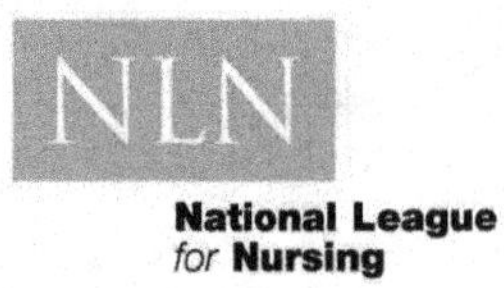

Report Students Will Receive Before Simulation

Time:

Joe Ramirez is a 25 year old Latino who identifies as a transgender female to male person (TGFtM). His name and gender at birth, and as identified on legal documents, is Josephine Ramirez and female. Joe presents at the clinic for a flu shot and a physical. His last visit with a primary care physician had been several years ago, and the only other healthcare professional he has seen lately and regularly is his endocrinologist.

Joe has been taking testosterone prescribed by the endocrinologist for well over a year now. Except for a surgical procedure at 22 (a mastectomy and chest reconstruction), he has avoided most doctors. No other masculinizing interventions have taken place or are planned at this time. Joe is in a committed relationship with his cisgender female partner.

The community clinic practice is relatively new--full of young, hardworking nurses and doctors, and unlicensed assistive personnel. The practice prides itself on a team-based approach to healthcare and is committed to addressing the needs of ALL patients in the community.

Significant Lab Values: none

Provider Orders: refer to chart

Home Medications: refer to chart

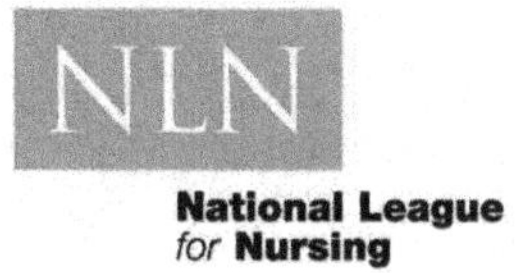

National League
for **Nursing**

Scenario Progression Outline

Timing (approx.)	**Manikin/SP Actions**	**Expected Interventions**	**May Use the Following Cues**
0-5 min	Waiting for name to be called for basic check-in at front desk. Responds to call. Waiting for name to be called by tech for set up for vital signs. Responds to the call.	Primary RN is observing the interaction between the patient and staff while completing other assignments.	**Role member providing cue:** From clerk: Josephine Ramirez. Repeat the calling of the name until there is a response by the patient. * From nursing student assistant: Josephine Ramirez. Repeat the calling of the name until there is a response by the patient. *
5-10 min	Patient is appropriate but initially reluctant to participate in care with nurse.	Primary RN introductions; hand hygiene, therapeutic communication, as appropriate for observable actions of colleagues, and proceeds in ascertaining the patient's purpose for visit, and with assessment, as appropriate.	

Note: The original source uses the deadname of the patient—Josephine Ramirez. For transgender patients who have changed their name, please remember to use the name and pronouns they chose and shared—in this case, Joe Ramirez (he/him).

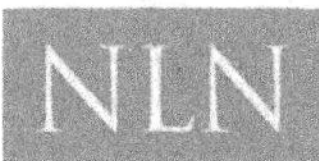

National League
for **Nursing**

10-15 min		Primary RN addresses concerns in ISBARR format with Doctor/NP	**Role member providing cue:** Cue: If RN omits sections of the ISBARR, then the Doctor/NP will ask: What is the situation? What is the background? What is your assessment? What do you recommend, etc., as appropriate.

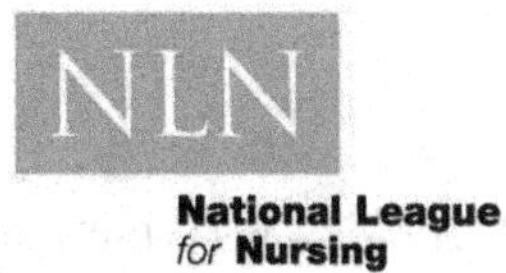

Debriefing/Guided Reflection Questions for This Simulation

(Remember to identify important concepts or curricular threads that are specific to your program)

1. How did you feel throughout the simulation experience?
2. Describe the objectives you were able to achieve.
3. Which ones were you unable to achieve (if any)?
4. Did you have the knowledge and skills to meet objectives?
5. Were you satisfied with your ability to work through the simulation?
6. To Observer: Could the nurse have handled any aspects of the simulation differently?
7. If you were able to do this again, how could you have handled the situation differently?
8. What did the group do well?
9. What did the team feel was the primary nursing diagnosis?
10. How were physical and mental health aspects interrelated in this case?
11. What were the key assessments and interventions?
12. What knowledge have you gained as a result of preparing for and engaging in this simulation that has helped you to understand the trans* and gender non-conforming community?
13. What are the skills, strategies, or interventions a nurse could use to address the barriers and inequities that affect trans* identified and gender non-conforming patients? In what ways did you see those skills utilized in this simulation?
14. What professional nursing values would apply to the situation identified in this scenario (altruism, autonomy, human dignity, integrity, honesty, social justice)? How were those values displayed in the context of this simulation?
15. How has this simulation helped to further develop your understanding of the meaning of nursing and the therapeutic use of self in assisting others—most particularly, the transgender and gender non-conforming population?
16. Is there anything else you would like to discuss?

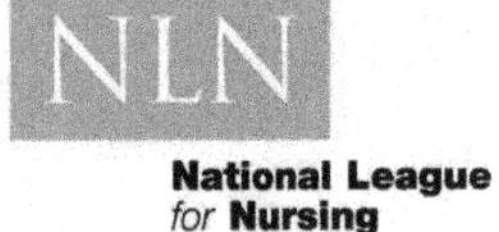

Complexity – Simple to Complex

Suggestions for Changing the Complexity of This Scenario to Adapt to Different Levels of Learners

With application of the NCLEX test plan to this simulation, student discussions can be further exploited as a way of expanding on the complexity of the current simulation as designed:

Safe and Effective Care and Environment: advocacy, case management, client rights, collaboration with interdisciplinary team members, confidentiality, ethical practice, performance improvement, to name a few.

Health Promotion and Maintenance: developmental stages and transitions, health promotion and screening, lifestyle choices, self-care, techniques of physical assessment, to name a few.

Psychosocial Integrity: coping mechanisms, cultural awareness and influences on health, family dynamics, support systems, therapeutic communication and therapeutic environment, to name a few.

Physiologic Integrity: non-pharmacologic comfort interventions, therapeutic procedures, to name a few.

The administration of an IM injection is one of the skills addressed in this simulation. This could be modified to address the IM injection of testosterone to this patient.

Discussion of the intersectionality issues that present in this simulation (Latino, African-American, Catholicism, Living with disabilities). For example, while there are particular health implications and social determinants that impact health affecting the transgender and gender non-conforming population, the goal of achieving optimal health may be further affected by ethnicities, faith, disabilities, etc. Thus, the fact that the patient identifies as transgender is simply one way to describe him/her. Engaging in a discussion about other factors impacting health outcomes can enhance the complexity of the simulation.

This simulation, while taking place in the community setting, is adaptable to the inpatient setting with some modifications.

Supplementing the discussion with additional required resources either before or after the simulation may also impact its complexity. Some of those resources are noted below:

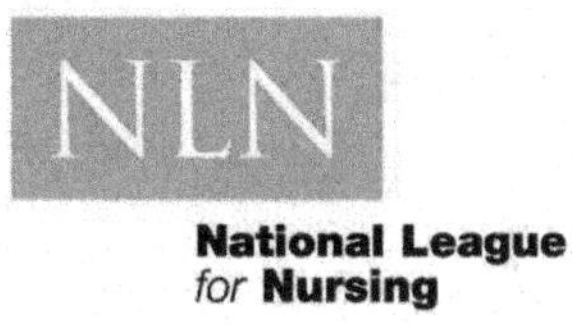

Online Video Resources to Access:

Re-Teaching About Gender & Sexuality from the Youth Perspective:
https://youtu.be/51kQQuVpKxQ

Buck Angel's PSA for Cervical Exams:
https://youtu.be/X_uNFmZHvO0

Buck Angel's PSA for Prostate Exam:
https://youtu.be/YK2fFjDlDE4

Southern Comfort Movie Trailer:
https://youtu.be/R6JIWD2DNyY

Southern Comfort: The Documentary:
https://youtu.be/IH0L3wlV0hg

Australian Rugby Team demonstrating testicular exams:
https://vimeo.com/74742259

The Trans* experiment at Montgomery College:
https://www.youtube.com/watch?v=JO3cIuBHf-U

Online Nursing Articles to Access:

Caring for....Transgender Patients:
http://www.nursingcenter.com/cearticle?an=00152258-201411000-00006

Culturally Sensitive Care for the Transgender Patient:
https://www.nursingcenter.com/CEArticle?an=01271211-201505000-00005&Journal_ID=682710&Issue_ID=3106455

Treating Transgender Patients With Respect:
http://www.americannursetoday.com/viewpoint-treating-transgender-patients-respect/

Nursing Care of Transgender Patients:
http://nursing.advanceweb.com/Features/Articles/Nursing-Care-of-the-Transgender-Patient.aspx

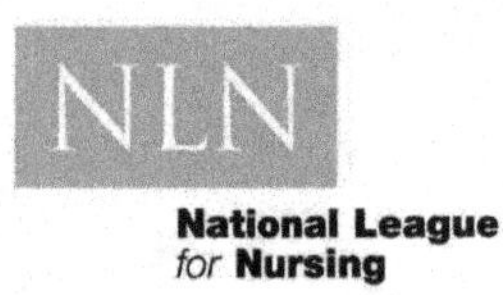

12 Tips for Nurses and Doctors in Treating Transgender Patients:
http://commonhealth.wbur.org/2014/11/treating-transgender-patients-tips

Caring for Transgender Patients at the Johns Hopkins ED:
http://www.hopkinsmedicine.org/news/articles/caring-for-transgender-patients

Movies in Popular Culture that Address the Topic of Transgender Issues:

The Danish Girl
The Dallas Buyers Club
Transamerica
Boys Don't Cry
Paris Is Burning
The Crying Game
The Adventures of Priscilla Queen of the Desert
All About My Mother

Television Programs in Popular Culture that Address Transgender Issues:

Orange Is the New Black

Transparent

Trade Books on the Topic of Being Trans* or Transgender Health:

Mock, J. (2014). *Redefining realness: My path to womanhood, identity, love & so much more.* New York, New York: Atria Paperback.

McKenzie, M. (2014). Black Girl Dangerous: On Race, Queerness, Class and Gender. Oakland, CA: BGD Press, Inc.

Schroth, L. (Ed.). (2014). Trans bodies, trans selves: A resource for the transgender community (1st ed.). New York, New York: Oxford University Press.

Teich, N. (2012). Transgender 101: A Simple Guide To A Complex Issue. New York: Columbia University Press.

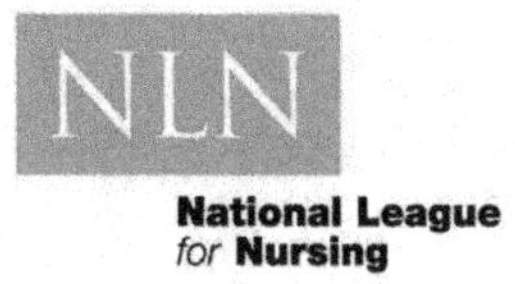

Selected Resources on Transgender Health:

National LGBT Health Education Center: www.lgbthealtheducation.org

The Fenway Institute: www.thefenwayinstitute.org

GLMA: Health Professionals Advancing LGBT Equality: www.glma.org

CDC: Lesbian, Gay, Bisexual, and Transgender Health: www.cdc.gov/lgbthealth

Center of Excellence for Transgender Health: www.transhealth.ucsf.edu

National Center for Transgender Equality: www.transequality.org

World Professional Association for Transgender Health: www.wpath.org

DC Trans Coalition: https://dctranscoalition.wordpress.com/about-dctc/

I AM Transpeople Speak: http://www.transpeoplespeak.org

Healthy People 2020: http://www.healthypeople.gov/2020/topics-objectives/topic/lesbian-gay-bisexual-and-transgender-health

C

Physician Assistant Program Simulation Scenarios

Asthma

Quinnipiac University
Dennis Brown, DrPH, MPH, PA-C

Zapletal, A. L., Baird, J. M., Van Oss, T., Hoppe, M. M., Prast, J. E., & Herge, E. A. *Clinical Simulation for Health Care Professionals* (pp. 231-247).

PHYSICIAN ASSISTANT PROGRAM SIMULATION SCENARIOS

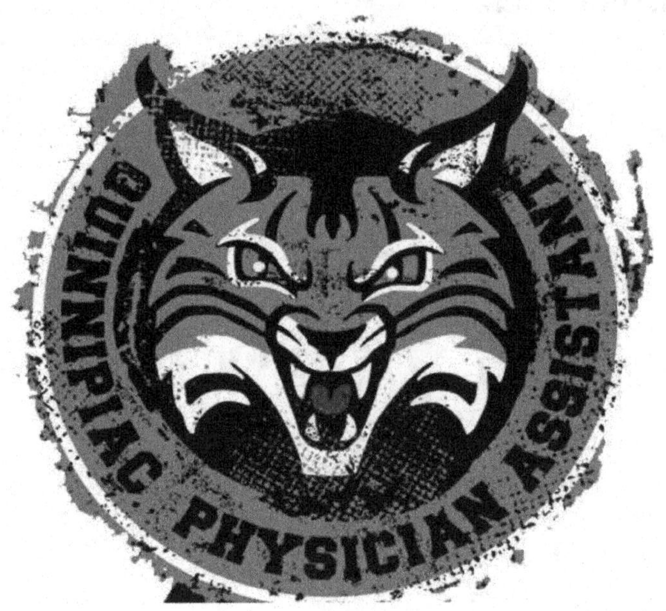

2014 Asthma

Simulation Scenarios

ASTHMA

AUTHOR

Dennis Brown, MPH, PA-C

TARGET AUDIENCE

Physician Assistant Students

Nursing Students

LEARNING OBJECTIVES

Primary

1) Work as an interprofessional team
2) Recognize the signs and symptoms of a patient with respiratory distress
3) Differentiate the difference between the causes of the respiratory illness
4) Obtain a quick and appropriate history
5) Perform an appropriate physical examination
6) Order and interpret appropriate diagnostic studies and be able to explain the reasoning
    a) Radiology
    b) Laboratory
    c) Cardiovascular & Pulmonary (EKG, Echo, ABG)
7) Initiate appropriate immediate, short acting and long term therapy
    a) Bronchodilators
    b) Steroids
    c) Other medical interventions (e.g. magnesium, epi SQ/racemic, theophylline, terbutaline, Heliox)
    d) Supplemental oxygen
    e) Criteria for admission/discharge
    f) Inhaled steroids
    g) Inhaled beta adrenergic
    h) Tapering steroid
8) Recognize the dynamics of a stable and unstable patient with respiratory disease
    a) Recognize need for intubation / ventilation (if warranted)
9) Continuous monitoring and evaluation of the patient for good or poor response to therapy
10) Demonstrate appropriate communications with:
    a) Interdisciplinary team
    b) Supervising physician
    c) Patient and family
11) Patient Education and Counselling
    a) About disease
        i) Triggers
        ii) Natural course
        iii) Pathophysiology
    b) Treatment and need for adherence to therapy
    c) Use of tests (e.g. PEFR/spirometer)

d) Follow up
 i) In office
 ii) Need for ER

Secondary/ Unique for situation

1. Ability to conduct a professional problem oriented history that is comprehensive and appropriate
2. Utilize multiple skills and techniques in obtaining a directed history
3. Ability to conduct a problem oriented directed physical examination utilizing proper techniques, and in a timely fashion
4. Ability to provide a comprehensive oral report to a preceptor which would enable the preceptor to understand the patient's severity, underlying diseases, risks, differential diagnosis, testing and treatment options

ENVIRONMENT

Lab setup

Emergency Department of a community hospital

Manikin setup

Laerdal 3G SimMan ™ in hospital gown in bed, head raised 90 degrees at the start of the scenario

Distractors

May be added for increasing complexity

ACTORS

RN

EQUIPMENT

Monitors required

X	Non-Invasive BP Cuff		12 lead EKG		
	Arterial Line				
	CVP				
	PA Catheter				
X	5 lead EKG				
X	Temperature Probe				
X	Pulse Oximeter				
X	Capnograph				
	BIS				
	Glucometer				

Other equipment required

	Anesthesia Machine	X	ETT		Ventilator
X	Pumps		LMA		
	Brochoscope	X	Laryngoscope		
	Defibrillator	X	Nebulizer		
	Hotline		Nasal Cannula		
	Nerve Stimulator	X	Non-rebreather mask		
	Echo Machine and Probe	X	PEFR (Peak Flow)		

Medications

X	Oxygen	X	IV fluids and admin set		Atropine
X	Epinephrine		SoluMedrol 125mg		Dextrose
X	Albuterol		Ketamine		Sodium Bicarbonate
X	Ipratropium		Propofol		Insulin
X	Magnesium Sulfate		Etomidate		

Supporting Files (cxr, ekg echo, assessment, handouts, etc)

1. file 1
2. file 2
3. etc

TIME DURATION

Set-up	10 minutes
Preparation	5 minutes
Simulation	15-20 minutes
Debrief	20 minutes

CASE NARRATIVE

History

25 year old male with history of asthma presents with cough and coryza symptoms for the past 3 days that significantly worsened 6 hours prior to arrival with increased wheezing and SOB. He took 2 puffs of his Pro-Air® inhaler every 30 minutes without relief. Patient is in significant distress.

Only if asked or if states review of old record

PMH: Asthma since childhood, with 6 previous admissions over the last 12 years; and last year required intubation

Meds: Pro-Air® and Flovent®, but stopped for past 6 months as he was feeling better

Allergies: PCN- as child told he had a rash

SH: Smokes ½ PPD, ETOH 3-4 beers on weekends or if gets together with friends, works as an accountant. Jewish religion

FH: Mom 58, healthy; dad 60, HTN; only child

ROS: Noncontributory

Physical Examination

General:	Well nourished well developed male in moderate respiratory distress
Weight, Height:	est. 185 lbs (84 kg), 70 inches
Vital Signs:	T 37.5; Pulse 100; Resp. 40; BP 106/72 S_aO_2 91% (room air)
Airway:	Patent, audible wheezes, unable to speak more than 3 words sentences, no perioral cyanosis
Lungs:	Diffuse expiratory wheezes and decreased air movement in the lower fields
Heart:	Tachycardic, RRR no murmur, gallops or rubs
Extremities:	No clubbing, edema or cyanosis
Neurologic:	CA&O X3 but starting to become lethargic

Diagnostic Studies

Laboratory:

Radiology:

CXR:

EKG:

See attached

SIMULATOR SETTINGS

Baseline Simulator State: What underlying alterations in physiology would this patient have when compared to "perfect" 70 kg man or woman? Include target numbers. This will comprise your baseline state:

Vitals:	T 37.5; Pulse 100; Resp. 40; BP 106/72 S_aO_2 91% (room air)
Neuro:	CA&O X3 but starting to become lethargic
Respiratory:	Wheezes and decreased air movement in the lower fields
Cardiovascular:	Normal
Gastrointestinal:	Decreased BS
Genitourinary:	NA
Metabolic:	NA
Environmental:	NA

State	Patient Status	Student learning outcomes or actions desired and trigger to move to next state	
1. BASELINE	*In distress, wheezing and only able to speak 3 word sentences*	Learner Actions: Elicit appropriate directed history from patient and/or family Recognition of distress, apply oxygen and get a nebulized treatment ordered ASAP	Operator: Wheezing and coughing Teaching Points: Recognition of distress and time to initiate actions with a focused hx Need to use any resource for information Short term immediate corrective actions Trigger: Breathing treatment initiated
2. Early response	*Continues to wheeze, SpO2 increases slightly with nebulizer* *Increased cough* *Pulse 118, Resp. 28, BP 142/92, Temp. 101.3*	Learner Actions: Initiate medium and long term plans: IV steroids, DuoNeb, supplemental O2 CXR r/o pneumonia +/- ABGs	Operator: Continue with wheeze, increase coughing, starting to have harder time breathing Teaching Points: Need to initiate medium and long term therapies Monitoring the patient Trigger:
3. Not responding to therapy	*Distress*	Learner Actions:	Operator: Teaching Points: ET Intubation

			Trigger:
4.		Learner Actions:	Operator: Teaching Points: Trigger:

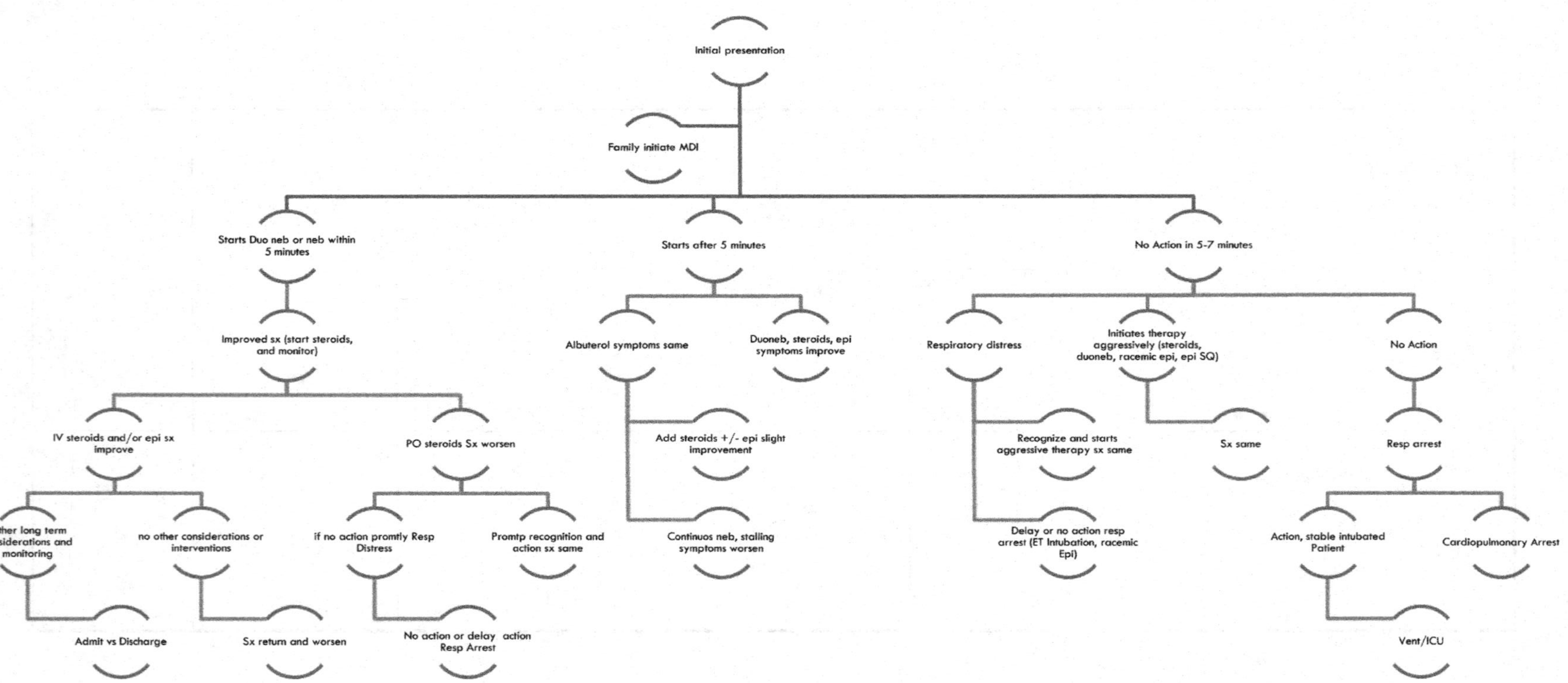

Initial presentation
Family initiate MDI
Starts Duo neb or neb within 5 minutes
Starts after 5 minutes
No Action in 5-7 minutes
Improved sx (start steroids, and monitor)
Albuterol symptoms same
Duoneb, steroids, epi symptoms improve
Respiratory distress
Initiates therapy aggressively (steroids, duoneb, racemic epi, epi SQ)
No Action
IV steroids and/or epi sx improve
PO steroids Sx worsen
Add steroids +/- epi slight improvement
Recognize and starts aggressive therapy sx same
Sx same
Resp arrest
Other long term considerations and monitoring
no other considerations or interventions
if no action promtly Resp Distress
Promtp recognition and action sx same
Continuos neb, stalling symptoms worsen
Delay or no action resp arrest (ET Intubation, racemic Epi)
Action, stable intubated Patient
Cardiopulmonary Arrest
Admit vs Discharge
Sx return and worsen
No action or delay action Resp Arrest
Vent/ICU

INSTRUCTOR NOTES

DEBRIEFING PLAN

1) Describe the initial treatment plans for asthma
   a) B2 agonist, short acting
      i) MDI mild to moderate
      ii) Nebulized moderate-severe
      iii) Continuous
      iv) Albuterol vs levalbuterol
         (1) Pure R-albuterol
         (2) S-albuterol may be weak bronchoconstriction
         (3) Not proven to be superior to racemic epinephrine
         (4) Higher cost
      v) Parenteral
         (1) Terbutaline SQ (0.01 mg/kg)
         (2) Epi 1:1000 SQ 0.3 mg
      vi) Steroids
         (1) Inhaled
         (2) Systemic
            (a) PO route equivalent to IV if tolerated
               (i) Prednisone 2 mg/kg
               (ii) Dexamethasone 0.6 mg/kg
               (iii) Side effects limit tolerance (taste, irritability, bloating)
            (b) IV
               (i) Methylprednisolone 1-2 mg/kg
         (3) Anticholinergic agent, relaxes smooth muscles
            (a) Ipratropium (250 mcg < 20 kg; 500 mcg > 20 kg)
            (b) Cheap and safe
            (c) Can use with nebulized and MDI albuterol (Duoneb)
         (4) Magnesium Sulfate
            (a) Cheap and safe
            (b) Class IIIb
         (5) Heliox (data inconclusive)
         (6) Ketamine (2 mg/kg IV)
            (a) Bronchodilator
            (b) Data limited
               (i) Some suggest may prevent ETT
            (c) Drug of choice for RSI
         (7) Noninvasive positive pressure ventilation
            (a) May prevent ETT
            (b) Must be able to protect airway, cooperative and stable patient
      vii) Mechanical Ventilation for asthma
         (1) High rate of complications due to hyperinflation
         (2) Poor reserve
         (3) Limit minute ventilation and allowance for expiration time
            (a) Tidal volumes 6-8 cc/kg

(b) Slower than usual rates (<10 in adults)

b) Patient Education
   i) Communication skills, at the right level for the patient and family to understand
   ii) Disease process, so patient and family understands
      (1) Pathophysiology
   iii) Treatments
      (1) Basic mode of action
      (2) Need for compliance
      (3) Risks vs benefits
      (4) Long term management of disease
      (5) Break through and action plans
   iv) Lifestyle and non-pharmacologic management
      (1) Restrictions/triggers/limitations
      (2) Tobacco use
      (3) NSAIDs
      (4) Exercise
   v) Monitoring status
      (1) PEFR
      (2) Symptoms
   vi) Need for emergent care

DEBRIEFING HANDOUT

PILOT TESTING AND REVISIONS

EVALUATION FORM ASTHMA

Name: ______________________ Date: ______________________

Simulation: ____

Evaluators: 1) ______________ 2) ______________ 3) ______________

4) ______________ 5) ______________

The form is objective, record only what was witnessed, there is no "benefit of doubt".

Action	Explanation	Completed	Not Done	Poor Technique	Comments
Obtains a comprehensive problem oriented history					
	Introduces self or alternative appropriate form of greeting and acknowledgement				
	Obtains a chief complaint				
	Elicits a pertinent HPI Onset, palliative/provoking (triggers)* factors, quality, radiation, severity, timing Pertinent PMH including previous treatments for asthma (meds, steroids, hospitalizations, ET intubations, home PEFR, spirometry)* Pertinent SH (tobacco*, ETOH, occupation and exposures) FH: Asthma, allergy, eczema ROS: Focused (including recent URI sx)				

Performs appropriate problem oriented directed physical exam					
	Washes hands*				
	Overall assessment of general status				
	Mentation (CA&OX3)				
	HEENT • Airway, oral pharynx • Posterior pharynx (noting +/- stridor) • Nares • TMs • Sinuses • Neck (JVD, tracheal deviation, lymph)				
	Chest • Work of breathing, retractions, accessory muscle use, Abd breathing • Respiratory excursion • Tactile fremitus				
	Lungs • Bilateral lung sounds anterior and posterior (min 4 areas each incl apex) • Egophony, whispered pectoriloquey				
	Heart • All areas sitting • Supine, squatting, lateral decub				

	Neurological ☐ Mental Status ☐ Cognitive Functions ☐ Cranial Nerves ☐ Motor ☐ Sensory ☐ DTRs ☐ Cerebellar				
Oral Presentation					
	Organized Follows a standard format of Hx, PE, Diff Dx.				
	History: Presents appropriate components including pertinent positives and negatives ☐ CC ☐ HPI ☐ PMH appropriate to case ☐ SH appropriate to case ☐ FH appropriate to case ☐ ROS appropriate to case				
	☐ Physical: Describes pertinent positive and negative findings to appropriate directed problem oriented exam				
	Diff Dx. ☐ Formulates at least 4 differentials of high likelihood, one of which should include the actual problem ☐ Discusses steps to rule in or out the differentials				
	☐ Preceptor can formulate a diagnosis based upon the presentation of the student				

Comments

QUINNIPIAC UNIVERSITY BEST MEDICAL CARE CENTER

PATIENT TRIAGE FORM

Patient: Ida Wanabreath **DOB: 6/7/1999**

Patient Id #: 098765 **PCP: Dr. I. Know**

Chief Complaint: "It is hard for me to catch my breath."

25 year old male with history of asthma presents with cough and coryza symptoms for the past 3 days that significantly worsened 6 hours prior to arrival with increased wheezing and SOB. He took 2 puffs of his Pro-Air® inhaler every 30 minutes without relief.

Non smoker, no flu shot

Medicines:

ProAir MDI

Tylenol prn

Nyquil

Allergies:

Unknown

Vital signs:

BP: **106/72** Pulse: **100** Respiration: **40** SpO2: **91% (room air)**

Weight: **86** kg Height: **71** inches Temp: **37.5**

D

Department of Physician Assistant Studies Simulation Scenario

Chest Pain Angina

Quinnipiac University
Dennis Brown, DrPH, MPH, PA-C

Zapletal, A. L., Baird, J. M., Van Oss, T., Hoppe, M. M., Prast, J. E., & Herge, E. A. *Clinical Simulation for Health Care Professionals* (pp. 249-263).

Dept. of Physician Assistant Studies

SIMULATION SCENARIO

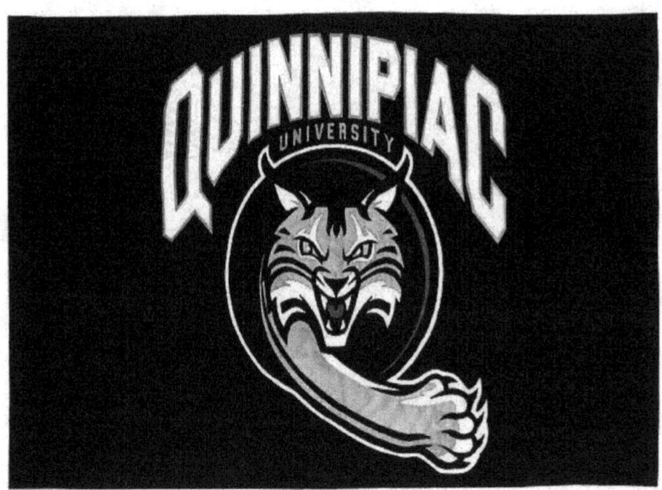

School of Health Sciences
Athletic Training
Cardio-Pulmonary Perfusion
Diagnostic Imaging
Occupational Therapy
Physical Therapy
Physician Assistant
Social Work

2016 Chest Pain-Angina

Simulation Scenario

CHEST PAIN-ANGINA

I. Author: Dennis Brown, MPH, PA-C

II. Target Audience
PA Student

III. Learning Objectives
A. Ability to obtain a problem oriented medical history that is pertinent and directed but comprehensive for the symptomatology
B. Ability to perform a directed physical examination that is problem oriented and directed and demonstrates proper technique
C. Ability to present a detailed, well organized oral presentation of the patient to a preceptor in time efficient manner, including a differential list and plan of action
D. Provide an approach to the care of the patient with utilization of appropriate diagnostic testing, treatment options, and education of the patient and family

Assessment Tool(s):

Rubric, direct observation, presentation to faculty member

Educational Rationale: Remediation experience based upon preceptor feedback, testing the student's competency in history, physical and oral presentations in a timely manner

Assessment Tool:

Specific rubric for remediation

IV. Equipment
Monitors required:

X	Non-Invasive BP Cuff				
	Arterial Line				

	CVP				
	PA Catheter				
X	5 lead EKG				
X	Temperature Probe				
X	Pulse Oximeter				
	Capnograph				
	BIS				

Other equipment required:

	Anesthesia Machine		ETT		
	Pumps		LMA		
	Brochoscope		Laryngoscope		
	Defibrillator				
	Hotline				
	Nerve Stimulator				
	Echo Machine and Probe				

Supporting Files (cxr, ekg echo, assessment, handouts, etc)

1. EKG: Sinus tach
2. CXR: Normal
3. Echo: Normal

Time Duration

Set-up	5 min
Preparation	10 min
Simulation	15 min
Debrief	15 min

V. Environment

Lab set-up: Emergency Department of a community hospital

Manikin set-up: Laerdal 3G SimMan™ in hospital gown in bed, head raised 90 degrees at the start of the scenario

Distractors: May be added for increasing complexity

VI. Case

Case Stem (one to two paragraphs on pertinent patient and scenario information-this should be the stem for the learner and should include location, physician/help availability, family present, etc.):

56 year old male presented to the ED with chest pains that have been intermittent for the past 3 months, he has no pain at the current time.

Only if asked or if states review of old record

Background and briefing information for facilitator/coordinator's eyes only:

Patient Data Background and Baseline State: *only made available when directly asked for or is performing proper exam techniques*

Patient History (should follow standard H and P format):

56 year old male with retrosternal chest pressure on and off for about 3 months now, started only with activity, recently has noticed with rest and when stressed at work. Relieved with resting and waiting it out. No radiation, severity moderate (6/10) but impacts what he is doing, scaring him to point he is less active than before. Timing as stated before, lasts about 10-15 minutes. No SOB, no diaphoresis, no lightheadedness or syncope, no edema of legs or ankles

PMH:

Borderline HTN no meds

SH:

(+) Tobacco, 1 PPD for 32 years (-) drugs, ETOH 2 mixed drinks a night, Occupation: account executive for a national insurance company

FH:

Father: deceased from lung CA age 68, +MI at 53

Mother: 78 HTN, DM

Brother: 59 MI

Review of Systems:

CNS: (-)h/a, - N/V/D, - vision changes, - tinnitus, - focal weakness or numbness

Cardiovascular: see HPI

Pulmonary: - SOB, - cough

Renal / Hepatic: - jaundice

Endocrine: - wt changes

Heme/Coag: - gingival bleeding

Derm: - rashes, - discoloration of nails or clubbing

Current Medications and Allergies:

Aspirin 81 mg a day (forgets at least 3 days a week)

Allergy: Shell fish - angioedema

Physical Examination:

General: Average build male in no discomfort

Weight, Height: 210 lbs, 70"

Vital Signs: BP: 172/98, HR: 88, R: 16, O_2 Sat 100% room air

Skin: Warm and dry

HEENT/Airway: PERRLA, EOMI, fundi normal. Patient airway, no specific findings.

Neck: Supple FROM – rigidity, - lymph, - bruits

Lungs: CTA

Heart: RRR, - murmurs/gallops/rubs

Abdomen: N/A (normal findings if tests)

GU/Rectal: N/A (normal findings if tests)

Musculoskeletal: N/A (normal findings if tests)

Neurologic: C,A& O X 3, MS and cognitive function appropriate for age and socioeconomic status. CN II-XII intact, 2+DTR = bilateral, = Bilat motor and sensory, - cerebellar testing

Flow Chart: *(Use flow chart for dynamic changes)*

4. State	Patient Status	Student learning outcomes or actions desired and trigger to move to next state	
1. BASELINE		**Learner Actions:** ○	**Operator:** ○ **Teaching Points:** ○ **Trigger:**
2.		**Learner Actions:** ○	**Operator:** ○ **Teaching Points:** ○ **Trigger:**

3.		**<u>Learner Actions:</u>** ○	**<u>Operator:</u>** ○ **<u>Teaching Points:</u>** ○ **Trigger:**
4.		**<u>Learner Actions:</u>** ○	**<u>Operator:</u>** ○ **<u>Teaching Points:</u>** ○ **Trigger:**

VII. Instructor Notes

VIII. Debriefing Plan

IX. References

X. Evaluation Form Headache/Chest Pain

Name: ______________________ Date: ______________________

Simulation: ____

Evaluators: 1) __________________ 2) __________________ 3) __________________

4) __________________ 5) __________________

The form is objective, record only what was witnessed; there is no "benefit of doubt".

Action	Explanation	Completed	Not Done	Poor Technique	Comments
Obtains a comprehensive problem oriented history					
	Introduces self or alternative appropriate form of greeting and acknowledgement				
	Obtains a chief complaint				
	Elicits a pertinent HPI • Onset, palliative/provoking (triggers)* factors, quality, radiation, severity, timing • Pertinent PMH (HTN*) • Pertinent SH (tobacco*, ETOH, occupation and exposures) • FH: CAD*, HTN, DM • ROS: Focused				
	Assesses cardiac risk factors				

Performs appropriate problem oriented directed physical exam					
	Washes hands*				
	Overall assessment of general status				
	Mentation (CA&OX3)				
	HEENT • Airway, oral pharynx • Neck (JVD, tracheal deviation, lymph, bruits)				
	Chest • Work of breathing • Gross exam of chest (lifts, heaves) • Palpates for tenderness and thrills				
	Lungs • Bilateral lung sounds anterior and posterior (min 4 areas each including apex)				
	Heart • Palpates PMI Sitting • Auscultates all areas with diaphragm and bell Supine • Auscultates all areas with diaphragm and bell Left lat decub • Auscultates with diaphragm				
	Neurological • Mental Status • Cognitive Functions • Optional				

	○ Cranial Nerves ○ Motor ○ Sensory ○ DTRs ○ Cerebellar				
	Skin and Extremities • Edema • Pulses • Cyanosis				
Oral Presentation					
	Organized Follows a standard format of Hx, PE, Diff Dx.				
	History: Presents appropriate components including pertinent positives and negatives • CC • HPI • PMH appropriate to case • SH appropriate to case • FH appropriate to case • ROS appropriate to case				
	Physical: Describes pertinent positive and negative findings to appropriate directed problem oriented exam				
	Diff Dx. • Formulates at least 4 differentials of high likelihood, one of which should include the actual problem • Discusses steps to rule in or out the differentials				
	Preceptor can formulate a diagnosis based upon the presentation of the student				

Comments

QUINNIPIAC UNIVERSITY BEST MEDICAL CARE CENTER

PATIENT TRIAGE FORM

Patient: Hal Tsetse

DOB: 6/7/1956

Patient Id #: 098767

PCP: Dr. Har Attick

Chief Complaint: "Chest Pain"

56 year old male with chest pain on and off for the past 3 months, no pain now.

Medicines:

ASA

Allergies:

Shellfish

Vital signs:

BP: **172/98** Pulse: **88** Respiration: **16** SpO2: **100% (room air)**

Weight: **210** lbs Height: **70** inches Temp: **98.5** F

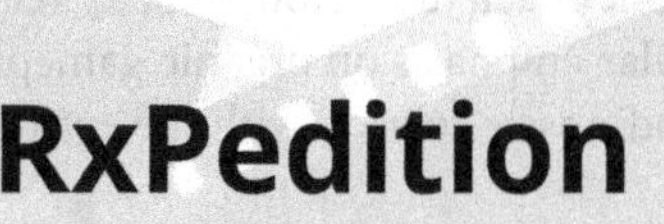

RxPedition

Gameful Simulation for Teaching Drug Development

Victoria L. B. Grieve, PharmD

- How the learners were prepared
  - Simulation takes place over 15 weeks. Learners are prepared throughout via just-in-time didactics covering elements of the drug development process. Student groups receive guidance in the simulation from the instructor/gamemasters as needed.
- Learning objectives
  - Understand the process of drug discovery and development, including the experimental nature of medication creation; biostatistics; applied pharmacokinetics/pharmacodynamics; and the business aspects of running a biotech company in the United States.
  - Enhance the learners' 21st century skills (e.g., critical thinking, creativity, communication, collaboration, resilience) through an immersive, gameful simulation.
- Clinical case overview
  - Student groups of five or six members take on the role of running a mock biotech startup company and proceed through a simulated metaphor of the actual process a company goes through to develop a medication. This involves researching active molecules through phase trials, acquiring investments to fund the process, managing the public image of the company, and finding their place in the market.
- Assessment measures used
  - Some traditional didactic assessments are deployed alongside the just-in-time training.
  - Certain metrics are gathered throughout the simulation as markers of performance. Most of these derive from presentations the students give to mock investors and coincide with feedback the student's receive.

Zapletal, A. L., Baird, J. M., Van Oss, T., Hoppe, M. M., Prast, J. E., & Herge, E. A. *Clinical Simulation for Health Care Professionals* (pp. 265-266).

- A *Grand Finale* assessment occurs at the very end that is a 2-hour assessment simulation. This is a scenario that embodies all the elements of the larger simulation. Group performance on this simulation helps determine mastery of important elements of the process throughout the 15 weeks.
- Debriefing questions or format
  - Debriefing occurs in the final session. The head instructor/gamemaster runs a simulation of company performance in the market to evaluate how much money each team would make. Teams are then highlighted who did outstanding work, with particular emphasis on organic gameplay between the groups. The instructor then leads a question-and-answer period with the entire group lasting roughly 1 hour to act as a mass debriefing.
- Simulation modality (standardized patient, task trainer, manikin, virtual, etc.)
  - Large-scale, in-person, gameful simulation with simulation software serving as a backbone.
- Materials, supply, equipment list, etc.
  - Learning management software, google sheets, SimCYP by Centura, gamemaster experience, typical classroom technology.
- Example schedules
  - 15 weeks of dual, 4-hour sessions in place of a traditional class.
- Training information (i.e., standardized patient training agenda)
  - Four instructor/gamemasters are required at minimum. Training is continuous throughout the process in the same way a tabletop role-playing game is run.

Pharmacy
Telephonic Standardized Patient Calls

Victoria L. B. Grieve, PharmD

- How the learners were prepared
  - Learners register their numbers with a staff member who programs them into the system. A brief lesson in class on appropriate phone communication techniques is given.
- Learning objectives
  - Enhance student skill and comfort with telephonic communication with patients.
- Clinical case overview
  - Usually done as an added task following a standardized patient (SP) case. Following the case, the instructor can have the patient follow up via telephone in a standardized way, recording the student's interactions for assessment.
- Assessment measures used
  - Simple rubrics that cover necessary elements of a telephonic patient conversation, as determined by instructor.
- Debriefing questions or format
  - Feedback is provided to the students directly in the form of completed rubrics.
  - Brief class-wide debrief occurs in the following class session to cover common mistakes and answer questions the students may have.
- Simulation modality (SP patient, task trainer, manikin, virtual, etc.)
  - SP.
- Materials, supply, equipment list, etc.
  - Google Voice account, SP or staff to provide patient voice to recorded message, rubric for assessing student messages.

Zapletal, A. L., Baird, J. M., Van Oss, T., Hoppe, M. M., Prast, J. E., & Herge, E. A. *Clinical Simulation for Health Care Professionals* (pp. 267-268).

- Example schedules
  - SP experience on Monday, call from patient released on Tuesday, students call back to leave their side of conversation by Friday.
- Training information (i.e., SP training agenda)
  - SP only has to record pre-written line once, system deploys same message to all students. Staff member monitoring system needs training on setting it up and pulling the student responses back down.

G

Standardized Patient Simulation for Mobility Training in the Intensive Care Unit

University of Pittsburgh
Andrea L. Hergenroeder, PhD, PT
Victoria Hornyak, PT, DPT

Use of Standardized Patient Simulation Experiences for Training in the Rehab Professions

Simulation-based learning experiences are used widely to complement the clinical training of students across health disciplines, including physical therapy. Using simulation, the instructor can incorporate various practice elements within a learning activity, assess student performance in a low-stakes environment, and allow the student to reflect on performance. There are numerous approaches to simulation and a variety of modalities that can range from low to high fidelity, depending on the extent to which the learning activity reproduces real world situations. High-fidelity human simulation (HFHS) is one health care education methodology that uses life-like manikins to simulate patients so that students can practice procedural and clinical decision-making skills in a realistic environment. Simulation with high-fidelity simulators is an effective modality for training in the health professions; however, there are several limitations for use with training for rehab professions such as physical and occupational therapy. HFHS manikins are expensive, often not readily available to programs that do not have a simulation center, and are limited in their ability to simulate human movement—which is an integral part of the examination and treatment in the rehab professions (e.g., patient movement in bed, transfers from one surface to another, and ambulation). For these reasons, standardized patients (SPs) are often used to facilitate training of students in the rehab professions. SP training experiences allow the student to practice communication skills with an SP while training the student in hands-on mobility skills and clinical decision making. The fidelity of the SP training experience can be enhanced using simulated environments (hospital settings) and simulation software such as Laerdal's SimMan to allow an immersive training experience.

Zapletal, A. L., Baird, J. M., Van Oss, T., Hoppe, M. M., Prast, J. E., & Herge, E. A. *Clinical Simulation for Health Care Professionals* (pp. 269-281).

Importance of Training Students in the Treatment of Patients in the ICU Setting

Rehabilitation providers have an important role in the examination and treatment of patients in critical care. In particular, a growing body of research has shown that early mobilization of patients in the intensive care unit (ICU) setting helps to improve physical function and reduce risk of adverse events in patients who are hospitalized. Students often have limited exposure to working in an ICU, given the complexity of the patient presentation and the lack of clinical experiences that may be available to students in this setting. In addition, the complexity of this hospital setting poses several challenges to students, which include the need for continuous assessment and monitoring of the patient's physiological status and the management of invasive and noninvasive monitoring equipment and medical devices (e.g., IV lines, catheters, supplemental oxygen delivery devices). In order for students to be competent and safe in treating patients in this setting, training experiences that allow students to demonstrate clinical decision making while performing "hands-on" clinical skills are critical.

Preparing the Learners (Prebriefing)

This simulation is delivered to first-year Doctor of Physical Therapy (DPT) students within the context of two required courses in the DPT plan of studies (Patient Management and Cardiopulmonary Physical Therapy). Prior to the simulation, students are taught the clinical skills required for participation in the simulation including patient chart review skills, assessment of vital signs, bed mobility, transfer, gait training, and varying aspects related to communication with the patient. Students are also provided practice in mobilizing a patient and managing hospital equipment such as the IV pole and portable oxygen tank.

The week of the simulation experience, students are provided written and verbal instructions about the simulation—including the schedule and sequence of events for the simulation, the learning objectives, and the role of the SP. The students are familiar with the environment in which the simulation is conducted because it is located within their clinical skills lab. Instructors emphasize that the purpose of the simulation activity is for formative assessment, and the students are informed that the activity is not a part of graded coursework for the course.

Description, Purpose, and Learning Objectives

The purpose of this simulation is for students to develop a physical therapy treatment session for a patient in the acute care setting using an SP and environment (ICU), in order to receive formative feedback from the instructor. This type of simulation is often referred to as a hybrid format—one in which two or more types of simulation are used together. In this case, the patient's physical presence, functional performance, and emotional tone are simulated by the SP's portrayal of the case, while the patient's physiologic status and responses to activity are simulated using computer-based technology. Additionally, the hospital environment is simulated using the department's clinical skills lab, which is discussed further in the materials and supplies section.

Students work in groups of two, acting as a physical therapy "team" to treat the SP—including developing the treatment plan before the session begins, implementing the plan, communicating with the patient, and making clinical decisions related to the patient. An instructor observes the treatment session and utilizes Laerdal's SimMan software to modify the patient's display on an ICU monitor in real time during the patient mobilization attempt. When the patient starts to mobilize out of bed and ambulate, the instructor is able to adjust the physiological parameters, including the heart rhythm, heart rate, respiratory rate, and oxygen saturation and observe how the student responds to the patient's physiological changes during the mobilization attempt.

The patient's blood pressure and heart rate are modified during the change in position from supine to sitting to reflect orthostasis. In addition, when the patient is ambulating with the student, the patient's vital signs are adjusted to reflect respiratory compromise from the patient's underlying medical condition and deconditioning associated with bedrest. These programmed vital sign responses include an increase in the patient's heart rate, blood pressure, and respiratory rate and a decrease in oxygen saturation while the patient is ambulating with the student.

During this simulation experience, students are expected to accomplish the following learning objectives:

- Using a simulated chart and documentation of a physical therapy examination, determine the patient's medical history and current functional status.
- Develop a mobility-focused treatment plan for the patient.
- Assess and monitor the patient's cardiovascular and pulmonary status during a treatment session.
- Use clinical reasoning to respond to cardiovascular and pulmonary changes within the treatment session.
- Demonstrate effective communication skills with the patient and the health care team.
- Maintain patient safety during the entire treatment session, which will focus on mobility skills.

Overview of the Clinical Case

The patient case was developed by board-certified clinical specialists in cardiovascular and pulmonary and geriatric physical therapy. The case includes physical therapy skills required for provision of a treatment session in a critical care setting, which are based on the Normative Model of Physical Therapist Education and the Core Competencies for Entry-Level Practice in Acute Care Physical Therapy.

The patient in this simulation is a 75-year-old woman who is admitted through the emergency department of an adult medical-surgical referral hospital due to fever, chills, progressive difficulty breathing, and generalized weakness and fatigue. The patient has a past medical history of diabetes, peripheral neuropathy, osteoarthritis, and a prior stroke that resulted in mild left-sided weakness. The patient is diagnosed with pneumonia on this hospital admission. The patient has fallen several times over the year and is fearful of falling.

The goal of the visit from the physical therapist is to perform a physical therapy treatment session with the patient that includes demonstration of vital sign assessment, monitoring of physiologic responses, and mobility training (e.g., bed mobility, transfer, and gait training).

The students are provided with information from the chart review as well as a summary of past medical history and findings from the initial physical therapy examination. Students are not required to ask questions related to the patient's past medical history and social history, as this information is provided by the instructor in the chart review. (Additional patient details can be found in the Student Materials for the Simulation section.)

Debriefing Form and Questionnaire for the Simulation

This simulation is conducted for formative assessment, and students are asked to reflect on their performance, but are not formally assessed by the instructor on clinical skills. After the simulation, the instructor completes a debriefing form and reviews the form with the students. The students are asked to complete an SP learning experience questionnaire that was developed by the instructors. This questionnaire asks the student to rate their level of agreement (from strongly disagree to strongly agree) using a five-point Likert scale on multiple aspects of the simulation, including the patient scenario provides the appropriate level of

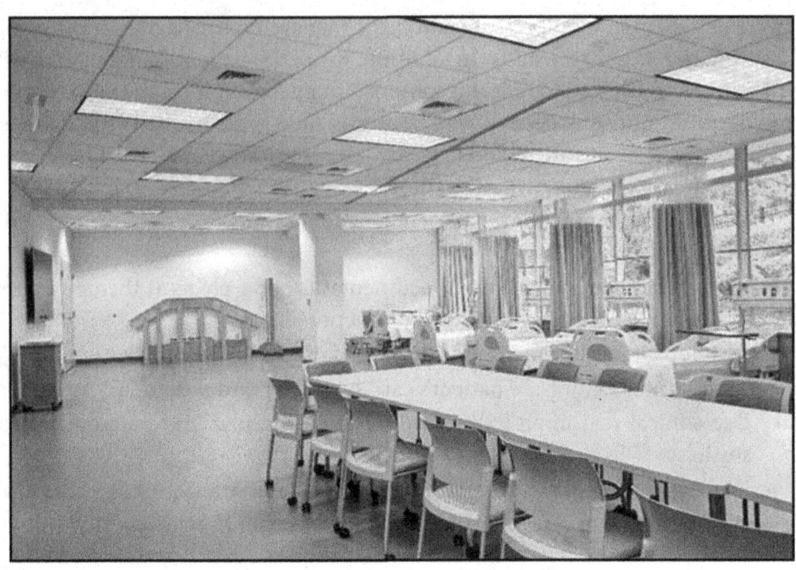

Figure G-1. Clinical skills training lab for the department of physical therapy.

fidelity, the level of complexity of the case is appropriate, the debriefing session is effective, the simulation is applicable to course material, the simulation contributes to the development of clinical reasoning and decision-making skills, and the simulation improves confidence in providing physical therapy care.

Environment and Equipment for the Simulation

The environment for the simulation activity is the physical therapy department's clinical skills training lab. The training lab contains five hospital beds that are separated by privacy curtains to simulate a hospital environment (Figure G-1). The hospital bed utilized in this simulation includes adjustable railings, a computer monitor to simulate an ICU monitor, and a head wall attached to the hospital bed that includes simulated oxygen, suction canisters with suction capabilities, and medical air. The ICU monitor is connected to a computer that contains Laerdal SimMan simulation software.

The equipment required for the simulation includes a bedside stool, an over-bed hospital table, a wheelchair, walker, straight cane, IV line and pole with a bag of normal saline solution, a nasal cannula, oxygen tubing, a portable oxygen tank, a foley catheter, hospital tape, a stethoscope, and a blood pressure cuff. For this simulation, the SP is wearing a hospital gown and is connected to the IV using medical tape and wearing a nasal cannula connected to a simulated oxygen port that is located on the head wall of the hospital bed (Figure G-2).

Students are asked to arrive at their scheduled time for the simulation. On arrival, students are provided with a paper patient chart that contains the information about the patient's past medical history, history of current illness, social history, and home set-up. The student team is provided with 10 minutes to review the patient care and prepare their treatment session for the simulation. The student team is permitted 15 to 20 minutes to conduct the treatment session with the SP. During the treatment session, the students are responsible for introducing themselves to the patient and conducting a physical therapy treatment session that includes mobilization of the patient out of bed. The instructor assists with monitoring the time of the session and informs students when they should end the treatment session. Afterward the students, the patient, and the instructor conduct a 10-minute debriefing session. At the end of the debriefing, the students are able to ask one question to the SP about their performance. At the end of the debriefing, students are asked to place all of the materials for the activity back in the folder and return to the classroom to complete the SP learning experience questionnaire. The example schedule for the simulation is shown in Table G-1.

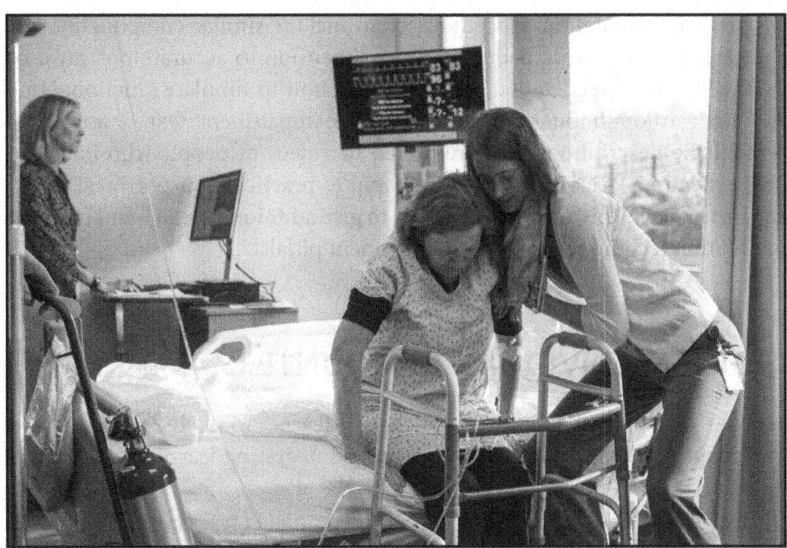

Figure G-2. Student, standardized patient, and instructor during the simulation.

Table G-1. Example Schedule for the Simulation

Schedule	Activity
10 minutes	Chart review and planning of treatment session for the students
15 to 20 minutes	Treatment session with students and SP
10 minutes	Debriefing of simulation event with instructor
10 minutes	Student completion of questionnaire

Standardized Patients in Physical Therapy Simulation

The Department of Physical Therapy works closely with the Standardized Patient Program (SPP), which is located in the School of Medicine. The SPP is a formal program that employs approximately 100 people who are specially trained to portray patient cases (known as SPs, or standardized patients). Most importantly, the SPs receive extensive training in how to provide detailed feedback to students from the patient perspective. The Department of Physical Therapy contracts with the SPP to utilize four SPs and an alternate for the event.

In order to adequately prepare for their roles, the SPs are given a portfolio of materials, including the student learning objectives, the student instructions and schedule, and a detailed patient profile. The patient profile includes the medical history; reason for hospitalization; background information such as a social history, family structure, and living arrangements; and guidelines for the emotional tone and presentation of the patient. Emotional tone is important because it allows for a range of responses and reactions that increase the realism of the interaction between the SP and the students.

The SPP at the University of Pittsburgh was developed for use in the medical school, and in the past several years has expanded its reach to all six schools of the health sciences including the School of Health and Rehabilitation Sciences, comprised of physical therapy, occupational therapy, speech-language pathology, physician assistant studies, and eight other health professions.

Traditionally, SPs are trained in accurate portrayal of typical encounters with physicians such as providing a medical history and chief complaint and submitting to office-related exam procedures (e.g., blood pressure assessment; auscultation of heart and breath sounds; inspection of eyes, ears, nose, and throat; and palpation of body parts). Rehabilitation procedures often include similar components, but also typically involve movement and exercise, which adds another dimension to accurate portrayal of the patient. To account for this, the SPs are given detailed descriptions of how to simulate functional impairments related to weakness, pain, cardiopulmonary distress, cognitive impairment, fear, or any other contributing factor. To supplement the descriptions, SPs are linked to videos of people who have the actual impairments of the case. Lastly, the SPs arrive early to the event to practice their portrayal of the movement dysfunction with the instructors. This allows instructors to give additional details and to make the SPs aware of accepted rehabilitation techniques and common student pitfalls.

Debriefing Individual Encounters

Debriefing is a critical part of any simulation activity and allows the learner to safely reflect on their performance, identify areas of strengths and weaknesses, and plan for integrating learning into future performance.

For this event, a 10-minute debriefing session is conducted after the simulated treatment session, and it includes the students, the SP, and a faculty facilitator. The communication skills and debriefing method used in our simulation are based on a teaching method used in the training of oncology and palliative care residents and fellows, called Oncotalk. The Oncotalk methodology uses learner-identified objectives and the use of a facilitator to guide the learner through difficult and often emotionally charged situations that are encountered in end-of-life discussions. The method lends itself well to any communication scenario that requires a clinician to skillfully use empathy. For this simulation, physical therapist students are often asking their patients to attempt movement that may cause physical distress, fear, or even pain. As such, the debriefing session often focuses on students learning how the patient (as portrayed by the SP) felt during the interaction, whether that involves specific verbal interactions or the hands-on techniques of therapeutic interventions.

The debriefing session begins with having the student self-identify areas of strength, which can be corroborated by their student partner, the SP, and/or the faculty facilitator. Students are then invited to identify areas of the encounter where they felt unsure or nervous about their skills. They are further invited to brainstorm aloud about what they might say or do differently if given the opportunity. If a student is unable to identify a better strategy, their peers are invited to offer suggestions. The student is then permitted to ask the SP one question about their performance in order to elicit constructive feedback. The SP, who has been listening closely to the debriefing thus far, gives specific feedback about their experience by providing a response to the question formulated by the student. Finally, the faculty facilitator elicits a take-home point from each student, with the intention of summarizing their learning in the encounter.

Feedback from the SP is a unique feature of the simulation. Because the SPs are given details about the learning objectives, standards of practice, and common student pitfalls, they are able to give feedback that is tailored to the experience. Students are given explicit instructions on how to formulate an effective question for the SP. For example, a question that is specific to a communication technique or manual skill that the student practiced will yield better feedback than a broad question such as "How did I do?" and in fact, that particular question is not permitted.

Each faculty facilitator is given a debriefing guide that outlines the steps of the debriefing process and a debriefing form on which to record notes for each phase of the debriefing process.

Evaluation of Performance and Learning

After all students have completed the activity, the course faculty conduct a debriefing session that includes all of the facilitators as well as the SPs. In this session, the instructors utilize a similar structure to the one used in the individual debriefing sessions: identifying what went well, what areas were difficult, and how the event could be improved for the next cohort. The SPs have been instrumental in this process, and over the course of 4 years have offered invaluable advice on how they can be used most effectively in giving feedback to the students.

During the facilitator debriefing, the team discusses the strengths and weaknesses of selected individual students and identifies trends in common errors among the class as a whole. The debriefing forms are a valuable tool in this process, helping facilitators to remember specific scenarios and take-home points.

This information is compiled by the course faculty and is presented to the students in a 20-minute debriefing of the class as a whole. Since the event is held near the end of the semester but before a graded, final skills evaluation, the students can use the information to practice specific communication and/or patient handling skills that were problematic during the event. Faculty use the information gained from the event debriefing to identify areas in the curriculum that are effective, as evidenced by strong student performance. Likewise, areas where the curriculum needs to be reinforced are identified and included in future instruction.

Limitations and Potential Enhancements to the Simulation

This simulation event is a high-fidelity simulation of an important aspect of physical therapy practice. It allows students to practice high stakes skills that are required when working in the ICU, in the low stakes format of a formative activity where it is "safe" to make mistakes.

There are several limitations of our simulation to consider. First, planning and executing the event requires significant time. In order for 60 DPT students to participate in the 30-minute event, it requires approximately 30 hours of facilitator time (i.e., 5 hours each for six facilitators on the day of the event). Case development represents many hours of work upfront, but results in cases that are used again each time the event is repeated in subsequent years. Second, budgeting must account for contracting the SPs through the SPP. For our event, four SPs are paid an hourly rate for the event, plus additional hours for rehearsal time. A fifth SP is paid as an alternate, in case of illness or unforeseen circumstances. Lastly, a 5-hour event, with four cases running simultaneously, only allows each student to participate for 30 minutes. In that 30-minute time frame, the students work in pairs, which decreases the time that each student individually practices any given skill. Student feedback about the event is very positive, but one common criticism is that students would like additional practice. More time and/or additional facilitators and SPs could increase an individual student's exposure to the simulation, but would need to be weighed against timing and cost.

There are several modifications to the simulation format that may enhance the learning experience. Each of these would require an evaluation of the additional time and resources required.

- *Video Recording of Each Student Encounter.* In its current form, the encounter is not recorded; however, video recording of simulation events is well described in the literature and allows students to see their own encounter and reflect on details that might not be remembered otherwise.
- *Including a "Time-Out" and "Rewind."* One teaching method that can be included in each student encounter is the opportunity to call a "time-out" when they are unsure what to do next. Once they have considered new options (formulated on their own or suggested by their peers or the facilitator), the student can rewind the interaction to the point of concern and try the skill again.
- *Increase the Complexity of the Case.* This event aims to provide formative feedback on foundational skills for managing patients in the ICU for first-year DPT students. The case could easily be modified to include more advanced skills by adding medical complexity, additional equipment considerations such as extensive tubes and lines attached to the patient, or the inclusion of a more serious adverse event to which the students must quickly and skillfully respond.

- *Add an Interprofessional Component.* This event could be expanded to include students of various professions, with objectives modified to include the Interprofessional Education Collaborative's Core Competencies.
- *Include Additional Outcome Measures.* This event is formative in nature and currently assesses student perceptions of the effectiveness of the event using a questionnaire. Skills checklists and before-and-after tests of self-efficacy or knowledge are additional options. Literature on objective structured clinical examinations (OSCEs) offers numerous ideas about measuring learner outcomes.

Lastly, the simulation uses a high-fidelity environment that closely replicates a room in an ICU, including the use of a simulated patient monitor. This event could be conducted in the absence of these enhancements. For example, instead of a simulated electronic patient monitor, students could verbally be told of vital sign changes in their patient. A simple mechanical adjustable bed or treatment table could be used, and teaching assistants, adjunct faculty, or other health professionals/colleagues could role play as the patient. All of these adjustments sacrifice some level of fidelity, but still allow for skill practice and acquisition of important clinical skills in a low-stakes environment.

Student Materials for the Simulation

Purpose

The purpose of this lab is for students to develop a treatment session for a hospitalized patient with a simulated patient and environment, in order to receive formative feedback.

Objectives

- Using a simulated chart and documentation of a physical therapy examination, determine the patient's medical history and current functional status.
- With your partner, develop a mobility-focused treatment plan for the patient.
- Assess and monitor the patient's cardiovascular status during the treatment session.
- Use clinical reasoning to respond to cardiovascular changes within the treatment session.
- Demonstrate effective communication skills with the patient and the health care team.
- Maintain patient safety during the entire treatment session, which will focus on mobility skills.

This activity is designed to give you an opportunity to practice some of the skills you learned in Patient Management 1 and Cardiopulmonary 1 in a realistic environment.

You will be working with an SP. SPs are actors who are specially trained through the University of Pittsburgh School of Medicine to portray patients in health care settings. *You should treat the SPs with the same respect and care you would with a patient in your clinic. Once you begin the session with the patient, you must stay in character in your role.*

You will work in groups of two, and you and your partner will act as a physical therapy team to treat the patient. You should work with your partner to conduct the treatment session, communicate with your patient, and make clinical decisions related to your patient. *You should attempt to distribute the patient-related duties equally so that you each have responsibilities during the patient encounter.* Consider making some of these decisions with your "physical therapy partner" during your planning meeting before the patient encounter.

- All students should dress in clinic-appropriate clothes. Although we are simulating inpatient cases, you can dress in outpatient-appropriate attire (since many of you do not have scrubs or other hospital attire).

As a group, you will have 10 minutes to prepare, 15 minutes to work with the patient, and 10 minutes to debrief. A physical therapy instructor or faculty member will observe your session and will participate in the debriefing and provide feedback.

During the debriefing, you and your partner will have the opportunity to ask the SP one question about your team's performance. The question should be related to the student's guarding techniques, hand placement for the treatment, effectiveness of instruction, and or concern/empathy for the patient's situation. Here are some examples of appropriate types of questions:

- "Did you feel safe when I was helping you to stand?"
- "Did you ever feel like you were going to fall when I was helping you walk?"
- "When you told me you were short of breath, did you feel like I addressed your concerns adequately?"
- "Did I cause you any pain during the treatment session from the way I was physically handling you?"
- "I was nervous and unsure of what to do when you said you were dizzy. Did you feel like I confidently handled the situation?"

Remember, you should *not* ask hypothetical questions: "Would it have worked better for you if I said my instructions differently?" Also, very general questions like "How did I do?" are not allowed.

Instructions

1. Arrive for your case at the designated time. You will meet in the first floor classroom and obtain the folder for your patient.
2. You will each spend the first 10 minutes in the classroom reviewing the patient's "chart" and the instructions. Your physical therapy team should plan your approach to the session and parcel duties during this time.
3. Together, you will also develop a mobility-based treatment session for your patient (bed mobility transfers, gait, etc.). You should decide who will take the lead during the mobility session. ***One of the goals of the interaction is to practice the mobility skills you learned previously.***
4. At the designated time, you can enter the hospital lab to begin working with your patient. Each group will gather around the patient's bed to begin the treatment session.
5. You will have 15 minutes to work with your patient. Enter the room, introduce yourself and the team, and explain why you're there.
6. Begin the session by taking vital signs, then proceed with your treatment as planned—responding to the patient's questions, functional performance, and cardiovascular response to activity as needed. You should decide who will take the lead in taking vital signs. ***Remember, another important goal of this activity is to assess and respond to vital signs.***
7. Your instructor will keep time and indicate when you should end the treatment session.
8. Your group, the SP, and the instructor will conduct a debriefing session. At the end of the debriefing, your team can ask one question to the SP about your performance.
9. At the end of the debriefing, place all of the materials for the activity back in the folder and return it to the classroom for the next group.
10. Return to the classroom and complete the evaluation form. You may leave when you are finished. Thank you!

Presenting Situation and Instructions to the Student: Mrs. Dorothy Brown

The patient, Mrs. Dorothy Brown, is a 75-year-old woman with diabetes, hypertension, osteoarthritis, and stroke who presented to the emergency department with progressive shortness of breath, fever, cough, fatigue, and weakness. She reports that she recently had the flu but does not seem to be getting better. She reports a history of falling in the past month. She is diagnosed with pneumonia on this hospital admission.

Refer to the records (see later) from chart review as well as a summary of past medical history and findings from the initial physical therapy examination. *You will not have to ask questions related to past medical history and social history since this is provided and this is a treatment session (not an examination).*

- Vital signs
  - Temperature: 100°F
  - Pulse: 96
  - Respiration: 26
  - Blood pressure: 152/88
  - O_2 saturation: 95% on 4 liters of oxygen
- Prescription medications
  - Lantus: 15 units at bedtime
  - Glipizide: 20 mg twice a day
  - Lisinopril: 10 mg daily
  - Hydrochlorothiazide: 12.5 mg daily
  - Aspirin: 81 mg daily
  - Lipitor: 80 mg daily
  - Neurontin: 900 mg three times daily
- Lab values and medical tests
  - Hematocrit: 28% (low)
  - Hemoglobin: 10 g/dL (low)
  - Platelets: 180,000 (normal)
  - White blood cells: 14,505 (high)
  - Chest x-ray: Left lower lobe infiltrates

As a team, you should:

- Review the patient information provided (you may refer to this information throughout the encounter). You will have 10 minutes to review this information.
- Perform an appropriate physical therapy treatment session to include assessment of the patient's *vital signs, bed mobility training, transfer training, and gait training while monitoring the patient's response to training on the patient monitor.* You should include all appropriate instruction/patient education for the activities that you are performing and make the appropriate clinical decisions about your patient based on their response to treatment. You should limit your session to these activities. You will have 15 minutes to perform the physical therapy treatment session.

Patient Profile for the Student

- *Diabetes:* The patient was diagnosed with diabetes about 15 years ago. Blood sugars run around 200 when the patient is able to check levels at home.
- *Peripheral Neuropathy:* The patient knows this is a complication of diabetes. She experiences numbness and tingling in her feet. She does not inspect her feet.
- *Stroke:* The patient was hospitalized about 1 year ago with a stroke that affected the left side of her body. She was in the hospital for a week and primarily had problems with weakness on the left side of the body and some mild memory problems. The weakness affected her walking, and she is not as steady as she used to be before the stroke.
- *High Blood Pressure:* This was diagnosed 30 years ago. She is taking medications for HTN but does not monitor BP at home.
- *Arthritis:* The patient has mild pain from arthritis in both knees for some time. Tylenol effectively relieves the pain.
- *Past Surgical History:* None
- *Allergies:* None
- *Family History:* Mother died of cancer, father died of heart disease. She cannot recall when, but both parents were older.
- *Social History:* The patient has been married for 50 years but has no children. She worked as an elementary school teacher for many years before retiring at age 60. She grew up in Pittsburgh and has stayed in the area. She has two sisters that live out of state. Her primary support is her husband.
- *A Typical Day for the Patient:* The patient wakes up at 9:00 a.m. and gets breakfast and gets dressed. The patient typically naps, reads, and watches TV during the day. The patient has dinner around 5:00 p.m. and goes to sleep around 11:00 p.m. The patient goes out to lunch with her husband or to the grocery store a few times per week.
- *Mental Status:* The patient is oriented to person, place, and time. She is able to recall recent events and discuss medical history. She is able to follow all simple commands, but may be a little bit slow to process multiple-step directions.
- *Functional Status Prior to Admission to the Hospital:* The patient does most things on her own, but uses a cane to walk outside of the house. She does not drive. She did not need help to get dressed, bathe, or walk around the house. She is able to walk a few blocks before becoming fatigued. She has fallen in the past.

Summary of Findings From Initial Physical Therapy Examination for the Student

- *Cognition:* The patient is alert and oriented x3 but had some problems following more complex multiple-step directions.
- *Resting Vitals:* Heart rate: 85/min, blood pressure: 132/82, oxygen saturation: 96% at rest on 4 liters of oxygen. With walking 10 feet, HR: 106/min, blood pressure 136/80, oxygen saturation 94%.
- *Range of Motion:* Within functional limits for bilateral upper and lower extremities.
- *Strength:* Grossly 3 to 4/5 on the left side and 4+/5 on the right side.
- *Sensation:* Decreased sensation to light touch in bilateral lower extremities in a stocking-glove distribution.
- *Pain:* Patient reports mild pain in both knees, 1 to 2/10 at rest.

- *Physical Function:* The patient was able to transfer supine to sit with minimal to moderate assistance, and ambulate 10 feet in her room with minimal assistance using a wheeled walker and 4 liters of oxygen via nasal cannula. Minimal shortness of breath was noted during ambulation but oxygen saturation was >94% throughout treatment. The patient had a slight loss of balance during ambulation due to left-sided leg weakness from prior CVA.
- *Assessment and Plan of Care:* The patient presents with deficits in functional mobility secondary to prior stroke and current deconditioning. The plan for physical therapy is to see the patient twice daily for transfer, gait training with least restrictive assistive device, instruction in therapeutic exercise, and balance training. The patient wishes to return home with husband at discharge. Would likely benefit from continued physical therapy upon discharge.

INSTRUCTOR MATERIALS

Debrief Instructions

Purpose

The purpose of this lab is for students to work in groups to develop a treatment session for a hospitalized patient with a simulated patient and environment, in order to receive formative feedback.

Objectives

- Using a simulated chart and documentation of a physical therapy examination, determine the patient's medical history and current functional status.
- Develop a mobility-focused treatment plan for the patient.
- Assess and monitor the patient's cardiovascular status during the treatment session.
- Use clinical reasoning to respond to cardiovascular changes within the treatment session.
- Demonstrate effective communication skills with the patient and the health care team.
- Maintain patient safety during the entire treatment session, which will focus on mobility skills. Students should be reminded that the debriefing component during the last 10 minutes of the activity is a valuable opportunity for formative feedback from faculty, peers, and the patient.

In order to facilitate the best feedback possible, consider the following techniques:

- *During the Treatment Session:* Faculty should take notes … it's helpful to have quotes of student-patient conversations—both successful and less-than-desirable examples. Also take note of handling skills that are done well vs. those that were awkward, unsafe, or those that could have benefited from better planning. The students should also be instructed to be observant in order to give feedback to their peer.
- *After the Treatment Session:* Start with the positive! Begin by asking the students what they did well. They should be able to identify something positive—even if it's only that the introductions went well. When the students can't come up with any other positives, the instructor takes a turn with positive feedback. Next, move to student-identified areas for improvement. Ask the students if there was any place in the interaction where they felt unsure, nervous, or believed they could have done better. Hopefully, the instructor can corroborate the difficult parts and give examples to support what the student noticed.

  Student: I messed up when it was time to transfer the patient to the chair and I realized that the chair was too far away. So I had to sit the patient back down and get the chair.

  Instructor: Yes, I noticed that too. The patient said, "Do I have to try to step over there?" and she seemed very unsure. What could you do differently to improve the situation next time?

  Student: Next time I will definitely get the chair closer to the patient before I start the transfer.

If the student can't come up with a way to improve the situation, ask permission to go to their peer for an idea. If there's a major safety issue that the student fails to bring up, the faculty member can do it here.

Next, a student can ask the SP one question about the interaction. It should be a focused, specific question about the communication or patient handling skills:

- "Did you feel safe when I was helping you to stand?"
- "When I explained your precautions, were the instructions too vague?"
- "Did you ever feel like you were going to fall when I was helping you walk?"
- "When you told me you were short of breath, did you feel like I addressed your concerns adequately?"
- "Did I cause you any pain during the treatment session from the way I was physically handling you?"
- "I was nervous and unsure of what to do when you said you were dizzy. Did you feel like I confidently handled the situation?"

Students should ***not*** ask hypothetical questions: "Would it have worked better for you if I said my instructions differently?" Also, very general questions like "How did I do?" are not allowed.

Finally, ask both students for a take-home point. Each student should be able to come up with a take-home point or summary statement about the interaction.

Bibliography

Back, A. L., Arnold, R. M., Baile, W. F., Fryer-Edwards, K. A., Alexander, S. C., Barley, G. E., Gooley, T. A., & Tulsky, J. A. (2007). Efficacy of communication skills training for giving bad news and discussing transitions to palliative care. *Archives of Internal Medicine, 167*(5), 453-460. https://doi.org/10.1001/archinte.167.5.453

Back, A. L., Arnold, R. M., Tulsky, J. A., Baile, W. F., & Fryer-Edwards K. (2003). Teaching communication skills to medical oncology fellows. *Journal of Clinical Oncology, 21*(12), 2433-2436. https://doi.org/10.1200/JCO.2003.09.073.

Hastings, S. N., Sloane, R., Morey, M. C., Pavon, J. M., & Hoenig, H. (2014). Assisted early mobility for hospitalized older veterans: Preliminary data from the STRIDE program. *Journal of the American Geriatric Society, 62*(11), 2180-2184. https://doi.org/10.1111/jgs.13095

Henneman, E. A., Cunningham, H., Roche, J. P., & Curnin, M. E. (2007). Human patient simulation: Teaching students to provide safe care. *Nurse Educator, 32*(5), 212-217.

Interprofessional Education Collaborative. (2016). *Core competencies for interprofessional collaborative practice: 2016 update.* Author.

Martinez-Villa, A., Casas-Herrero, A., Zambom-Ferraresi, F., Sáez de Asteasu, M. L., Lucia, A., Galbete, A., García-Baztán, A., Alonso-Renedo, J., González-Glaría, B., Gonzalo-Lázaro, M., Iráizoz, I. A., Gutiérrez-Valencia, M., Rodríguez-Mañas, L., & Izquierdo, M. (2019). Effect of exercise intervention on functional decline in very elderly patients during acute hospitalization: A randomized clinical trial. *JAMA Internal Medicine. 179*(1), 28-36. https://doi.org/10.1001/jamainternmed.2018.4869

Mori, B., Carnahan, H., & Herold, J. (2015). Use of simulation learning experiences in physical therapy entry-to-practice curricula: A systematic review. *Physiotherapy Canada, 67*(2), 194-202.

Ohtake, P. J., Lazarus, M., Schillo, R., & Rosen, M. (2016). Simulation experience enhances physical therapist student confidence in managing a patient in the critical care environment. *Physical Therapy, 93*(2), 216-228.

Pritchard S. A., Felicity, C., Blackstock, D. N., & Keating, J. L. (2016). Simulated patients in physical therapy education: Systematic review and meta-analysis. *Physical Therapy, 96*(9), 1342-1353. https://doi.org/10.2522/ptj.20150500

Sabus, C., & Macauley, K. (2016). Simulation in physical therapy education and practice: Opportunities and evidence-based instruction to achieve meaningful learning outcomes. *Journal of Physical Therapy Education, 30*(1), 3-13.

Silberman, N., Litwin, B., Fernandez-Fernandez, A., Ng, G., & Dornbaum, M. (2019). Development and evaluation of a simulation-based acute care course in a physical therapist education program. *Journal of Physical Therapy Education, 34*(1), 1. https://doi.org/10.1097/JTE.0000000000000122

Zang, K., Chen, B., Wang, M., Chen, D., Hui, L., Guo, S., Ji, T., & Shang, F. (2020). The effect of early mobilization in critically ill patients: A meta-analysis. *Nursing in Critical Care, 25*(6), 360-367. https://doi.org/10.1111/nicc.12455

Portions of Appendix G are reproduced with permission from the University of Pittsburgh.

H

Occupational Therapy in a Skilled Nursing Facility/Long-Term Care

Virginia Commonwealth University
Carole Ivey, PhD, OTR/L, FAOTA
Jaime Smiley, MS, OTR/L

Zapletal, A. L., Baird, J. M., Van Oss, T., Hoppe, M. M., Prast, J. E., & Herge, E. A. *Clinical Simulation for Health Care Professionals* (pp. 283-310).

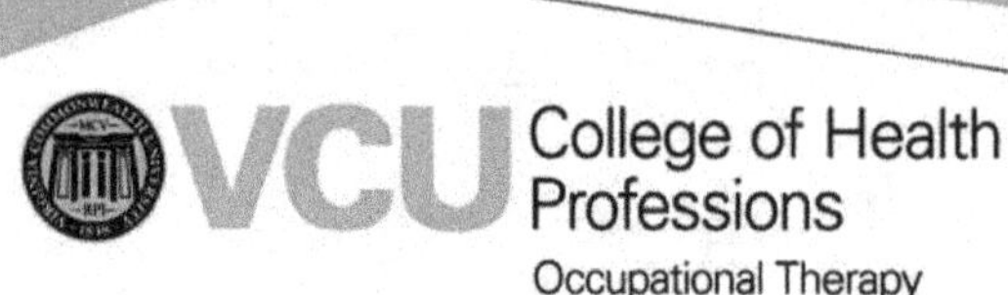

Appendix A Standardized Patient Lab – Prebrief

Educational Objectives

By the end of this standardized patient module, students will be able to:

1. Apply relevant medical and social information from a chart review during a patient evaluation.
2. Select relevant assessment methods on the basis of client needs, contextual factors, and psychometric properties of assessments.
3. Perform an initial occupational therapy evaluation on a patient with a CVA, demonstrating appropriate safety standards and client-centered evaluation techniques.
4. Document results of initial evaluation, including formulation of an appropriate intervention plan using a standard medical reporting technique.

Our assumption – we believe that everyone (SPs and students) participating in this lab is intelligent, capable, cares about doing their best, and wants to improve.

Logistics

Check in with instructor at table by first floor classrooms (by snack machines).

Schedule:

30 minutes for the student to complete a chart review, answer three written questions, and gather assessment materials;

20 minutes of the SP evaluation lab session;

15 minutes debriefing with the SP;

10 minutes to clean up materials;

1 hour to write a SOAP note.

We will gather a variety of assessments for you to look over and choose what you want to bring in to the room. Included in these assessments will be manual blood pressure cuffs & stethoscope, pulse oximeter, dynamometer, pinchometers, goniometers, standardized tests, and adaptive equipment (e.g., reachers, long handled sponges, button hooks). If there is a specific assessment you want from the assessment cabinet, please let the coordinator know ahead of time.

Patient & Environment

Patient diagnosis: MCA CVA

Setting: Skilled Nursing Facility

Patient room with basic toiletries (comb, toothbrush, toothpaste, razor, shaving cream, cup, washcloth, hand towel, deodorant, and soap), clothes for dressing

See sample

Roles

Standardized patients (SPs) have all been trained, worked from a rubric, and are random assignment.

The SPs will stay in character for the duration of the patient evaluation. When you are finished, say goodbye and start walking out as if you are leaving session. That will be the clue for the SP to switch to their debriefing role debrief with you.

You are responsible for monitoring your time.

We ask for you to accept direct and critical feedback, practice skills, and work outside your comfort zone.

Expectations

- ☐ No live tweets or social media posts
- ☐ No sharing any information to other classes about this lab

Fiction Contract

- This is a standardized patient but it is based on a real patient and the intent is to simulate a real patient encounter
- There is much fiction in our environment
- With these fictional elements, we ask for your buy-in

You will be evaluated on

- Initial Questions from chart review - knowledge of information and planning
- Evaluation lab with SP
    - Communication – clearly and effectively communicate verbally and nonverbally with clients
    - Fundamentals of practice – safety
    - Carries out appropriate evaluation techniques correctly
- SOAP note
    - Ability to thoroughly and accurately document occupational performance using standardized and nonstandardized assessment tools
    - Accurately document occupational therapy services in an efficient and timely manner
- Thoughtful self-evaluation of your skills during the lab (through observation and reflection of your video)

Things to Bring

- Device to video record your lab session (or contact coordinator if you don't have one)
- Anything that you would/could normally bring in with you to help you

Joe #1 Chart Review

You are an occupational therapist in a skilled nursing/long-term care facility. You have completed a chart review on your patient and have talked to the patient's son in the admission director's office prior to initiating your evaluation. Below is the information you have gathered.

Chart review findings:
Name: Joe Smith
Age: 85
Gender: M
Primary Diagnosis: (L) middle cerebral artery (MCA) CVA
Insurance: Medicare / United Healthcare
Hospital Admission Date: 5 days ago
SNF Admission Date: yesterday
Height: 5'9"
Weight: 180 lbs
Hand Dominance: Right

PMH: hypertension (HTN), coronary artery disease (CAD), gastroesophogeal reflux disease (GERD), hypothyroidism, dementia, (L) total hip arthroplasty (THA) 2011, type II diabetes

Precautions: PEG tube: bolus feedings. NPO.

From the hospital notes: Pt was found at home by son. Pt has expressive aphasia and right hemiparesis.

Medications	Dose:	Treatment of:
Aspirin	81mg	Deep vein thrombosis (DVT)
Docusate	100mg	Constipation
Esomoprazole (before breakfast)	20mg	GERD
Hydrochlorothiazide	125mg	HTN
Levothyorine	75mg	Thyroid
Metoprolol	50mg q12h	HTN
Prednisone	5mg p breakfast	
Ropinirole	1mg @bedtime	Restless leg syndrome (RLS)
Tylenol	q4h prn	Pain/temperature
Milk of magnesia (MOM)	30cc prn	Constipation
Mylanta	30cc prn q4h	Indigestion

From interview with patient's son:
Pt is 85 year old retired paper mill worker. Pt's father worked as a mail loader/unloader of trains. He passed away when Joe was 3 years old from a massive heart attack. His mother raised 9 children and passed away from cancer when Joe was 16 years old.

Joe met his wife in a nearby town where he grew up. They married young and had 3 children: Jane, Joe Jr, and Lorraine. All of his children are married. He has 11 grandchildren and 13 great grandchildren.

Joe and his wife resided in the city and his wife passed away 12 years ago. Joe stills lives in the same home. All of his children live locally.

Joe attends church at Mt. Tabor Baptist Church every week. He has many friends and neighbors. He enjoys doing puzzles and doing house repairs.

Home situation and prior level of function (PLOF): Joe resides in a one-story home with 5 steps to enter (STE) with rail on both sides. Pt was independent with ADLs and IADLs prior to admission. Pt previously used straight point cane (SPC) for community ambulation. Pt drove his own car short distances.

Pre-Evaluation Questions from chart review (2 pts each)

1. What do you expect to see with aphasia?

2. What considerations do you have knowing the patient has type II diabetes?

3. How is hemiplegia different from hemiparesis?

Joe #2 Chart Review

You are an occupational therapist in a skilled nursing/long-term care facility. You have completed a chart review on your patient and have talked to the patient's son in the admission director's office prior to initiating your evaluation. Below is the information you have gathered.

Chart review findings:
Name: Joe
Age: 85
Gender: M
Primary Diagnosis: R CVA
Insurance: Medicare / United Healthcare
Hospital Admission Date: 5 days ago
SNF Admission Date: yesterday
Height: 5'9"
Weight: 180 lbs
Hand Dominance: Right

PMH: hypertension (HTN), coronary artery disease (CAD), gastroesophogeal reflux disease (GERD), hypothyroidism, dementia, (L) total hip arthroplasty (THA) 2011, type II diabetes

Precautions: PEG tube: bolus feedings. NPO.

From the hospital notes: Pt was found at home by son. Pt has (L) hemianopsia and (L) hemiparesis.

Medications	Dose:	Treatment of:
Aspirin	81mg	Deep vein thrombosis (DVT)
Docusate	100mg	Constipation
Esomoprazole (before breakfast)	20mg	GERD
Hydrochlorothiazide	125mg	HTN
Levothyorine	75mg	Thyroid
Metoprolol	50mg q12h	HTN
Prednisone	5mg p breakfast	
Ropinirole	1mg @bedtime	Restless leg syndrome (RLS)
Tylenol	q4h prn	Pain/temperature
Milk of magnesia (MOM)	30cc prn	Constipation
Mylanta	30cc prn q4h	Indigestion

From interview with patient son:
Pt is 85 year old retired paper mill worker. Pt's father worked as a mail loader/unloader of trains. He passed away when Joe was 3 years old from a massive heart attack. His mother raised 9 children and passed away from cancer when Joe was 16 years old.

Joe met his wife in a nearby town where he grew up. They married young and had 3 children: Jane, Joe Jr, and Lorraine. All of his children are married. He has 11 grandchildren and 13 great grandchildren.

Joe and his wife resided in the city and his wife passed away 12 years ago. Joe stills lives in the same home. All of his children live locally.

Joe attends church at Mt. Tabor Baptist Church every week. He has many friends and neighbors. He enjoys doing puzzles and doing house repairs.

Home situation and prior level of function (PLOF): Joe resides in a one-story home with 5 steps to enter (STE) with rail on both sides. Pt was independent with ADLs and IADLs prior to admission. Pt previously used straight point cane (SPC) for community ambulation. Pt drove his own car short distances.

Pre-Evaluation Questions from chart review (2 pts each)

1. Describe neglect vs hemianopsia.

2. What considerations do you have knowing the patient has type II diabetes?

3. How is hemiplegia different from hemiparesis?

Joe #3 Chart Review

You are an occupational therapist in a skilled nursing/long-term care facility. You have completed a chart review on your patient and have talked to the patient's son in the admission director's office prior to initiating your evaluation. Below is the information you have gathered.

Chart review findings:
Name: Joe
Age: 85
Gender: M
Primary Diagnosis: R CVA
Insurance: Medicare / United Healthcare
Hospital Admission Date: 5 days ago
SNF Admission Date: yesterday
Height: 5'9"
Weight: 180 lbs
Hand Dominance: Right

PMH: hypertension (HTN), coronary artery disease (CAD), gastroesophogeal reflux disease (GERD), hypothyroidism, dementia, (L) total hip arthroplasty (THA) 2011, type II diabetes

Precautions: PEG tube: bolus feedings. NPO.

From the hospital notes: Pt was found at home by son. Pt has (L) neglect and (L) hemiplegia.

Medications	Dose:	Treatment of:
Aspirin	81mg	Deep vein thrombosis (DVT)
Docusate	100mg	Constipation
Esomoprazole (before breakfast)	20mg	GERD
Hydrochlorothiazide	125mg	HTN
Levothyorine	75mg	Thyroid
Metoprolol	50mg q12h	HTN
Prednisone	5mg p breakfast	
Ropinirole	1mg @bedtime	Restless leg syndrome (RLS)
Tylenol	q4h prn	Pain/temperature
Milk of magnesia (MOM)	30cc prn	Constipation
Mylanta	30cc prn q4h	Indigestion

From interview with patient son:
Pt is 85 year old retired paper mill worker. Pt's father worked as a mail loader/unloader of trains. He passed away when Joe was 3 years old from a massive heart attack. His mother raised 9 children and passed away from cancer when Joe was 16 years old.

Joe met his wife in a nearby town where he grew up. They married young and had 3 children: Jane, Joe Jr, and Lorraine. All of his children are married. He has 11 grandchildren and 13 great grandchildren.

Joe and his wife resided in the city and his wife passed away 12 years ago. Joe stills lives in the same home. All of his children live locally.

Joe attends church at Mt. Tabor Baptist Church every week. He has many friends and neighbors. He enjoys doing puzzles and doing house repairs.

<u>Home situation and prior level of function (PLOF)</u>: Joe resides in a one-story home with 5 steps to enter (STE) with rail on both sides. Pt was independent with ADLs and IADLs prior to admission. Pt previously used straight point cane (SPC) for community ambulation. Pt drove his own car short distances.

Pre-Evaluation Questions from chart review (2 pts each)

1. Describe neglect vs hemianopsia.

2. What considerations do you have knowing the patient has type II diabetes?

3. How is hemiplegia different from hemiparesis?

Joe #1: Notes/Guidelines for the Standardized Patient

Set-Up Notes

- Have only regular (not hospital "grip") socks on – shoes off but in room.
- Take off wheelchair footrests – place a few feet from w/c.
- Have sweater/jacket off – in room.
- Present sitting in **unlocked** w/c, leaning to the right with right arm dangling over the right armrest with arm dangling down by wheel.
    - **NOTE** Do they fix your position upon entering? (both centering and upright) Are they aware of safety precautions with arm by wheel? Do they lock your brakes? If needed, do they put on footrests?

Patient Level of Function

- Able to follow basic 1-2 step verbal commands, but slowly
- Able to understand simple gesturing (pointing); able to manipulate common objects/complete basic tasks when presented (wash cloth, toothbrush, hairbrush, clothing, etc.) with left hand
- Unable to complete basic tasks using tactile cueing with affected (R) side (due to diminished sensation on the hemiparetic side)
- Unable to complete written responses or drawings – due to the right-handed weakness (and you are right-hand dominant) and the aphasia
- Unable to legibly write with left hand, but can point to something
- Alert and not oriented (seems to recognize name when addressed)
- Use common objects appropriately
- Weakness on right side of body but able to move all body parts (hemiparesis)
    - Full PROM; decreased AROM on right side due to weakness (> half and < less than full AROM)
    - Right side strength – movement against gravity but will break with any resistance – grade
    - Sit to stand – mod A: look at technique e.g. encourage Joe to weight bear on (L) leg and push up with (L) arm
    - In standing, mod A for balance, stability; tires after 1 minute. "Plop" back in chair. If they get you walking, you have greater loss of balance and stability with each step (ideally they should not because you can hardly stand)
    - Inconsistent responses with sensation due to expressive aphasia and mild cognitive deficits due to onset of dementia and general aging **NOTE** Do students visually check legs (due to diabetes)?
    - **NOTE** If students try to have you stand, do they put shoes or gripper socks on you? Did they test sensation and strength in LEs? Do they put on a gait belt (ideally they should)?
- Difficulty maintaining upright in sitting, tend to lean (slump) to the right and back
- Attempt verbalizations ("ta ta ta, da da da") but unable to produce functional language
- Emotional lability and unable to manage emotions, may break out in crying or crying for no apparent reason
- Please note you are on a PEG tube with bolus feedings and are NPO
    - **NOTE** Any safety precautions with this – do they offer you a drink of water? Brush your teeth? If so, you cough uncontrollably

Other things to note

- If student proceeds with grooming task - observe how she/he gives instructions **NOTE** If tactile cueing on (R) side
- For dressing (putting on shirt) **NOTE** For correct instructions and technique
- **NOTE** Which side student stands for sit – stand or attempting to walk (for safety). Student should stand on affected side
- IF students decides to do a transfer (stand pivot transfer with mod A) **NOTE** If they lead with affected (R) side (should lead with unaffected side)
- If students takes BP **NOTE** If BP taken on right arm (should be left arm)

Joe #2: Notes/Guidelines for the Standardized Patient

Set-Up Notes

- Have only regular (not hospital "grip") socks on - shoes off but in room.
- Take off wheelchair footrests – place a few feet from w/c.
- Have sweater/jacket off – but in room.
- Present sitting in **unlocked** w/c with left side facing door, leaning slightly to left (you have left hemianopsia and left hemiparesis) and left hand wedged between armrest and body.
    - **NOTE** Do they fix your position upon entering? Do they lock your brakes? Do they put on footrests if needed?

Patient Level of Function

- Alert and oriented to name only, unable to identify that you're in a skilled nursing facility or had a stroke. If asked where you are, he will look around, pick up cues from the room, and in a questioning voice, say "hospital? Or something?" Think it was just Valentine's Day a day or so ago (or a recent holiday).
- Very impulsive and unsafe; attempt to get up without assistance 3-4 times in the first 5 minutes or so (you may say things like, "I need to find my son. He's here to take me home"). If they do not keep you engaged (long wait time), then attempt to get up without assistance.
- Unable to see anything in left visual field. Once you turn your head to the left, you can see and interact with person/object. (If student approaches and talks on left side, use head to scan to find them.)
    - **NOTE** Do students adjust their body position to allow you to see them better?
- Weakness on left side of body but able to move all body parts (hemiparesis) –
    - Full PROM; less than full AROM on left side due to weakness
    - Left side strength – movement against gravity with some resistance
    - Sit to stand – supervision to min A
    - In standing, able to bear weight for 2-3 minutes before becoming tired, with slight lean to right (bearing more weight on right leg) – needs min A for balance and stability. Main issue is impulsivity – with weakness on left, walking independently would be unsafe
    - Sensation present on left side **NOTE** Do students visually inspect legs/feet (due to diabetes)?
    - **NOTE** If students try to have you stand, do they put shoes or gripper socks on you? Did they test sensation and strength in LEs?
- Perceptual difficulty. If asked to dress self, you are unable to put arm in sleeve. With set-up you can complete simple ADLs (like brush teeth), but perceptually you have difficulty putting paste on toothbrush and sequencing multiple steps. You can comb hair **NOTE** If they have you shave – impulsivity and perception issues will make shaving dangerous
- Please note you are on a PEG tube with bolus feeding and are NPO **NOTE** Any safety precautions with this – do they offer you a drink of water?
- Have mild/beginning stages of dementia –
    - Memory – knows wife passed away ("10 years or so ago?" –even though it was 12 years); good long term memory, but unable to do immediate recall or short term recall on cognitive screening test. Unable to recall recent news events.
    - Paying bills – initially say "I get my bills paid on time", etc. but upon further questioning, say things like "my son needs to help," "I had some problems a few years ago," "got some in late" or "added wrong"

- Remember things based on routine – "Wednesday night is Men's club at church…'Frank' usually takes me", "Sunday at church" but otherwise has some difficulty describing days and plan ("Drink my coffee; work on my puzzle")
- Food preparation – "kids leave food for me to microwave or I just pop in a frozen dinner or make an egg, spaghetti, soup"
- If they do a clock drawing test, complete like this:

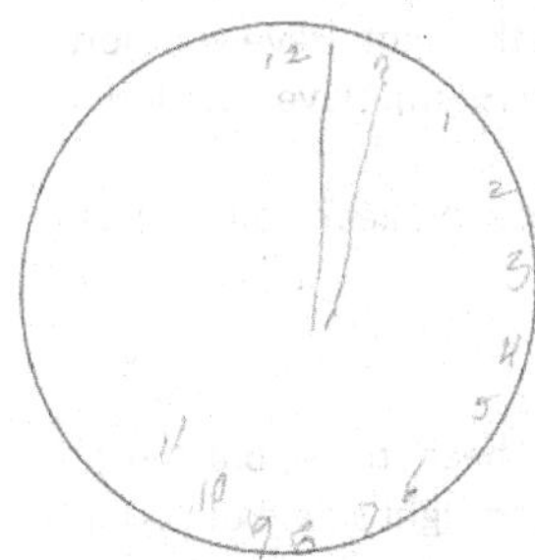

Home Environment

- Lives alone in one-story home.
- 5 steps to enter with rail on both sides.
- All children live locally – his son, Joe Jr, works nearby and stops in once or twice a week on way home from work. They all try to get together about once a month for dinner but "it's hard with grandchildren – they're so busy".
- Was independent with ADLs and IADLs prior to admission.
- Previously used straight point cane (SPC) for community ambulation.
- Drove his own car short distances.

Social

- Attends church at Mt. Tabor Baptist Church every week. He has many friends and neighbors. He enjoys doing puzzles and house repairs.

Joe #3: Notes/Guidelines for the Standardized Patient

Set-Up Notes

- Have only regular (not hospital "grip") socks on - shoes off but in room.
- Take off wheelchair footrests – place a few feet from w/c.
- Have sweater/jacket off – but in room.
- Present sitting in **unlocked** w/c, with body and head angled/leaning to the right. Have your left side facing door (so with your neglect you do not see student enter the room). Have your left hand hanging over armrest by wheel.
    - **NOTE** Do they fix your position upon entering? Do they lock your brakes? Do they put on footrests if needed?

Patient Level of Function

- Complete inattention (neglect) to anything on L side of body. You may "hear" them, but can't figure out where noise is coming from, so you may look around briefly on right side, but you don't respond until they come with your right field of vision.
    - **NOTE** Whether they stay on your left side and if they are aware that you have neglect on that side.
- Flaccid L UE and LE (no tone) –
    - Full PROM; no AROM on left side (**NOTE** Do they palpate to check for subluxed shoulder?)
    - No movement on left – not even gravity eliminated
    - No responses on left to light touch (**NOTE** Do they visually inspect legs/feet due to diabetes?)
    - Sit to stand – dependent. If they have you stand, you would present as a "pusher" – you would lean/push to right due to neglect on left.
    - **NOTE** Do they try to have you stand? Is this safe with their MMT? If so, do they put shoes and gripper socks on you?
- Keep head turned to right side and lean to the right – when student tries to re-position you upright, lean to the right. If they keep pushing you toward a central, upright position, ask "why are you pushing me over? Stop pushing me."
- Alert and oriented to name and can figure out he's in a "hospital" by his surroundings (look around – yes, "I'm in the hospital" but you don't know name of the place). Don't know why you are in the skilled nursing facility. Is unaware of the date.
- ADLs – you can put R arm in sleeve but only dress one side. You comb hair, wash face, brush teeth only on right side.
- Please note you are on a PEG tube with bolus feedings **NOTE** Any safety precautions with this – do they offer you a drink of water?
- Have mild/beginning stages of dementia –
    - Memory – knows wife passed away ("10 years or so ago?" – even though it was 12 years); good long term memory, but unable to do immediate recall or short term recall on cognitive screening test. Unable to recall recent news events.
    - Paying bills – initially say "I get my bills paid on time", etc. but upon further questioning, say things like "my son needs to help," "I had some problems a few years ago," "got some in late" or "added wrong"

- Remember things based on routine – "Wednesday night is Men's club at church…'Frank' usually takes me", "Sunday at church" but otherwise has some difficulty describing days and plan ("drink my coffee; work on my puzzle")
- Food preparation – "kids leave food for me to microwave or I just pop in a frozen dinner or make an egg, spaghetti, soup"
- If they do a clock drawing test, complete like this:

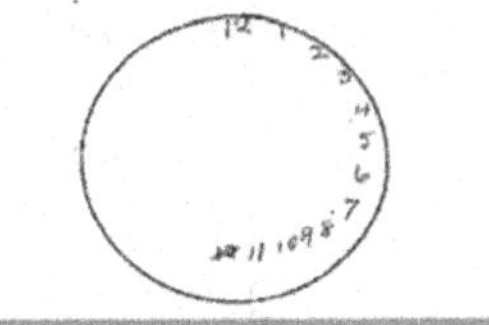

Home Environment

- Lives alone in one-story home.
- 5 steps to enter with rail on both sides.
- All children live locally – his son, Joe Jr, works nearby and stops in once or twice a week on way home from work. They all try to get together about once a month for dinner but "it's hard with grandchildren – they're so busy".
- Was independent with ADLs and IADLs prior to admission.
- Previously used straight point cane (SPC) for community ambulation.
- Drove his own car short distances.

Social

- Attends church at Mt. Tabor Baptist Church every week. He has many friends and neighbors. He enjoys doing puzzles and doing house repairs.

Standardized Patient Lab Rubric: Pre-Evaluation Questions and Soap Note

Student Name ____ Date________________
Version (circle) __Joe #1 Joe #2 Joe #3

Pre-Evaluation Questions from chart review (2 pts each)	
Question 1 Question 2 Question 3	_____/ 6

SOAP Note Documentation		
	GENERAL	_____/ 34
___/ 2	• Note is written legibly.	
___/ 2	• Note is written in black ink.	
___/ 2	• Note is dated and signed legibly with your last name and legal first name or initials, followed by OTS.	
___/ 2	• If a mistake is made in charting, a line is drawn through the error, "error" is written above the mistake, along with the date and initials.	
___/ 2	• No open lines in note.	
	ORGANIZATION	
___/ 3	• Information is organized.	
___/ 2	• Subjective information is relevant to patient needs.	
___/ 5	• Accurate, objective reporting of tests and measures in "O."	
___/ 5	• Interprets subjective and objective information to determine client's occupational performance strengths, challenges, and rehab potential.	
___/ 5	• Occupation-based measurable goals.	
___/ 4	• Accurate and appropriate plan based on the evaluation results.	

Total Pre-Questions	**_____/ 6**
Total Evaluation Session Criteria	**_____/ 60**
SOAP Note	**_____/ 34**
Total Lab Practical Grade	**_____/ 100**

Standardized Patient Lab Rubric – Evaluation Session (to be completed by SP)

Student Name ______________________________ Date______________

Scenario (circle) Joe #1 Joe #2 Joe #3 SP: ______________

Communication – Clearly and effectively communicates verbally and nonverbally with clients	
Yes No 1) Introduces self (2 pts)	____/10
2) Appropriate patient interview Yes No • Considers instruction method, body language, etc. (2 pts) Yes No • Adjusts body position based on patient condition/needs (e.g., due to hemianopsia or neglect) (2 pts)	
Yes No 3) Instructions to patient in terms patient can understand (2 pts)	
Yes No 4) Use of open body language and good eye contact (2 pts)	
Comments:	

Fundamentals of Practice: Safety	
***items must be successfully completed or retake of practical may be required.**	____/25
1) Completes environmental scan upon entering room Yes No • Correctly positioned pt in w/c (3 pts) Yes No • *Locks wheelchair/leaves pt with wheelchair locked (4 pts)	
2) Adheres to safety precautions/regulations Yes No • Uses proper body mechanics (3 pts) Yes No • *Uses gait belt if stands or transfers (4 pts) □ did not stand or transfer Yes No • *Appropriate guarding (3 pts)	
Yes No 3) *Takes steps to prevent accidents (e.g., gets another therapist for difficult transfer, puts shoes on or non-skids socks, not shave if pt is impulsive) (4 pts)	
Yes No 4) Follows NPO precautions (no water offered, did not brush teeth) (4 pts)	
Comments:	

Carries out appropriate evaluation techniques correctly	
Yes No 1) Selects appropriate assessment(s)/assessment techniques (5 pts) **List assessment(s)/techniques used:** **Considerations (check box if completed)** □ visual inspection of legs/feet □ assesses both sides of body □ sensory testing/MMT on LEs before standing □ use of ADLs in evaluation	____/15
Yes No 2) Administers assessment(s) appropriately (5 pts)	
Yes No 3) Adjusts assessment procedures as needed (5 pts)	
Comments:	

Post-Treatment	
Yes No 1) Leaves client properly and safely positioned (3 pts)	____/10
Yes No 2) Provides client with education (3 pts)	
Yes No 3) Cleans up room/takes equipment (3 pts)	
Yes No 4) Addresses any concerns of patient (1 pt)	
Comments:	

______/60

Appendix F Scoring Guidelines Pre-Evaluation Questions

Question 1		
For Joe #1: What do you expect to see with aphasia?		
0 – Does not include communication/language issues	1 – Indicates a global expectation that communication will be an issue with the patient	2 – Indicates a deeper understanding of the communication deficits that may occur with the patient, such as difficulty producing language, understanding language, or reading and writing
For Joe #2 and #3: Describe neglect vs hemianopsia.		
0 – Describes both terms incorrectly	1 – May describe neglect or hemianopsia correctly, but not both. May describe one or both in general terms, but does not show a deeper understanding of neglect being a cognitive/ perceptual issue and hemianopsia as a visual issue	2 – Describes neglect as a cognitive and/or perceptual inattention in which the patient does not attend, is unaware of, or does not perceive one side of the body or environment. Describes hemianopsia as a visual field deficit in which the patient may not see ½ of the visual field in each eye
Question 2: What considerations do you have knowing the patient has type II diabetes?		
0 – Lists only 1-2 considerations and does not include considerations of peripheral neuropathy, decreased sensation in feet/lower extremities, or weakness in feet/lower extremities	1 – Identifies some important considerations (such as decreased sensation, blood sugar testing, possible diet restrictions, vision) but does not include considerations of peripheral neuropathy, decreased sensation in feet/lower extremities, or weakness in feet/lower extremities	2 – Identifies more than 2 important considerations (such as decreased sensation, blood sugar testing, possible diet restrictions, vision) and includes considerations of peripheral neuropathy, decreased sensation in feet/lower extremities, or weakness in feet/lower extremities
Question 3: How is hemiplegia different from hemiparesis?		
0 - Incorrect definitions or switched the definitions	1 - Describes hemiplegia or hemiparesis correctly, but not both	2 – Correctly identifies hemiplegia as “paralysis” or similar description on one side of the body, and hemiparesis as “slight paralysis” or “weakness” on one side of the body

Scoring Guidelines SOAP Note Documentation

<table>
<tr><th colspan="5">General Documentation</th></tr>
<tr><th>Scoring
Criteria</th><th>0</th><th>1</th><th colspan="2">2</th></tr>
<tr><td>Legibility</td><td>Very hard to read/illegible</td><td>Few places hard to read</td><td colspan="2">Written legibly</td></tr>
<tr><td>Written in black ink</td><td>Written in pencil</td><td>Written in colored ink</td><td colspan="2">Written in black ink</td></tr>
<tr><td>Note is dated & signed</td><td>Missing 2 or more elements</td><td>Missing either date, legible legal name, or OTS</td><td colspan="2">Note is dated and signed legibly with legal name, followed by OTS</td></tr>
<tr><td>Errors lined through correctly</td><td>Scribbles and no initials throughout</td><td>Error is scribbled through or student does not initial it</td><td colspan="2">If a mistake is made in charting, a single line is drawn through the error, "error" is written above the mistake, along with the date and initials of the OTS</td></tr>
<tr><td>No open lines</td><td>Leaves open lines</td><td></td><td colspan="2">Does not leave open lines or draws line through open spaces</td></tr>
<tr><th colspan="5">SOAP Note Organization</th></tr>
<tr><td>Organization</td><td>(0) note not organized by sections and/or very disorganized</td><td>(1) multiple errors with information in sections</td><td>(2) some information put in wrong section</td><td>(3) information is put in the right section</td></tr>
<tr><td>"S" section</td><td>(0) information is not relevant to patient needs</td><td>(1) information is tangentially relevant to patient needs</td><td>(2) information in "S" is relevant to patient needs</td><td></td></tr>
<tr><td>"O" section</td><td colspan="4">Score a range of 0-5 looking at accurate reporting of tests and measures in the "O" section of the note. Take away at least one point each (or more if occurs frequently) if data
□ is not objectively and accurately reported
□ is not focused on occupation
□ is not concise, specific, and organized
□ is not focused on client's response to treatment (rather than what therapist did)
□ is not specific about assist levels
□ does not include information about length, purpose, and initial positioning of the client</td></tr>
<tr><td>"A" section</td><td colspan="4">Score a range of 0-5 looking for ability to interpret subjective and objective information ("A" section) to determine client's occupational performance strengths, challenges, and rehab potential
□ Take away 1 point each if strengths, challenges, and rehab potential are not included
□ Take away 1 point if new information is introduced in this "A" section</td></tr>
<tr><td>Goals</td><td colspan="4">Score a range of 0-5 looking at ability to write occupation based, measurable goals related to areas identified in the "A" section. Take away 1 point each if goal
□ overlaps with a potential PT or SLP goal
□ addresses oral hygiene or feeding (due to NPO precautions)
□ is not reimbursable (e.g., not ADL or IADL focused)
□ is not occupation based
□ does not include time frames</td></tr>
<tr><td>"P" section</td><td colspan="4">Score a range of 0-4 looking at establishment of an accurate and appropriate plan ("P") based on the evaluation results and goals. Take away at least 1 point each if they do not
□ specify the frequency and duration of future OT sessions
□ describe the purpose of future OT sessions
□ include brief information on intervention strategies to address goals
□ include possible discharge information</td></tr>
</table>

Scoring Guidelines Evaluation Session

<table>
<tr><th colspan="4">Communication – Clearly and effectively communicates verbally and nonverbally with clients</th></tr>
<tr><th>Scoring / Criteria</th><th>0</th><th>1</th><th>2</th></tr>
<tr><td>Introduces self</td><td>Does not introduce self by name or OT</td><td>Introduces self by name or as an OT, but not both</td><td>Introduces self by name and as an OT</td></tr>
<tr><td rowspan="2">Appropriate patient interview</td><td>Does not adjust instruction or body language in response to patient's needs</td><td>Attempts to adjust instructions or body language, but is not proficient; may adjust after well into the evaluation session</td><td>Uses appropriate instruction method, body language, etc. (Ex., may be more firm with Joe #2, empathetic for Joe #3, try non-verbal methods for Joe #1)</td></tr>
<tr><td>Does not adjust body position (e.g., positions self on left side for most of session for Joes #2 & 3)</td><td>Attempts to adjust body position but may not do so immediately or consistently throughout the session</td><td>Adjusts body position based on patient/condition/needs throughout the session</td></tr>
<tr><td>Instructions patient can understand</td><td>Uses professional jargon and does not define OT</td><td>Uses some jargon but attempts to explain terms or does not define OT clearly</td><td>Gives instructions and defines OT in terms patient can understand</td></tr>
<tr><td>Body language and eye contact</td><td>Does not make eye contact or use open body language</td><td>Periodic use of open body language and good eye contact, but not consistent throughout session</td><td>Makes eye contact, gets on patient's level, asks open questions</td></tr>
<tr><th colspan="4">Fundamentals of practice - safety</th></tr>
<tr><td rowspan="2">Completes environmental scan upon entering room</td><td colspan="3">Score a range of 0-3 looking at whether student correctly positions pt in w/c. Consider:
□ timeliness (e.g., did they reposition immediately or did it occur after 10 minutes)
□ success (e.g., did they attempt it but it was not successful. NOTE: Joe #3 may be harder to position successfully)</td></tr>
<tr><td colspan="3">Score a range of 0-4 looking at whether student locks wheelchair. Consider:
□ timeliness (e.g., did they lock brakes immediately or not until well into session)
□ consistency (e.g., did they lock brakes once, but not left them unlocked after moving)
□ safety (e.g., did a potential safety hazard occur before student realized brakes were unlocked)</td></tr>
<tr><td rowspan="3">Adheres to safety precautions/ regulations</td><td colspan="3">Score a range of 0-3 looking at student use of proper body mechanics. Consider:
□ body mechanics across a variety of positions (e.g., sitting, standing, reaching)
□ consistency (e.g., use proper mechanics through the session or just some of session)</td></tr>
<tr><td colspan="3">Score a range of 0-4 looking at whether student uses gait belt appropriately and safely. Consider whether:
□ gait belt is used safely and appropriately for standing, transfers, and/or repositioning
□ ease with which student places gait belt on patient
□ consideration of PEG with gait belt placement</td></tr>
<tr><td colspan="3">Score a range of 0-3 looking at whether student appropriately guards patient. Consider:
□ guarding during reaching, transfers, or movements
□ safety (e.g., effectiveness of guarding)
If patient falls (during a transfer or out of chair/bed) due to poor guarding, score a 0.</td></tr>
<tr><td>Takes steps to prevent accidents</td><td colspan="3">Score a range of 0-4 looking at whether student takes appropriate steps to prevent accidents. Consider whether they:
□ put on shoes or non-skid socks prior to standing or transfers
□ use safe materials (e.g., not use razor for Joe #2)</td></tr>
<tr><td>Follows NPO precautions</td><td colspan="3">Score a range of 0-4 looking at whether NPO precautions are followed. Consider if student:
□ offered water
□ brushed teeth with water
□ did not monitor patient when using a wet washcloth</td></tr>
</table>

Carries out appropriate evaluation techniques correctly				
Selects appropriate assessment techniques	Score a range of 0-5 looking at whether appropriate assessment method were selected based on client diagnosis, setting, and time to gather necessary information needed to develop an initial OT plan. Take away at least one point each they did not: □ perform sensory testing/MMT on LEs before standing patient □ assess both sides of the body Take away at least two points if they did not assess ADLs in the evaluation session			
Administers assessments appropriately	Score a range of 0-5 looking at whether assessments were administered appropriately. Consider whether: □ assessment was administered in a standardized manner (if standardized assessment) □ positioning was appropriate during the assessment □ instructions were understandable			
Adjusts assessment procedures as needed	Score a range of 0-5 looking at whether adjustments were made as needed. Consider whether: □ they appropriately made adjustment or if they made adjustments that are not standardized □ they continued with an assessment that was not working (e.g., using a verbal questionnaire with Joe #1 with aphasia)			
Post-Treatment				
Scoring / Criteria	**0**	**1**	**2**	**3**
Leaves client properly and safely positioned	Client is not left in safe and proper position	Client may be positioned well, but not safely	Client is left in a safe position, but positioning is not ideal	Client is left in room in safe (e.g., w/c locked, not near water) and proper position
Provides client with education	Does not educate client	Attempts to educate client, but not clearly or effectively	Educates client on area, but technique is not most effective	At some point during session, educates client on setting, safety, diagnosis, etc. using effective technique
Cleans up room/takes equipment	Does not clean up room and leaves equipment in room	Does not clean up room or leaves equipment in room	Cleans up and takes equipment out of room, but does not put away correctly	Cleans up materials (e.g., around sink), takes equipment out of room, puts away correctly
Addresses patient concerns	Does not address patient concerns or questions	Appropriately addresses concerns of patient at some point during session		

Standardized Patient Lab Signup

Date

Total Lab Time	**Chart Review/ Questions**	**SP Lab/ Debrief Time**	**Room 1**		**Room 2**		**Room 3**		**Room 4**	
			SP (Joe version)	**Student Name**	**SP (Joe version)**	**Student Name**	**SP (Joe version)**	**Student Name**	**SP (Joe version)**	**Student Name**
8-10:15	8-8:30	8:30-9:15								
8:45-11	8:45-9:15	9:15-10								
9:30-11:45	9:30-10	10-10:45								
10:15-12:30	10:15-10:45	10:45-11:30								
11-1:15	11-11:30	11:30-12:15								
Built in short break										
12-2:15	12-12:30	12:30-1:15								
12:45-3	12:45-1:15	1:15-2								

30 min for chart review, answer questions, gather materials
20 min for SP evaluation session
15 min debrief with SP
10 min clean up materials/SP evaluate
1 hour SOAP note
Total Lab Time: 2 hr 15

Sample SP Recruitment Letter

Dear

I wanted to ask you if you or any of the therapists would be interested and available to come help with our standardized patient lab. This lab is to develop students' knowledge and skills of information and planning an initial evaluation, client safety, knowledge and skills in an evaluation session, documentation, and client rapport. I am seeking help for this lab – we need clinicians to play the role of the "patient" for this lab and to provide feedback to the students on their session.

Each student will be given a "chart review" of a client. Following the chart review, they will need to answer a few questions about the client, then they will proceed to complete a short evaluation session (about 20 minutes) on a "standardized patient" (a therapist or faculty member simulating the patient's symptoms in a standardized manner). Following the evaluation session, the students will have one hour to complete an evaluation SOAP note.

We need therapists who are willing and able to come be our "standardized patients." We will provide you with information about the client ahead of time – their diagnosis (we already know they will all be CVA), their presentation of symptoms, functional level, etc. We will also provide you with a rating scale that you will use to evaluate the students.

Students will be doing this over 2 days – all day on date (hours) and date (hours). If you have any time on these days to participate, even if it's just an hour, we would really appreciate it - just let me know the time frame that you are available. Last year the students really enjoyed this experience and learned a lot. We would really like to offer it again, but need assistance to manage this for 42 students.

Thank you for your support of our students.

Sample Confirmation Letter

Dear

Thank you so much for agreeing to help with the standardized patient lab for Clinical Reasoning. The students are very excited by this hands-on opportunity to try out their skills - and they are very nervous! I have you scheduled for this Friday date (hours). Please arrive 30 minutes early so we can review important information with all of our "patients." Please let me know if there are any changes you need to make to this time.

Attached is information on the case (Joe #3) that you will be "acting out".

- The Chart Review and Pre-Evaluation Questions – This is the information that will be provided to the student, along with the 3 questions that they have to answer prior to evaluating you.
- Joe Standardized Patient Notes – This includes information on how to position yourself, your functional level (the students will NOT have this information) and some information to guide your responses during the evaluation.
- Joe Case Template –This provides background information on "Joe" to understand other aspects of your role.
- Joe Standardized Patient Lab Rubric – Evaluation Session – This is the rubric that you will use to grade student performance at the completion of each student's evaluation session. We would like for you to provide us feedback on the student's skills in the areas of communication, safety, evaluation, and post-session as outlined on the rubric. Please review this prior to coming to the lab.

The students will have about 20 minutes to perform an OT evaluation on you. Following this time, you can *briefly* provide them with general feedback. They will then proceed to another room to write an evaluation SOAP note (so make sure your feedback does not include information for their SOAP note).

Please wear socks and shoes on this day and if you can, dress in layers (t-shirt with cardigan or top shirt), so students can work on "dressing" you if needed.

Please let us know if you have any questions. Thank you so much for your help!

Appendix I: Joe Lab Debrief Guide

Debriefing general process guidelines

(based on the PEARLS Healthcare Debriefing Tool: https://debrief2learn.org/pearls-debriefing-tool/)

	Objective	Task	Example Script
Setting the Scene	Create a safe context for learning	State the goal of debriefing; articulate the basic assumption	Let's spend 10 minutes debriefing. Our goal is to improve care for our patients and we want to work with you to improve.
Reactions	Allow for a brief decompression; explore feelings	Solicit initial reactions and emotions	• Any initial reactions? OR • How do you feel that went? OR • How are you feeling?
Description	Clarify facts	Develop shared understanding of case	Can you share a short summary of Joe?
Analysis	Encourage participation and build rapport Allow learners to explain their perspective	**Plus-Delta**	• What went well? • What would you do differently?
	Explore variety of performance domains Help the learner find ways to improve performance	**Advocacy-Inquiry** Observe a particular event or result	• You notice e.g. (Joe #1) that student does not know how to respond to or deal with Joe's expressive aphasia.
		Comment on observation from your perspective	• I noticed that you were not sure how to respond when Joe could not answer your question.
		Explore the student's thinking and actions for that observed event	• What were you thinking when you were not able to get a verbal response from Joe? OR Were you surprised by Joe's response?
		Discover with the student ways to attend to the issues that arose and ways to attain positive results	• I understand how difficult it is when one is not able to get the desired response. What could you have done to move on to the next step of the evaluation?
Any Outstanding Issues/Concerns?			
Application/ Summary	• Invite reflection on the experiences as a whole – reinforce learning • Identify take-aways	• Inquire what learning they will take away	• How are you feeling about the evaluation now? • What is the biggest thing that you will take away from the simulation?

Joe # 1 Debriefing Script

Phase	Student event/result	Example script
Set Scene		Let's spend 10 minutes debriefing. Our goal is to improve care for our patients and we want to work with you to improve
Reaction	Reaction following the scenario	How was that? Any initial reactions?
Description	Shared summary of case	Tell me about Joe #1.
Analysis	Start with these two questions **(Plus-Delta)**	What went well? What would you do differently?
Analysis		**Advocacy-Inquiry**
	OTS does not introduce themselves and perform an environmental scan for safety purposes at the start of the evaluation	• I noticed that you started the evaluation before checking the environment for safety. • I know there is a lot to do in 20 minutes, but you missed some important safety issues (locking brakes, socks, etc.). • Walk me through what you were thinking. What was your reason for not doing that right at the beginning?
	OTS performs functional ROM and MMT while Joe is improperly positioned	• I notice that you did a functional ROM and MMT of Joe's UE while he was slumped down and leaning on his side in the wheelchair. • I liked that you considered testing ROM and MMT. • How do you think the positioning could have impacted results?
	OTS does not know how to respond to or deal with Joe's expressive aphasia	• I noticed that you were not sure how to respond when Joe could not answer your questions. • I understand how difficult it is when one is not able to get the desired response. • What could you have done to move on to the next step of the evaluation?
	OTS attempts to walk Joe without testing LE sensation and strength	• I noticed you tried to get Joe from sit to stand and then attempt to walk. • I understand why you were surprised when Joe could not balance on both feet and could stand only very briefly. • What was your reasoning for wanting him to stand and walk? Why do you think he had difficulty standing?
	OTS spent a large majority of the time asking questions, rather than getting ADL baseline	• I noticed that you asked a lot of questions for your evaluation. • I liked that you were working to get information from Joe – being client centered, but it seems like you ran out of time to gather baseline information on ADLs. • Can you walk me through your evaluation plan?
Summary	Invite reflection on the experience as a whole – reinforce learning	• How are you feeling about the evaluation now? • What is the biggest thing that you will take away from the simulation? • Direct students to something to observe in their video for reflection.

Joe # 2 Debriefing Notes

Phase	Student event/result	Example script
Debrief (start with this)	Reaction following the scenario	• How was that? Feelings?
Debrief	SP will start with these two questions **(Delta-Plus Process)**	• What went well? • What would you do differently?
Debrief	**Advocacy-Inquiry**	
	OTS does not introduce themselves and perform an environmental scan for safety purposes at the start of the evaluation	• I noticed that you started the evaluation before checking the environment for safety. • I know there is a lot to do in 20 minutes, but you missed some important safety issues – like locking brakes, socks. • Walk me through what you were thinking. What was your reason for not doing that right at the beginning?
	OTS performs functional ROM and MMT while Joe is leaning to one side and slumped in sitting position in the w/c	• I notice that you did a functional ROM and MMT of Joe's UE while he was slumped down and leaning on his side in the wheelchair. • I liked that you considered testing ROM and MMT. • How do you think the positioning could have impacted results?
	OTS spent a large majority of the time asking questions, rather than getting ADL baseline	• I noticed that you asked a lot of questions for your evaluation. • I liked that you were working to get information from Joe – being client centered, but it seems like you ran out of time to gather baseline information on ADLs. • Can you walk me through your evaluation plan?
Wrap up	Invite reflection on the experience as a whole – reinforce learning	• How are you feeling about the evaluation now? • What is the biggest thing that you will take away from the simulation? • Direct students to something to observe in their video for reflection.

Joe # 3 Debriefing Notes

Phase	Student event/result	Example script
Debrief	SP will start with these two questions **(Delta-Plus Process)**	• What went well? • What would you do differently?
Debrief	**Advocacy-Inquiry**	
	OTS does not introduce themselves and perform an environmental scan for safety purposes at the start of the evaluation	• I noticed that you started the evaluation before checking the environment for safety. • I know there is a lot to do in 20 minutes, but you missed some important safety issues – like locking brakes, socks. • Walk me through what you were thinking. What was your reason for not doing that right at the beginning?
	OTS performs functional ROM and MMT while Joe is leaning to one side and slumped in sitting position in the w/c	• I notice that you did a functional ROM and MMT of Joe's UE while he was slumped down and leaning on his side in the wheelchair. • I liked that you considered testing ROM and MMT. • How do you think the positioning could have impacted results?
	OTS positions self on left side out of your vision area	• I noticed that you positioned yourself on my/Joe's left side. When you stood there, I was unable to see you, see your cues, know that you were here. • Can you walk me through your thought process?
	OTS repeatedly works to re-position Joe and doesn't seem to understand the pusher syndrome	• I noticed that you repeatedly tried to reposition me. • I liked that you tried to reposition me, but I saw this was hard for you/frustrating. • What was going through your mind? Why was it hard to reposition him? (may need to explain/remind about pusher syndrome)
	OTS spent a large majority of the time asking questions, rather than getting ADL baseline	• I noticed that you asked a lot of questions for your evaluation. • I liked that you were working to get information from Joe – being client centered, but it seems like you ran out of time to gather baseline information on ADLs. • Can you walk me through your evaluation plan?
Wrap up	Invite reflection on the experience as a whole – reinforce learning	• How are you feeling about the evaluation now? • What is the biggest thing that you will take away from the simulation? • Direct students to something to observe in their video for reflection.

Using Standardized Patients in the Occupational Therapy Curriculum

Audrey L. Zapletal, OTD, OTR/L, CLA
Madeleine Clements, MS, OTR/L
Pari Kumar, OTD, OTR/L
Jennifer A. Merz, OTD, OTR/L
Chalia Bellis, MS, OTR/L

Occupational therapy programs are increasingly using medical simulations as an instructional method; 70% reported using simulation, including standardized patients (SPs; Bethea et al., 2014). High-fidelity simulations, including using SPs, provides learners with the opportunity to apply assessment and treatment knowledge in a structured and safe environment with trained individuals, depicting the roles of patients, family members, or other members of the health care team (VanPuymbrouck et al., 2017). Simulation experiences reportedly have various benefits for learners, including the ability to increase clinical reasoning, cultural competence, and self-confidence as it relates to the role as a future practitioner, and the opportunity to analyze all aspects of a patient's health and well-being comprehensively (Bahreman & Swoboda, 2016; Bosek et al., 2007; Ozkara San, 2018; Sahu et al., 2019). When interacting with SPs, students have a chance to engage in the Intentional Relationship Model, a conceptual model that offers a practical set of skills and interpersonal reasoning approaches that relies on communication styles to promote the client's occupational engagement (Taylor, 2020). Simultaneously, the students critically appraise how their own therapeutic use of self, the deliberate and artful use of personal attributes and behaviors, may support or impede a client's participation in meaningful occupations (Taylor, 2020). This is facilitated through various educational tools (e.g., video recordings, feedback sessions, the student's own dynamic interactions with the SP; Molitor & Nissen, 2020; Wilbanks et al., 2020).

In general, simulation is used as a method to prepare learners for fieldwork (Giesbrecht et al., 2014; Molitor & Nissen, 2020) and ultimately, to assist with the transition to entry-level practice (Bethea et al., 2014). In recent years, the occupational therapy profession has faced a shortage of fieldwork sites and, as a result, has searched for ways to meet the "early experiential needs" (VanPuymbrouck et al., 2017, p. 7) of learners. In addition, the Accreditation Council for Occupational Therapy Education (ACOTE®) allows SP experiences to augment Level I Fieldwork (ACOTE, 2018). ACOTE Standard C.1.9 states that Level I Fieldwork may be met through one of the following instructional methods:

Zapletal, A. L., Baird, J. M., Van Oss, T., Hoppe, M. M., Prast, J. E., & Herge, E. A. *Clinical Simulation for Health Care Professionals* (pp. 311-316).

SPs, simulated environments, faculty-led site visits, faculty practice, or supervision by a fieldwork educator in a practice environment (ACOTE, 2018). However, for the accreditation standard to be met, these experiences must be comparable to the rigor of a traditional Level I experience (ACOTE, 2018). These experiences should include opportunities to practice client-centered care and engagement in occupation-based practice to highlight the distinct value of occupational therapy (American Occupational Therapy Association, [AOTA], 2015; 2020) and include opportunities for assessment and self-reflection.

This article explains strategies for instructors and learners who are involved with SP experiences, as well as how scaffolding SP experiences can contribute to skill development preparation for Level II Fieldwork.

Standardized Patient Experiences

SP experiences provide the opportunity for learners to practice being client-centered and occupation based, which is key to the distinct role of the profession of occupational therapy (AOTA, 2015, 2020). However, despite the benefits, SP experiences can be stressful for learners. To optimize the SP experience, Table 1 provides some tips for learners and their instructors.

Standardized Patients at Thomas Jefferson University (Jefferson)

Jefferson's Department of Occupational Therapy Program (Center City campus) uses a *spiral curriculum*, or an educational structure that continues to revisit topics in increasing complexity to promote understanding and competence (Coelho & Moles, 2016). SP experiences are integrated throughout the curriculum with goals and expectations following the spiral model. SP experiences at Jefferson are developed and implemented incorporating evidence-based guidelines, including pre-briefing and preparation materials, debriefing sessions, and feedback for each student. Before each SP experience, educators provide learners with an occupational profile, medical history, the context of the SP experience, and any other information relevant to a case. Learners are also provided the opportunity to practice with their peers, using similar equipment and techniques anticipated for the SP experience as part of their preparation. Learners are encouraged to study, practice, and plan for the experience using the occupational therapy process and applicable elements of the curriculum. Directly after the experience, learners engage in debriefing sessions to interpret their own experience and learn from the experiences of classmates. All sessions are video recorded to allow learners to review and understand any feedback they receive and to provide the opportunity for the learner to self-reflect. Table 2 demonstrates the developmental progression of high-fidelity simulations through the curriculum, with a brief description of the simulation.

Conclusion

After completing their Level II Fieldwork, four Jefferson occupational therapy student authors met to reflect on their SP experiences. The students reported various benefits associated with participating in the SP experience beyond clinical skills, including developing the therapeutic use of self, improving observation skills, advancing multi-tasking abilities, and increasing awareness of skills that needed to be improved before embarking on Level II Fieldwork.

Table 1. Tips for Learners and Instructors for Standardized Patient (SP) Experiences

Tips for Learners	
Before the Simulation	• Practice working through the scenario with your classmates as much as possible. • Take advantage of resources provided by your school (e.g., open lab, videos). • Write out key points to remember during the SP experience. You may not use it but it is a good security blanket in case you get nervous!
During the Simulation	• Use your therapeutic use of self and ask SPs about themselves. This is your time to build rapport! • Peer observation can be intimidating, but remember that you are all learning together. • Don't be afraid to take a moment to think and breathe throughout the simulation. Take your time!
Always Remember	• SP encounters are learning experiences. During fieldwork, you will get additional opportunities to practice these skills.
Tips for Instructors to Prepare Learners	
Before the Simulation (Pre-Briefing Period)	Familiarize learners with the simulation environment, video recording process, and materials/objects needed in the official simulation encounter to increase comfort before the actual encounter occurs (INACSL Standards Committee, 2016; Li et al., 2016).
	Encourage learners to practice skills among family members and peers to increase familiarity with uncertainty and decrease feelings of being "put on the spot" during the actual simulation (Carey et al., 2018; Sahu et al., 2019).
	Provide instructor-approved resources so learners have access to accurate information (INACSL Standards Committee, 2016) and to practice skills required in the simulation. • Design "learning bundles" or materials such as self-paced videos and organize by theme/topic (Blazeck & Zewe, 2013; Carey et al, 2018).
	Provide learners with opportunities to practice clinical skills in environments that are as realistic as possible (Bosek et al., 2007; INACSL Standards Committee, 2016; Sahu et al., 2019). Consider: • Environmental set-up. • Using SPs trained in depicting appropriate behaviors and emotions. • Clothing and/or moulage related to the role and timing of the encounter (e.g., session length, time between sessions).
	Remember learners may be nervous before the simulation experience. • Inform learners before the experience who will be observing and why. Describing the benefit of peer observers or faculty may ease some of the stress (O'Regan et al., 2016). • Explain that SPs are trained to simulate medical conditions to provide an opportunity to practice before fieldwork to enhance critical reasoning and clinical thinking skills (Lasater, 2007; Molitor & Nissen, 2020).

During the Simulation	Recognize the various support roles needed to operate the simulation experience (Bosek et al., 2007). Recruit faculty and staff to: • Operate camera and ensure the video is recording. • Help the learners locate patient rooms or materials. • Observe the encounter from the video monitoring station to assist with evaluating the students and/or simulation encounter.
After the Simulation (Debriefing and Feedback Period)	Arrange time for debriefing. • Structure debriefing sessions to promote learning, decrease feelings of anxiety post-encounter, validate successes, and highlight opportunities for growth (Evain et al., 2017; Fanning & Gaba, 2007).
	Provide video recordings of each learner's encounter. • Facilitate additional opportunities for self-reflection through structured questions and/or assignments (Giles et al., 2014; Zhang et al., 2019).
Best Practice Guidelines: Additional Considerations	Scaffolding simulation encounters allows learners to practice new and complex skills, and gain exposure to new populations. • Consider progressing from low- to high-fidelity simulations to improve practice performance (INACSL Standards Committee, 2016; Mills et al., 2016).

Table 2. Developmental Progression of High-Fidelity Simulations

Simulation		Scenario
1	Interview and administer standardized assessment.	Interviewed and administered standardized cognitive assessment.
2	Administer an evaluation in a group.	Administered wheelchair evaluation for client with spinal cord injury.
3	Provide a treatment session in pairs.	Participated in instructor-guided session focused on learning how to complete bed mobility, functional mobility, and dressing/undressing activities for a client with hemiparesis.
4	Deliver 35-minute 1:1 treatment session with peer observers.	Participated in a 3-hour hospital simulation, which included preparing for treatment sessions focused on ADLs and IADLs for four patients with chronic or acute physical disabilities.
5	Implement 10-minute treatment session with peer observer.	Delivered meal-prep OR craft activity for patient with schizophrenia depicting either positive or negative symptoms.
6	Summative assessment with 30-minute 1:1 treatment session and documentation.	Prepared six different treatment sessions for clients with chronic and/or physical conditions in a medical setting; implemented one 30-minute session graded by trained lab instructor and completed relevant documents post-session.

References

Accreditation Council for Occupational Therapy Education. (2018). 2018 Accreditation Council for Occupational Therapy Education (ACOTE®) Standards and Interpretive Guide (effective July 31, 2020). *American Journal of Occupational Therapy, 72*(Suppl. 2), 7212410005. https://doi.org/10.5014/ajot.2018.72S217

American Occupational Therapy Association. (2015). Articulating the distinct value of occupational therapy. https://www.aota.org/Publications-News/AOTANews/2015/distinct-value-of-occupational-therapy.aspx

American Occupational Therapy Association. (2020). Occupational therapy practice framework: Domain and process (4th ed.). *American Journal of Occupational Therapy, 74*(Suppl. 2), 7412410010. https://doi.org/10.5014/ajot.2020.74S2001

Bahreman, N. T., & Swoboda, S. M. (2016). Honoring diversity: Developing culturally competent communication skills through simulation. *Journal of Nursing Education, 55*, 105–108. https://doi.org/10.3928/01484834-20160114-09

Bethea, D. P., Castillo, D. C., & Harvison, N. (2014). Use of simulation in occupational therapy education: Way of the future? *American Journal of Occupational Therapy, 68*(Suppl. 2), S32–S39. https://doi.org/10.5014/ajot.2014.012716

Blazeck, A., & Zewe, G. (2013). Simulating simulation: Promoting perfect practice with learning bundle-supported videos in an applied, learner-driven curriculum design. *Clinical Simulation in Nursing, 9*(1), E21–E24. https://doi.org/10.1016/j.ecns.2011.07.002

Bosek, M., Li, S., & Hicks, F. (2007). Working with standardized patients: A primer. *International Journal of Nursing Education Scholarship, 4*. https://doi.org/10.2202/1548-923X.1437

Carey, M. C., Kent, B., & Latour, J. M. (2018). Experiences of undergraduate nursing students in peer assisted learning in clinical practice: A qualitative systematic review. *JBI Database of Systematic Reviews and Implementation Reports, 16*, 1190–1219. https://doi.org/10.11124/JBISRIR-2016-003295

Coelho, C. S., & Moles, D. R. (2016). Student perceptions of a spiral curriculum. *European Journal of Dental Education, 20*, 161–166. https://doi.org/10.1111/eje.12156

Evain, J.-N., Zoric, L., Mattatia, L., Picard, O., Ripart, J., & Cuvillon, P. (2017). Residual anxiety after high fidelity simulation in anaesthesiology: An observational, prospective, pilot study. *Anaesthesia Critical Care & Pain Medicine, 36*, 205–212. https://doi.org/10.1016/j.accpm.2016.09.008

Fanning, R. M., & Gaba, D. M. (2007). The role of debriefing in simulation-based learning. *Simulation in Healthcare, 2*, 115–125.

Giesbrecht, E., Wener, P., & Pereira, G. (2014). A mixed methods study of student perceptions of using standardized patients for learning and evaluation. *Advances in Medical Education and Practice, 241*, 241–255. https://doi.org/10.2147/amep.s62446

Giles, A. K., Carson, N. E., Breland, H. L., Coker-Bolt, P., & Bowman, P. J. (2014). Use of simulated patients and reflective video analysis to assess occupational therapy students' preparedness for fieldwork. *American Journal of Occupational Therapy, 68*(Suppl. 2), S57–S66. https://doi.org/10.5014/ajot.2014.685s03

INACSL Standards Committee. (2016). INACSL standards of best practice: SimulationSM simulation design. *Clinical Simulation in Nursing, 12*(Suppl.), S5–S12. https://doi.org/10.1016/j.ecns.2016.09.005

Lasater, K. (2007). High-fidelity simulation and the development of clinical judgment: Students' experiences. *Journal of Nursing Education, 46*, 269–276.

Li, H., Jin, D., Qiao, F., Chen, J., & Gong, J. (2016). Relationship between the Self-Rating Anxiety Scale score and the success rate of 64-slice computed tomography coronary angiography. *International Journal of Psychiatry in Medicine, 51*, 47–55. https://doi.org/10.1177/0091217415621265

Mills, B., Carter, O., Rudd, C., Claxton, L., & O'Brien, R. (2016). An experimental investigation into the extent social evaluation anxiety impairs performance in simulation-based learning environments amongst final-year undergraduate nursing students. *Nurse Education Today, 45*, 9–15. https://doi.org/10.1016/j.nedt.2016.06.006

Molitor, W. L., & Nissen, R. (2020). Correlation between simulation and fieldwork performance in adult physical rehabilitation. *Journal of Occupational Therapy Education, 4*(2). https://doi.org/10.26681/jote.2020.040209

O'Regan, S., Molloy, E., Watterson, L., & Nestel, D. (2016). Observer roles that optimise learning in healthcare simulation education: A systematic review. *Advances in Simulation, 1*, Article 4. https://doi.org/10.1186/s41077-015-0004-8

Ozkara San, E. (2018). Effect of the diverse standardized patient simulation (DSPS) cultural competence education strategy on nursing students' transcultural self-efficacy perceptions. *Journal of Transcultural Nursing, 30*, 291–302. https://doi.org/10.1177/1043659618817599

Sahu, P., Chattu, V., Rewatkar, A., & Sakhamuri, S. (2019). Best practices to impart clinical skills during preclinical years of medical curriculum. *Journal of Education and Health Promotion, 8*, 57. https://doi.org/10.4103/jehp.jehp_354_18

Taylor, R. R. (2020). *The intentional relationship: Occupational therapy and use of self (2nd Ed.)*. F.A. Davis.

VanPuymbrouck, L., Heffron, J. L., Sheth, A. J., The, K. J., & Lee, D. (2017). Experiential learning: Critical analysis of standardized patient and disability simulation. *Journal of Occupational Therapy Education, 1*(3), Article 5. https://doi.org/10.26681/jote.2017.010305

Wilbanks, B., McMullan, S., Watts, P., White, T., & Moss, J. (2020). Comparison of video-facilitated reflective practice and faculty-led debriefings. *Clinical Simulation in Nursing, 42*, 1–7. https://doi.org/10.1016/j.ecns.2019.12.007

Zhang, H., Mörelius, E., Goh, S, & Wang, W. (2019). Effectiveness of video-assisted debriefing in simulation-based health professions education: A systematic review of quantitative evidence. *Nurse Educator, 44*(3), E1–E6. https://doi.org/10.1097/NNE.0000000000000562

Financial Disclosures

Dr. Joanne M. Baird has no financial or proprietary interest in the materials presented herein.

Chalia Bellis has no financial or proprietary interest in the materials presented herein.

Dr. Dennis Brown has no financial or proprietary interest in the materials presented herein.

Madeleine Clements has no financial or proprietary interest in the materials presented herein.

Leslie Cody has no financial or proprietary interest in the materials presented herein.

Dr. Victoria L. B. Grieve has no financial or proprietary interest in the materials presented herein.

Dr. E. Adel Herge has no financial or proprietary interest in the materials presented herein.

Dr. Andrea L. Hergenroeder has no financial or proprietary interest in the materials presented herein.

Dr. Maureen M. Hoppe has no financial or proprietary interest in the materials presented herein.

Dr. Victoria Hornyak has no financial or proprietary interest in the materials presented herein.

Dr. Carole Ivey has no financial or proprietary interest in the materials presented herein.

Dr. Pari Kumar has no financial or proprietary interest in the materials presented herein.

Dr. Jennifer A. Merz has no financial or proprietary interest in the materials presented herein.

Dr. Susan Norkus has no financial or proprietary interest in the materials presented herein.

Dr. John M. O'Donnell has no financial or proprietary interest in the materials presented herein.

Dr. Jean E. Prast has no financial or proprietary interest in the materials presented herein.

Jaime Smiley has no financial or proprietary interest in the materials presented herein.

Dr. Tracy Van Oss has no financial or proprietary interest in the materials presented herein.

Dr. Audrey L. Zapletal has no financial or proprietary interest in the materials presented herein.

Index

Printed in the United States
by Baker & Taylor Publisher Services

Printed in the United States
by Baker & Taylor Publisher Services